Endoscopy in Pancreatic Disease:
Diagnosis and Therapy

Endoscopy in Pancreatic Disease:
Diagnosis and Therapy

Pier Alberto Testoni MD

Assistant Professor of Medicine
Institute of Internal Medicine
University of Milan
IRCCS Policlinico, Milan
Chief of Gastroenterology and Gastrointestinal Endoscopy
Policlinico San Marco, Zingonia
Italy

Alberto Tittobello MD

Professor of Medicine
Chief of Gastroenterology and Gastrointestinal Endoscopy
Institute of Biomedical Sciences
University of Milan
IRCCS San Raffaele, Milan
Italy

M Mosby-Wolfe

Chicago London Philadelphia St. Louis Sydney Tokyo

Copyright © 1997 Times Mirror International Publishers Ltd.

Published in 1997 by Mosby-Wolfe, a division of Times Mirror International Publishers Ltd.

Printed by Grafiche Alma, Milan (Italy)

ISBN 0 7234 2481 0

For full details of all Mosby International titles, please write to Mosby International, Lynton House, 7–12 Tavistock Square, London WC1H 9LB, England, UK. Tel: +44 (0) 171 388 7676; Fax: +44 (0) 171 391 6559.

A CIP catalogue record for this book is available from the British Library.

Library of Congress Cataloging-in-Publication Data applied for.

Preface

The introduction of endoscopic retrograde cholangiopancreatography (ERCP) as a diagnostic procedure was rapidly followed by its adoption as a powerful therapeutic tool; in fact, no other endoscopic procedure has made such an impact on the management of diseases of the gastrointestinal tract. Biliary sphincterotomy was introduced in clinical practice in 1974 as a therapeutic application of ERCP. This procedure gained wide acceptance in the 1980s because of its efficacy, relative safety and low cost, and over the last 20 years it has become the procedure of choice for the treatment of biliary tract diseases.

A wealth of literature addressing all aspects of ERCP has appeared, and several books are available on diagnostic ERCP and biliary sphincterotomy, written by internationally known authorities in the field. However, new developments in this ever-expanding area have enabled endoscopists in the 1990s to enhance their knowledge of the pathophysiology of the papillary region and adopt new approaches to the treatment of pancreatic diseases, with encouraging results. As a result of this technical evolution, we now have a clearer understanding of the pathological mechanisms that are involved in most cases of recurrent 'idiopathic' pancreatitis, and can provide more successful endoscopic treatment. Furthermore, the developments have also resulted in greater diagnostic accuracy of pancreatic lesions, a means of treating obstructive chronic pancreatitis and its complications, and, finally, have provided ways of minimizing the risk of postprocedure complications – mainly acute pancreatitis.

Because pancreatic therapeutic endoscopy still remains an evolving technique, at present there is no comprehensive state-of-the-art reference text available. Therefore, the goal of this volume is to provide, in one volume, a comprehensive, critical review of the present status of diagnostic and therapeutic ERCP in pancreatic diseases addressed not only to those who perform these procedures but to all physicians and surgeons who care for patients with pancreatic disease. For this purpose, experienced authorities have been entrusted to contribute reviews of specific fields in which they have worked extensively and, in many cases, have played a major developmental role.

Pier Alberto Testoni, MD
Alberto Tittobello, MD

Contents

Section 5
Complications

Contributing Authors

Chapter 1

Glen A. Lehman, MD, Professor of Medicine and Radiology, Indiana University Medical Center, University Hospital, Indianapolis, IN, USA.

Stuart Sherman, MD, Associate Professor of Medicine and Radiology, Indiana University Medical Center, University Hospital, Indianapolis, IN, USA.

Chapter 2

Giorgio Cavallini, MD, Professor of Gastroenterology and Head of Gastroenterology Unit, University of Verona, Policlinico di Borgo Roma, Verona, Italy.

Paola Bovo, MD, Gastroenterology Unit, University of Verona, Policlinico di Borgo Roma, Verona, Italy.

Luca Frulloni, MD, PhD, Gastroenterology Unit, University of Verona, Policlinico di Borgo Roma, Verona, Italy.

Vincenzo Di Francesco, MD, PhD, Gastroenterology Unit, University of Verona, Policlinico di Borgo Roma, Verona, Italy.

Bruna Vaona, MD, Gastroenterology Unit, University of Verona, Policlinico di Borgo Roma, Verona, Italy.

Marco Filippini, MD, Gastroenterology Unit, University of Verona, Policlinico di Borgo Roma, Verona, Italy.

Chapter 3

Walter J. Hogan, MD, Professor of Medicine and Radiology and Chief, Division of Gastroenterology, Medical College of Wisconsin, Froedtert Memorial Lutheran Hospital, Milwaukee, WI, USA.

Chapter 4

Niels Ebbehøj, MD DMSc, Associate Professor, Department of Occupational Medicine, H:S Rigshospitalet, University of Copenhagen, Copenhagen N, Denmark.

Peter Funch-Jensen, MD DMSc, Associate Professor of Surgery, Department of Surgical Gastroenterology, H:S Hvidovre Hospital, University of Copenhagen, Hvidovre, Denmark.

Chapter 5

T. Lok Tio, MD, PhD, Professor of Medicine, Division of Gastroenterology, Georgetown University Medical Center, Washington, DC, USA.

Chapter 6

Charles Duckworth, MD, Assistant Professor of Internal Medicine, Emory University School of Medicine, Division of Digestive Diseases, Atlanta, GA, USA.

Robert Kiss, PhD, Senior Research Associate at the Fonds National de la Recherche Scientifique, Laboratory of Histology, Faculty of Medicine, Universite Libre de Bruxelles, Brussels, Belgium.

Paul Yeaton, MD, Assistant Professor of Internal Medicine, Division of Gastroenterology and Hepatology, University of Virginia Health Sciences Center, Charlottesville, VA, USA.

Chapter 7

Pier Alberto Testoni, MD, Assistant Professor of Medicine, Institute of Internal Medicine, University of Milan, IRCCS Policlinico, Milan and Chief of Gastroenterology and Gastrointestinal Endoscopy, Policlinico San Marco, Zingonia, Italy.

Alberto Tittobello, MD, Professor of Medicine, Chief of Gastroenterology and Gastrointestinal Endoscopy, Institute of Biomedical Sciences, University of Milan, IRCCS San Raffaele, Milan, Italy.

Chapter 8

José Sahel, MD, Professor and Head of Department of Hepatogastroenterology, Hopital Sainte Marguerite, Marseille, France.

Marc Barthet, MD, Praticien Hospitalier Universitaire, Department of Hepatogastroenterology, Hopital Sainte Marguerite, Marseille, France.

Chapter 9

Marc Barthet, MD, Praticien Hospitalier Universitaire, Department of Hepatogastroenterology, Hopital Sainte Marguerite, Marseille, France.

José Sahel, MD, Professor and Head of Department of Hepatogastroenterology, Hopital Sainte Marguerite, Marseille, France.

Chapter 10

Antonio Russo, Professor of Surgery, Chief of Surgical Endoscopy Unit, Department of Surgery, University of Catania, Italy.

Clara Virgilio, MD, Department of Surgery, University of Catania, Italy.

Francesco Russo, Medical Student, University of Catania, Italy.

Chapter 11

Khay Guan Yeoh, MBBS, MMed, Visiting Fellow in Therapeutic Endoscopy, Medical University of South Carolina, Senior Lecturer, Department of Medicine, National University of Singapore, Singapore.

Robert H. Hawes, MD, Professor of Medicine and Chief of Endoscopy, Digestive Disease Center, Division of Gastroenterology, Medical University of South Carolina, Charleston, SC, USA.

Chapter 12

Michel Cremer, MD, Professor of Medicine and Head of Department of Gastroenterology, Universite Libre de Bruxelles, ULB-Erasme, Brussels, Belgium.

Jacques Devière, MD, PhD, Associate Clinical Professor, Department of Gastroenterology, Universite Libre de Bruxelles, ULB-Erasme, Brussels, Belgium.

Chapter 13

Kees Huibregste, MD, PhD, Chief of Endoscopy, Department of Gastroenterology and Hepatology, Academic Medical Center, Amsterdam, The Netherlands.

Chi Pong Kwan, MBBS, MRCP, Department of Medicine, Princess Margaret Hospital, Kowloon, Hong Kong.

Chapter 14

Seth A. Cohen, MD, FACP, Assistant Clinical Professor of Medicine, Columbia College of Medicine, New York, New York, and Attending Physician, Endoscopy, Beth Israel Medical Centre, New York, NY, USA.

Jerome H. Siegel, MD, FACP, FACG, Associate Clinical Professor of Medicine, Albert Einstein College of Medicine, Bronx, New York, and Chief, Endoscopy, Beth Israel Medical Centre, North Division, New York, NY, USA.

Chapter 15

Paul G. Wilson, MB, ChB, MRCP, Clinical Research Fellow, Department of Surgery, University of Birmingham, Queen Elizabeth Hospital, Edgbaston, Birmingham, UK.

James D Evans, MB, ChB, FRCS, Clinical Research Fellow, University Department of Surgery, Royal Liverpool University Hospital, Liverpool, UK.

Ogunju Ogunbiyi, MD, FRCS, Lecturer in Surgery, Department of Surgery, University of Birmingham, Queen Elizabeth Hospital, Edgbaston, Birmingham, UK.

John P Neoptolemos, MA, MB, BChir, MD, FRCS, Professor of Surgery, University Department of Surgery, Royal Liverpool University Hospital, Liverpool, UK.

Chapter 16

Pier Alberto Testoni, MD, Assistant Professor of Medicine, Institute of Internal Medicine, University of Milan, IRCCS Policlinico, Milan and Chief of Gastroenterology and Gastrointestinal Endoscopy, Policlinico San Marco, Zingonia, Italy.

Alberto Tittobello, MD, Professor of Medicine, Chief of Gastroenterology and Gastrointestinal Endoscopy, Institute of Biomedical Sciences, University of Milan, IRCCS San Raffaele, Milan, Italy.

Chapter 17

Jonathan Cohen, Therapeutic Endoscopy Fellow, The Centre for Advanced Therapeutic Endoscopy and Endoscopic Oncology, The Wellesley Hospital, University of Toronto, Toronto, Ontario, Canada.

Gregory B. Haber, MD, FRCP(C), The Centre for Advanced Therapeutic Endoscopy and Endoscopic Oncology, The Wellesley Hospital, University of Toronto, Toronto, Ontario, Canada.

Chapter 18

Judy Dorais, Therapeutic Endoscopy Fellow, The Centre for Advanced Therapeutic Endoscopy and Endoscopic Oncology, The Wellesley Hospital, University of Toronto, Toronto, Ontario, Canada.

Gregory B. Haber, MD, FRCP(C), The Centre for Advanced Therapeutic Endoscopy and Endoscopic Oncology, The Wellesley Hospital, University of Toronto, Toronto, Ontario, Canada.

Chapter 19

Guido Costamagna, MD, Associate Professor of Surgery, Istituto Clinica Chirurgica, Università Cattolica S. Cuore, Policlinico 'A Gemelli', Rome, Italy.

Chapter 20

Stuart Sherman, MD, Associate Professor of Medicine and Radiology, Indiana University Medical Center, University Hospital, Indianapolis, IN, USA.

Glen A. Lehman, MD, Professor of Medicine and Radiology, Indiana University Medical Center, University Hospital, Indianapolis, IN, USA.

Chapter 21

Stuart Sherman, MD, Associate Professor of Medicine and Radiology, Indiana University Medical Center, University Hospital, Indianapolis, IN, USA.

Glen A. Lehman, MD, Professor of Medicine and Radiology, Indiana University Medical Center, University Hospital, Indianapolis, IN, USA.

Chapter 22

Ulricke von Arnim, MD, Department of Gastroenterology, Otto-von-Guericke University, Magdeburg, Germany.

J Enrique Dominguez-Muñoz, MD, Department of Gastroenterology, Otto-von-Guericke University, Magdeburg, Germany.

Peter Malfertheiner, MD, Professor of Medicine, Chief of Department of Gastroenterology, Otto-von-Guericke University, Germany.

New concepts
in aetiopathogenesis
of pancreatitis

1

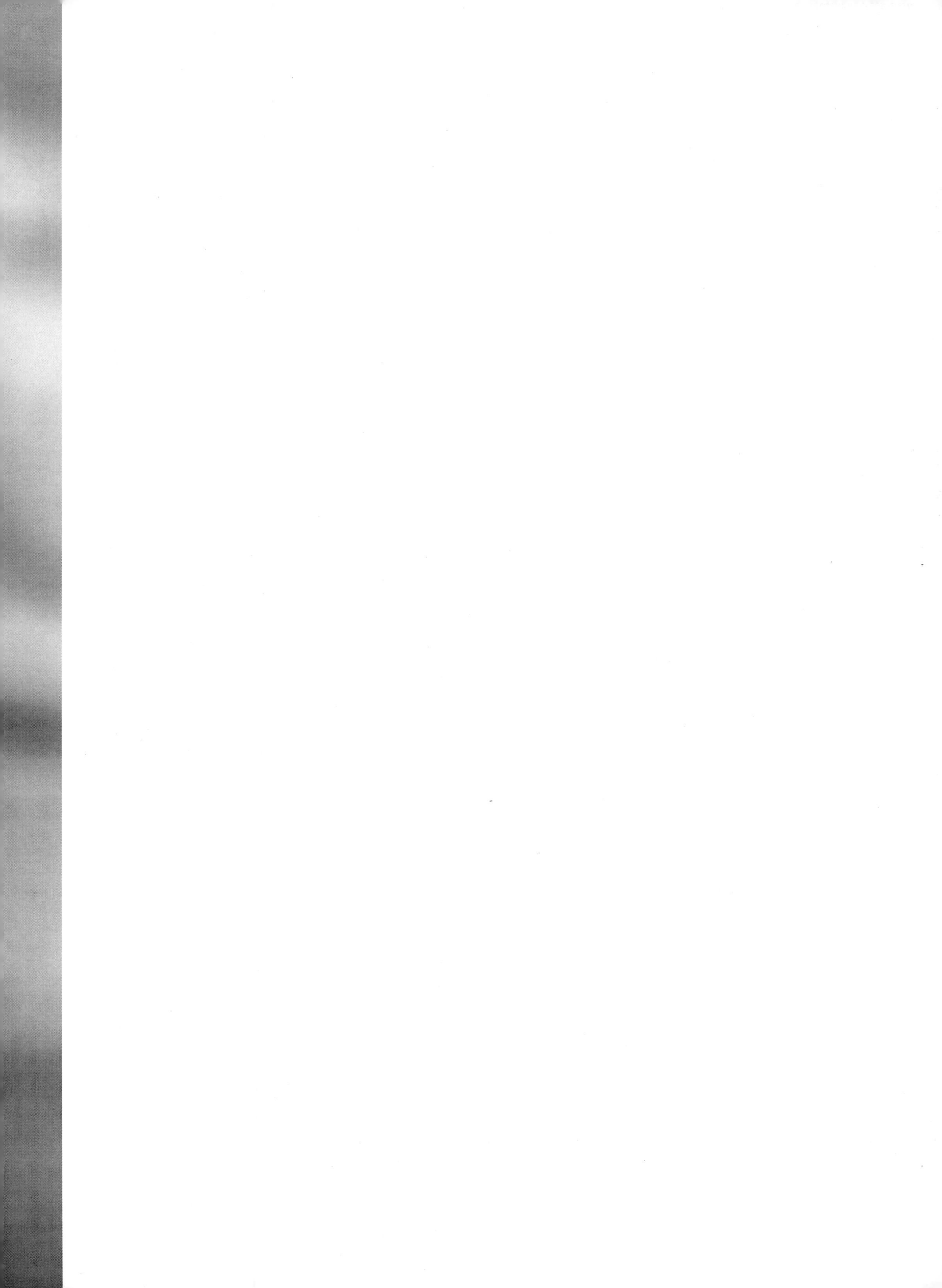

1

Aetiologies of relapsing pancreatitis

Glen A. Lehman & Stuart Sherman

INTRODUCTION

Acute relapsing pancreatitis generally refers to that entity in which the patient has clinical acute pancreatitis on more than one occasion. The severity of the bouts may vary from trivial to devastating, but most bouts are mild to moderate and result in hospitalizations of 3–10 days. Clinically, affected patients have upper abdominal pain with or without nausea or vomiting, associated with serum amylase and/or lipase elevation usually greater than three times the upper limits of normal. Pancreatic oedema may or may not be found to be present on ultrasound or computed tomography (CT) scan evaluation. Only rarely do such patients have more devastating pancreatitis with CT evidence of necrosis, haemorrhage or other serious consequences. Occasionally pseudocysts occur. While the emphasis with the above is on self-limited oedematous changes within the pancreas, such patients may, in reality, have varying degrees of established chronic pancreatitis with all its typical radiographical and histological criteria (i.e. morphological changes of chronic pancreatitis with clinical bouts of acute pancreatitis). Despite the inaccuracies attached to this diagnosis, the term 'acute relapsing pancreatitis' continues to be used clinically. Appropriate differential diagnoses and patient management plans need to be engendered by the managing physician. Since the aetiology of pancreatitis is often key in the ultimate management, this chapter will emphasize predominantly the differential diagnosis of acute relapsing pancreatitis and key points in sorting out the true aetiology. As many patients with clinical acute pancreatitis have already developed the structural and functional changes of chronic pancreatitis[1,2], this chapter will overlap considerably with subsequent chapters on chronic pancreatitis.

Figure 1.1 lists a broad categorization of conditions causing clinical acute relapsing pancreatitis. Virtually any cause of acute pancreatitis, e.g. viral, drug, metabolic condition, tumour, may cause recurrent disease if the original underlying factor is not corrected[3]. Almost any cause of chronic pancreatitis may result in more than one bout of clinical pain and therefore may present as acute recurrent pancreatitis. Comments in this chapter are restricted to the more common causes of clinical acute relapsing pancreatitis. Figure 1.2 shows a recommended evaluation for patients presenting with relapsing pancreatitis.

Figure 1.1 Causes of acute relapsing pancreatitis.*

1. Alcohol: > 40g/day
2. Gall stones: > 2mm or microlithiasis
3. Consequences of pancreatitis (pseudocyst, stricture, stones, leaks, ascites, fistula, pseudoaneurysm with intraductal bleed)
4. Sphincter of Oddi dysfunction
5. Idiopathic (gross, minimal change, tropical)
6. Congenital: Pancreas divisum, annular pancreas, anomalous pancreatobiliary junction
7. Neoplasms: Benign and malignant
8. AIDS (and associated infections: cryptosporidia, microsporidia, cytomegalovirus)
9. Drugs (if recurrent or continued exposure)
10. Metabolic diseases (e.g. hypercalcaemia or hyperlipidaemia)
11. Hereditary
12. Duodenal diverticula
13. Choledochocoele
14. Duodenal obstruction (e.g. Crohn's disease/afferent limb obstruction in Billroth II, atresia)
15. Chronic renal disease (includes dialysis-related)
16. Cystic fibrosis
17. Collagen vascular disease
18. Duodenal duplicate cyst
19. Parasites (e.g. *Ascaris*)

Many patients have histological or radiological criteria for chronic pancreatitis also.

The aetiologies are listed in approximately the order of frequency seen by the authors in their referral practice.

Figure 1.2 Evaluation of patients with acute relapsing pancreatitis.

1. Detailed history and physical examination, including query of family members about surrepticious alcohol or drug use.

---

2. Serological evaluation to include liver chemistries, amylase, lipase, calcium, lipids, cystic fibrosis gene testing (if less than 40 years of age), alpha-1 antitrypsin level (if less than 40 years of age), tumour markers (CEA and CA 19-9 if > 40 years of age).

---

3. Non-invasive imaging, preferably CT scanning, but include ultrasonography if higher suspicion of gall bladder stones.

---

4. If upper endoscopy is being done for other reasons, include duodenal aspiration of bile after magnesium sulphate- or CCK-stimulated bile flow.

---

5. If patient has had two or more bouts of unexplained recurrent pancreatitis, ductography (ERCP) is generally recommended, unless other more obvious pathology is seen on non-invasive images, such as gallstones in the gall bladder. Manometry is recommended during this ERCP.

BILIARY CALCULOUS DISEASE

Macrolithiasis

The presence of gallstones is one of the two most common causes of recurrent pancreatitis[4,5]. Often, this aetiology of the pancreatitis is obvious once serum liver chemistries and/or non-invasive imaging of the gall bladder or bile ducts are obtained. Long-standing biliary obstruction results in elevations of gamma-glutamyl transpeptidase (gamma-GT) and alkaline phosphatase to 2–10 times the normal level, along with bilirubin elevation in more severe cases. Acute obstruction commonly results in alanine aminotransferase (ALT) or aspartate aminotransferase (AST) elevations to 2–5 times normal levels. Occasionally such elevations exceed 1000 IU/l (but there should not be confusion with hepatitis because these levels quickly drop over 1–3 days to near normal). Patients with rapidly resolving liver test abnormality have usually passed a stone through the sphincter of Oddi and on into the duodenum. Less often, the stone(s) will have disimpacted from the papilla and migrated more cephalad. Persistent liver test abnormalities usually indicate residual ductal stones. The severity of pancreatitis and frequency of complications (cholangitis, necrosis, pseudocyst, abscess and multiorgan system failure) are related to the duration of stone obstruction of both the bile duct and pancreas. Therefore, prognosis is improved in patients undergoing early duct evacuation by endoscopic retrograde cholangiopancreatography (ERCP)[6–8]. The rapidity of intervention is related to the time the patient arrives at the health care facility. Patients who stay at home for the first few days may have a worse outcome because prolonged gallstone obstruction may have resulted in more advanced pancreatic necrosis.

Microlithiasis

The gallstone disease may be more subtle and manifest only by the presence of: (a) very tiny stones, less than 2mm in diameter; (b) sludge in the gall bladder (visualized by ultrasonography or cholangiography[9]; or (c) the presence of calcium carbonate, cholesterol monohydrate crystals or calcium bilirubinate crystals seen in bile aspirated from the gall bladder, bile duct or duodenum. It is unlikely that these microscopic crystals actually cause pancreatitis, but they are signs that larger stones have passed through the sphincter. Reported series vary greatly as to the frequency of such microlithiasis in patients with 'idiopathic' or relapsing (range: 5–75%) pancreatitis. Patient selection bias almost certainly accounts for this difference. Patients with abnormal serum liver tests detected during pancreatitis, especially those whose liver tests improve promptly over the first few days, should not be designated as having 'idiopathic pancreatitis' but rather 'probable gallstone pancreatitis'[10]. An appropriate search for microscopic or macroscopic lithiasis should be carried out. Collection of bile from the duodenum may be performed via nasoduodenal tube placed by fluoroscopy or by upper gastrointestinal endoscopy. Gall bladder or ductal bile may be sampled during ERCP, or less commonly, percutaneously[11]. Aspirated bile is centrifuged for analysis of the sediment or may be analysed unspun. Quantitation as to the definition of a 'positive' specimen is not well standardized but probably even a small number of crystals is abnormal.

The finding of crystals in bile has been shown to be predictive of the presence of small stones in the gall bladder based on evaluation of cholecystectomy specimens or follow-up ultrasonography (demonstrating macroscopic stones)[10].

CONGENITAL DUCT VARIANTS AND ANOMALIES

Approximately 10% of the general population has some congenital variant anatomy of the pancreatic duct system that could predispose to pancreatitis.

Pancreas divisum

Pancreas divisum, the most common congenital variant of pancreatic duct anatomy, occurs when the ductal systems of the dorsal and ventral buds fail to fuse during the second month of gestation, with non-union of the ducts. The major portion of the pancreatic exocrine juice must flow through the relatively small orifice of the minor papilla. This may result in congestive pancreatopathy, manifest by chronic pain or frank pancreatitis. Most cases of pancreatitis are mild but necrosis with pseudocyst formation occurs infrequently. The diagnosis can generally not be established without pancreatography and is generally easily recognized by major papilla cannulation showing the typical short terminally tapered ventral pancreatic duct (Figure 1.3). Alternatively, about one third of pancreas divisum patients have no ventral pancreas identified via the major papilla and the diagnosis must be made by cannulation of the minor papilla with dorsal duct filling. The development of needle-tip catheters, 0.018 inch (0.46mm) diameter guide wires and highly tapered catheters has helped make cannulation of the minor papilla more routine. When pancreas divisum is identified in patients with recurrent pancreatitis, the therapy generally recommended is to open the minor papilla[12–15] (sphincterotomy, sphincteroplasty), although long-term follow-up of such patients after medical therapy has not been well defined. Patients with saccular dilatation of the terminal dorsal duct (Santorinicoele) (Figure 1.4) or those with pain-free intervals between attacks are most likely to respond to treatment.

Figure 1.3 Normal delicate ventral ductogram of pancreas divisum.

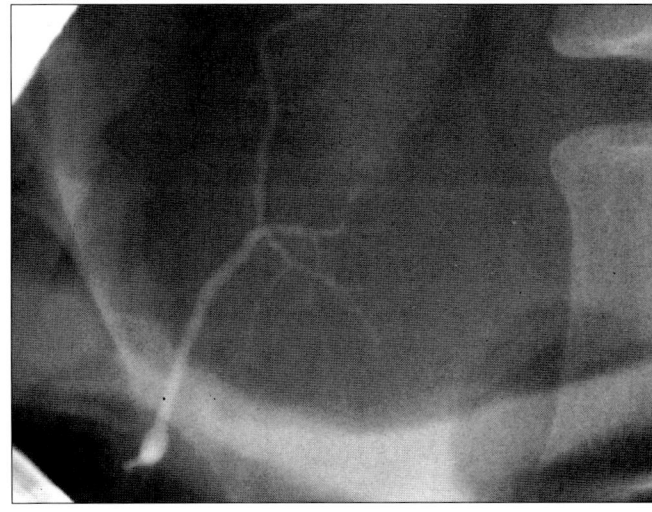

Figure 1.4 Dorsal ductogram of pancreas divisum showing diffuse main duct dilatation of the head and body. Saccular dilatation of the terminal duct (Santorinicoele) is present.

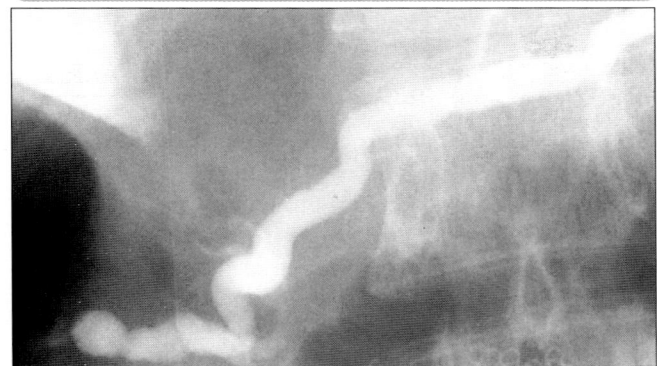

Figure 1.5 Incidence of abnormal sphincter of Oddi manometry in pancreatitis.*

Author (Ref)	Year	n	Incidence
Toouli (42)	85	14/28	50%
Catalano (43)	93	10/18	56%
Guelrud (44)	83	17/42	40%
Sherman (45)	92	15/49	31%
Gregg (46)	89	28/125	22%
Geenen (47)	89	17/116	15%
		101/378	27%*

Figure 1.6 Incidence of abnormal basal pressure of both ducts in sphincter of Oddi dysfunction.

Author (Ref)	Year	n	Incidence of abnormalities in both ducts*
Silverman (44)	91	43	65%
Rolny (43)	89	17	47%
Raddawi (42)	91	15	33%

Abnormal is greater than 40mmHg.

Annular pancreas

An annular pancreas typically causes symptoms of gastric outlet obstruction but occasionally it presents with pancreatitis of the annulus or of the remaining pancreas[16]. Indeed, one third of patients with annular pancreas also have pancreas divisum and therefore the aetiology of any pancreatitis needs to be determined using careful ductography.

Anomalous pancreatobiliary junction

In this condition the common pancreatobiliary channel is anomalously long (generally greater than 15mm) and there are no sphincters that separate the biliary and pancreatic ducts. As a result, free reflux of bile and pancreatic juice is possible into the alternative duct. Bile entering the pancreas is a known pancreatic irritant and pancreatic juice entering the biliary tree is thought to increase the frequency of biliary cancer. The diagnosis is usually obvious on ERCP as initial cannulation results in filling of both ductal systems. Choledochal cysts are commonly associated with such a junction. Sphincter ablation will theoretically result in appropriate directional flow of biliary and pancreatic juices; however, a large series of studies on sphincter ablation therapy has not been reported.

SPHINCTER OF ODDI DYSFUNCTION

An abnormally narrow sphincter segment to the biliary channel, to the common ampullary channel, or to the pancreatic sphincter are well recognized causes of recurrent pancreatitis[17,18]. The aetiology of sphincter of Oddi dysfunction is generally not known. The frequency of finding sphincter dysfunction as documented by sphincter of Oddi manometry in patients presenting with idiopathic pancreatitis varies in reported cases from 10 to 60%, but overall, approximately one quarter of such patients have sphincter dysfunction (Figure 1.5). Patient selection remains a major factor in the incidence of such pathology. In patients with recurrent pancreatitis undergoing manometry, evaluation of both the biliary and pancreatic sphincter segments is suggested (Figure 1.6). Non-invasive tests for sphincter dysfunction (e.g. transcutaneous ultrasound-monitored pancre-

atic duct diameter after fatty meal or secretin stimulant) probably have low sensitivity and are not widely used. Use of an aspiration-type catheter appears to add to the safety of manometry[19]. Resolution of pancreatitis after biliary sphincterotomy alone has been reported, while there is increasing evidence that most such patients with abnormal pancreatic sphincter manometry also need pancreatic sphincter therapy[20]. Passage of microliths in such patients (the large majority) may provide a better explanation for their improvement following biliary sphincterotomy alone.

NEOPLASMS

Benign and malignant tumours of the pancreatobiliary tree[21–24] present as acute pancreatitis in 5–7% of cases. The possibility of the presence of a neoplasm should be considered in any such patient over 40 years of age or in whom a mass lesion or duct dilation is seen by non-invasive imaging. Careful evaluation of the papillae, and ductograms for mass lesions, strictures, duct cut-off and intraductal casts are needed. Infiltrating neoplasms (especially islet cell tumours) occasionally present as idiopathic pancreatitis and non-specific ductal narrowings, even in the absence of an overt mass. Endoscopic ultrasonography with guided fine-needle aspiration may be helpful in identifying the underlying neoplasm.

Cystic neoplasms (including mucinous duct ectasia) may present as acute recurrent pancreatitis and, especially, be confused with pseudocysts. Concern for cystic neoplasms should be heightened in patients who: (a) present with peripancreatic fluid collection without a history of prior pan-

Figure 1.7 ERCP of a 48-year-old male with recurrent pancreatitis. (a) A filling defect (mucus) is seen in the main duct in the head. (b) After aspiration of mucus from the main duct and orifice to the uncinate branch, the uncinate branch shows cystic dilatation with a residual strand of mucus. Surgical resection showed intraductal papillary carcinoma. Peripancreatic lymph nodes were negative for cancer.

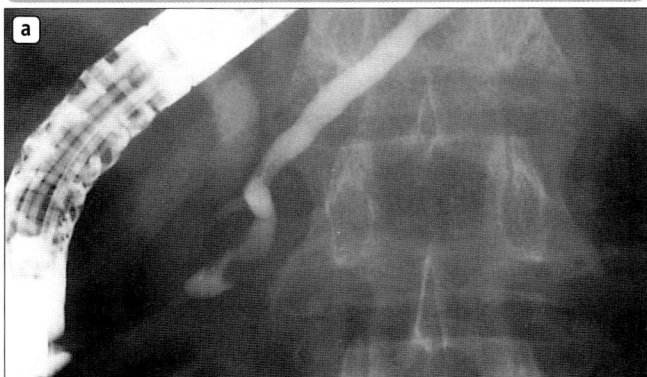

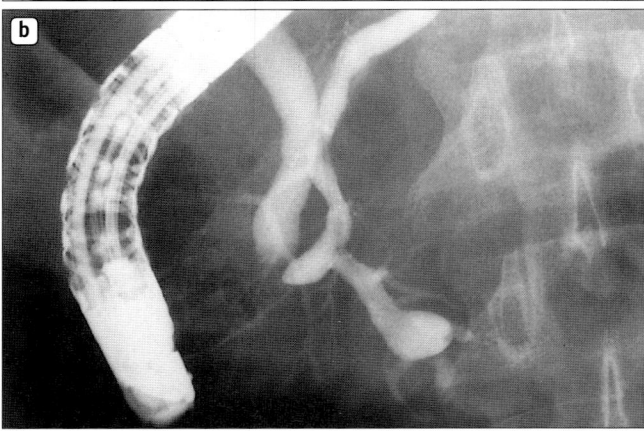

creatitis; (b) have a thick wall to the cyst; (c) have high serum CA 19-9; or (d) have multiloculated cysts with little or no adjacent inflammation. On ERCP, a dilated papillary orifice with exiting mucus is diagnostic. Identification of cast-like intraductal filling defects is almost diagnostic of a mucin-producing tumour. Cystic neoplasms arising in the side branches may not communicate with the main duct nor have mucus in the main duct (Figure 1.7). Intraductal aspiration of juice or mucus for cytology is suggested. The cancer detection sensitivity of such cytology has not been defined for mucinous tumours.

CHOLEDOCHOCOELE

Cystic dilatation of the terminal segment of the pancreato-biliary ductal system (choledochocoele) may cause recurrent pancreatitis with or without the presence of stones within the choledochocoele. Choledochocoele may be suspected from ultrasonography or CT scan findings but is usually diagnosed at ERCP or with other definitive-type ductography. Choledochocoeles must be separated from duodenal duplication cysts, which may appear quite similar but have Brunner's glands within the walls. Endoscopic unroofing of

the choledochocoele or duodenal duplication cyst is usually therapeutic without surgical intervention[25–28].

PARASITIC DISEASE

Worldwide, *Ascaris lumbricoides* is the most common parasite to gain access into the pancreatobiliary ductal system and cause obstructive pancreatitis. Transcutaneous ultrasonography or CT scans may suggest the diagnosis by finding linear filling defect(s) in the bile duct or pancreatic duct. On ERCP, adult worms may be observed in the duodenum, papilla, or within the biliary ducts or pancreas.

ACQUIRED IMMUNODEFICIENCY SYNDROME (AIDS)

Relapsing pancreatitis in AIDS patients is due to a variety of causes, including drugs used to treat the disease (e.g. didanosine). CMV (cytomegalovirus), cryptosporidia or microsporidia may invade the periampullary or ductal tissue causing oedema and perhaps obstructive pancreatitis[29–33]. Whether the human immunodeficiency virus (HIV) itself causes pancreatitis remains uncertain. Barthet[34] and colleagues reported that more than half of AIDS patients with recurrent pancreatitis had ductographic changes of chronic pancreatitis. More detailed culture, endoscopic biopsy, and histological autopsy data are needed to define these conditions further.

FAMILIAL PANCREATITIS

Hereditary pancreatitis may cause acute relapsing or chronic pancreatitis and ductograph findings vary from normal to advanced changes. The family history is key. A worldwide registry of such families is being developed.

CYSTIC FIBROSIS

Cystic fibrosis may cause acute relapsing or chronic pancreatitis with changes seen on ductograms varying from normal to advanced disease. Genetic testing has facilitated this diagnosis. Such testing is recommended for all patients with recurrent pancreatitis presenting at under 40 years of age. Sweat chloride testing may alternatively be used. Genetic testing will identify numerous heterozygotes (5% of the Caucasian European and North American populations) and raises the interesting, but uncertain, question as to whether the heterozygous state is associated with any pathology.

CONSEQUENCES OF PRIOR PANCREATITIS OR PANCREATIC TRAUMA

Once pancreatitis has occurred, a variety of sequelae may follow, including stricture, pseudocyst formation, stones,

Figure 1.8 There is non-specific diffuse stricturing of the main duct throughout the pancreas in this alcoholic patient.

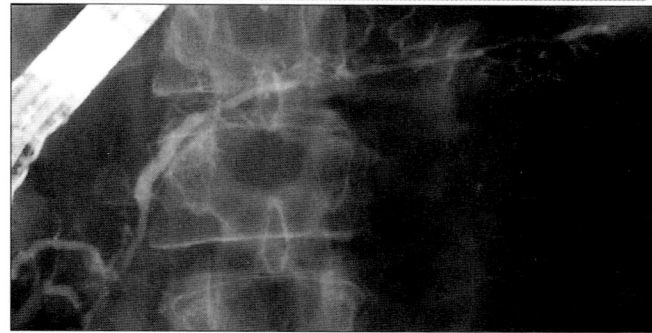

duct leaks, ascites, fistulae and pseudoaneurysms (Figure 1.8)[35–41]. Each may then cause additional pain or pancreatitis. Usually there is some suspicion of these sequelae from non-invasive imaging, especially CT scan, although the correct diagnosis is often not established without detailed ductography. Appropriate therapy varies according to the aetiology, ductography and other pathology findings.

MISCELLANEOUS

A variety of other metabolic and anatomical factors are listed in Figure 1.1. Many are uncommon and will be seen infrequently by the clinician.

Acknowledgment

The authors are grateful to Joyce Eggleston for the technical preparation of this document.

References

1. Sarles H, Sahel J, Staub JL, Bourry J, Laugier R. Chronic pancreatitis. In *The Exocrine Pancreas*. Edited by HT Howatt, H Sarles. WB Saunders, Philadelphia; 1979: 402–39.
2. Steer ML, Waxman I, Freedman S. Chronic pancreatitis. *New Engl J Med* 1995; 335:1482–90.
3. Venu RP, Geenen JE, Hogan W, Stone J, Johnson K, Sorgel K. Idiopathic recurrent pancreatitis. An approach to diagnosis and treatment. *Dig Dis Sci* 1989; 34:56–60.
4. Carr-Locke DL. Endoscopic treatment of biliary acute pancreatitis. In *Standards in Pancreatic Surgery*. Edited by Beger HG, Buchler MW, Malfertheiner P. Springer-Verlag, Heidelberg; 1933: 127–34.
5. Steinberg WM. Acute pancreatitis – never leave a stone unturned. *New Engl J Med* 1992; 326:635–7.
6. Neoptolemos JP, Carr-Locke DL, London NJ, Bailey IA, James D, Fossard DP. Controlled trial of urgent ERCP and endoscopic sphincterotomy versus conservative treatment for acute pancreatitis due to gallstones. *Lancet* 1988; ii:979–83.
7. Fan ST, Lai ECS, Mok FP, Lo CM, Zhang S-S, Wong J. Early treatment of acute biliary pancreatitis by endoscopic papillotomy. *New Engl J Med* 1993; 328:228–32.
8. Nowak A, Nowakowska-Dulawa E, Marek TA et al. Final results of the prospective, randomized, controlled study on endoscopic sphincterotomy versus conventional management in acute biliary pancreatitis. *Gastroenterology* 1995; 108:A380.
9. Lee SP, Nocholls JE, Park HZ. Biliary sludge as a cause of acute pancreatitis. *New Engl J Med*, 1992; 326:589–93.
10. Ros E, Navarros S, Bru C et al. Occult microlithiasis in idiopathic acute pancreatitis: prevention of relapses by cholecystectomy or ursodeoxycholic acid therapy. *Gastroenterology* 1991; 101:1701–9.
11. Buscail L, Escourrou J, Delvaux M et al. Microscopic examination of bile directly collected during endoscopic cannulation of the papilla. Utility in patients with suspected microlithiasis. *Dig Dis Sci* 1992; 37:116–20.
12. Carr-Locke DL. Pancreas divisum: the controversy goes on? *Endoscopy* 1991; 23:88–90.
13. Siegel JH, Ben-zvi JS, Polano W, Cooperman A. Effectiveness of endoscopic drainage for pancreas divisum, endoscopic and surgical results in 31 patients. *Endoscopy* 1990; 22:129–33.
14. Lans JI, Geenen JE, Johanson, JF, Hogan, WJ. Endoscopic therapy in patients with pancreas divisum and acute pancreatitis: a prospective, randomized, controlled trial. *Gastrointest Endosc* 1992; 38:430–4.
15. Nisi R, Sherman S, Hawes R, Jamidar P, Lehman GA. Controlled trial of minor papilla sphincterotomy (MiES) in pancreas divisum (Pdiv) patients with pain only. *Gastrointest Endosc* 1992; 38:257.
16. Urayania S, Kozarek R, Ball T et al. Presentation and treatment of annular pancreas in an adult population. *Am J Gastroenterol* 1995; 90:995–9.
17. Okazaki Y, Yamamoto Y, Nishimori I et al. Motility of the sphincter of Oddi and pancreatic main ductal pressure in patients with alcoholic, gallstone-associated and idiopathic chronic pancreatitis. *Am J Gastroenterol* 1988; 83:820–6.
18. Gilbert DA, DiMarino AJ, Jensen DM et al. Status evaluation: sphincter of Oddi manometry. *Gastrointest Endosc* 1992; 38:757–9.
19. Sherman S, Hawes RH, Troiano FP, Lehman GA. Pancreatitis following bile duct sphincter of Oddi manometry: utility of the aspirating catheter. *Gastrointest Endosc* 1992; 38:347–50.
20. Guelrud M, Plaz J, Mendoza S, Beker B, Rojas O, Rossiter G. Endoscopic treatment in Type II pancreatic sphincter dysfunction. *Gastrointest Endosc* 1995; 41:A398.
21. Binmoeller K, Soehendra N. Endoscopic therapy of ampullary adenomas. *Gastrointest Endosc* 1993; 39:127–31.
22. Parsons WG, Carr-Locke DL. Tumors of the main duodenal papilla. In *Gastroenterologic Endoscopy*, 2nd edition. Edited by M Sivak. WB Saunders, Philadelphia; 1997 (In press).
23. Ohta Y, Nagakawa, T, Akiyama T et al. The "duct-ectatic" variant of mucinous cystic neoplasm of the pancreas: clinical and radiologic studies of seven cases. *Am J Gastroenterol* 1992; 87:300–4.
24. Lichtenstein DR, Carr-Locke DL. Mucin secreting tumors of the pancreas. *Gastroenterol Clin North Am* 1995; 5:237–58.
25. Lopez RR, Pinson CW, Campbell JR, Harrison M, Katon RM. Variation in management based on type of choledochal cyst. *Am J Surg* 1991; 161:612–15.
26. Martin RF, Biber BP, Bosco JJ, Howell DA. Symptomatic choledochoceles in adults. ERCP recognition and management. *Arch Surg* 1991; 161:612–15.
27. Johanson JF, Geenen JE, Hogan WJ, Huibregtse K. Endoscopic therapy of a duodenal duplication cyst. *Gastrointest Endosc* 1992; 38:64–5.
28. Al-Mofarreh MA, Laajam, MA. Periampullary cysts: endoscopic management. *Am J Gastroenterol* 1992; 87:211–13.
29. Murthy UK, Degregorio F, Oates RP, Blair DC. Hyperamylasemia in patients with the acquired immunodeficiency syndrome. *Am J Gastroenterol* 1992; 87:332–6.
30. Cappell MS, Marks M. Acute pancreatitis in HIV-seropositive patients: a case-control study of 144 patients. *Am J Med* 1995; 98:243–7.
31. Kapemba MS, Fleming SC, Griffin GE, Sewankambo N, Serwadda D, Goodgame R. Spectrum of pancreatic disorders in patients with the acquired immunodeficiency syndrome. *Am J Gastroenterol* 1990; 85:475–8.
32. Torre D, Montanari M, Fiori GP. HIV and the pancreas. *Lancet* 1987; ii:1212.
33. Baskerville A, Ramsay AD, Millward-Sadler GH, Cook RW, Cranage MP, Greenaway PJ. Chronic pancreatitis and biliary fibrosis associated with cryptosporidiasis in Simian AIDS. *J Comp Pathol* 1991; 105:415–21.

34. Barthet M, Chauveau E, Bonnet E *et al*. Pancreatic ductal changes in HIV patients. *Gastrointest Endosc*; 1997 (in press).

35. Kozarek RA, Patterson DJ, Ball TJ, Traverso, IW. Endoscopic placement of endoscopic drains in the management of pancreatitis. *Ann Surg* 1989; 209:261–6.

36. Sherman S, Lehman GA, Hawes RH *et al*. Pancreatic ductal stones, frequency of successful endoscopic removal and improvement in symptoms. *Gastrointest Endosc* 1991; 37:511–17.

37. Kozarek RA, Ball TJ, Patterson DJ. Endoscopic approach to pancreatic duct calculi and obstructive pancreatitis. *Am J Gastroenterol* 1992; 87:600–3.

38. Delhaye M, Vandermeeren A, Baize M, Cremer M. Extracorporeal shockwave lithotripsy of pancreatic calculi. *Gastroenterology* 1992; 102:610–20.

39. Binmoeller KF, Seifert H, Walter A, Soehendra N. Transpapillary and transmural drainage of pancreatic pseudocysts. *Gastrointest Endosc* 1995; 42:219–24.

40. Lehman GA. Endoscopic management of pancreatic pseudocysts continues to evolve. *Gastrointest Endosc* 1995; 42:273–5.

41. Smits ME, Rauws EAJ, Tytgat GNJ, Huibregtse K. The efficacy of endoscopic treatment of pancreatic pseudocysts. *Gastrointest Endosc* 1995; 42:202–7.

42. Toouli J, Bushall M, Iannos J, *et al*. Per operative sphincter of Oddi manometry: motility disorder in patients with cholelithiasis. *Aust NZ J Surg* 1986; 56:625–9.

43. Catalano MF, Sivak MV, Falk G, *et al*. Idiopathic pancreatitis (IP): diagnostic role of sphincter of Oddi manometry (SOM) and response to endoscopic sphincterotomy (ES). *Gastrointest Endosc* 1993; 39:310.

44. Guelrud M, Mendoza S, Vincent S, *et al*. Pressures in the sphincter of Oddi in patients with gallstones, common duct stones, and recurrent pancreatitis. *J Clin Gastroenterol* 1983; 5:37–41.

45. Sherman S. Idiopathic acute recurrent pancreatitis (RP): endoscopic approach to diagnosis and therapy. *Gastrointest Endosc* 1992; 38:261.

46. Gregg JA. Function and dysfunction of the sphincter of Oddi. In *ERCP: Diagnostic and Therapeutic Applications*. Editred by IM Jacobson. Elsevier Science, New York; 1989:139–70.

47. Venn RP, Geenen JE, Hogan W, *et al*. Idiopathic recurrent pancreatitis; an approach to diagnosis and treatment. *Dig Dis Sci* 1989; 34:56–60.

2

Chronic pancreatitis

*Giorgio Cavallini, Paola Bovo, Luca Frulloni,
Vincenzo Di Francesco, Bruno Vaona & Marco Filippini*

INTRODUCTION

When considering chronic pancreatitis, the tendency recently has been to distinguish between two main forms, namely chronic calcifying pancreatitis (CCP), more recently termed pancreatic lithiasis1, and chronic obstructive pancreatitis (COP). Together these two forms account for all or almost all the cases of chronic pancreatitis observed, since the third form of the disease, the form known as inflammatory chronic pancreatitis (IPC), has been reported only sporadically, and pancreatic fibrosis is actually no more than an anatomopathological finding of little or no clinical significance, at least in Western countries.

The terms chronic calcifying pancreatitis and chronic obstructive pancreatitis, as we see it, are no longer valid, and a major review of the terminology is called for on the basis of the latest aetiopathogenetic observations[2]. The latter, in fact, suggest that: (a) stone formation is an event which, with a certain frequency, may also affect patients with so-called chronic obstructive pancreatitis; and (b) the obstruction phenomenon is probably the main pathogenetic event, or key factor, not only in COP but also in CCP.

In this connection, it is curious that it is the advocate of chronic pancreatitis as a lithiasic disease, Professor Henri Sarles of Marseilles, who states: '... in advanced stages of the disease (CCP), the ultrastructural modifications are no different from those observed in obstructive pancreatitis; CCP is, in reality, obstructive pancreatitis of multiple small areas of the gland ...!'[3]. It would thus perhaps be more correct to distinguish, at least provisionally, between primary (PCP) and secondary (SCP) chronic pancreatitis[2], using the former term to embrace those forms of the disease in which the precise aetiological factor still escapes us, while the term 'secondary' should be reserved for all those cases in which there is a marked and indisputable presence of an extra- or intrapancreatic factor capable of causing outflow obstruction at the level of the main pancreatic duct.

The pathogenesis of PCP and SCP are, in actual fact, very similar, and what differentiates the two forms is the aetiology which, in turn, conditions the level at which the obstructive factors operate and determines a different topography of the lesions, which are sparse and irregularly distributed in PCP and more evenly distributed in SCP. A review of the various hypotheses proposed for the pathogenesis of PCP (see below) reveals that, whatever the sequence postulated, the central event is the occurrence of ductal stenotic lesions and that these are the crucial anatomopathological factors responsible for the progressive chronic inflammatory lesions leading to the destruction of first the exocrine and then the endocrine parenchyma.

The various pathogenetic hypotheses diverge only with regard to the primary factor they suggest as being responsible for the onset of ductal stenosis. According to the Marseilles School, this is the biochemical alteration of the pancreatic juice (protein plug hypothesis); in the other three theories (necrosis–fibrosis, toxic–metabolic, primary duct disease) the primary factors are identified as inflammatory and/or necrotic lesions with periductal fibrotic scarring of the pancreatic parenchyma.

PRIMARY CHRONIC PANCREATITIS

The protein plug hypothesis

According to this theory, proposed by Sarles and his team several years ago[4,5], the pathophysiological events are thought to begin with the precipitation of eosinophilic protein aggregates within the ducts. These aggregates consist of a fibrillary insoluble peptide (LS-H2) that is a fragment of the protein secretory lithostatin (LS-S); lithostatin is very unstable and therefore readily subject to degradation (spontaneous or induced). Lithostatin is produced by the acinar cells and its function is to stabilize the calcium with which the pancreatic juice is supersaturated. The precipitation of calcium on the plugs, i.e. the formation of stones, is thought to be the result of impoverishment of the juice due to a deficiency of lithostatin caused by its inappropriate or defective synthesis and/or excessive degradation. According to this theory, hereditary (congenital) and acquired factors (e.g. alcohol, cigarette smoking) are regarded as responsible for the lithostatin abnormalities. The plugs and stones are believed to be capable of ulcerating the epithelium of the ducts, triggering a periductal inflammatory reaction with fibrotic scarring. This causes ductal stenosis with dilatation upstream of the stenosis and stasis of the juice which, in turn, is thought to facilitate further precipitation of plugs and atrophy upstream of the undrained acini. In other words, the pathophysiological chain of events forms a vicious circle with the following primary sequence: plugs/stones > stenosis > plugs/stones.

Exogenous factors such as alcohol (and also the composition of the diet and cigarette smoking) are thought to potentiate protein precipitation by modifying the biochemical composition of the pancreatic juice in such a way as to promote lithogenesis. It has been abundantly demonstrated that alcohol is capable of increasing the protein secretion of the acinar cells, of increasing the secretion of lactoferrin, of reducing the production of bicarbonates and citrates, of altering the pH of the juice, and of reducing the concentration of pancreatic secretory trypsin inhibitor and increasing that of cationic trypsinogen[4]. It has also been reported that alcohol, through its direct action on the acinar cell, may adversely affect the concentration of LS-S in pancreatic juice[5].

The apparent conclusions that can be drawn on the basis of this theory are that in some cases defective LS synthesis may be exclusively of a genetic/hereditary type, as in so-called hereditary chronic pancreatitis, whereas in others the congenital defect can be identified above all as a greater susceptibility to alcohol (and perhaps a greater susceptibility to lithostatin itself) as in adult calcifying pancreatitis. For the tropical forms of the disease, on the other hand, it has been suggested that the composition of the diet of the child or intrauterine foetus exerts a significant influence on the pancreas, and the lithogenetic mechanisms are believed to be similar to those postulated for alcohol in chronic pancreatitis in the Western world.

This hypothesis, though fascinating, tends to overlook the fact that chronic pancreatitis does not present calcifications in the early stages of the disease[6–8], that the plugs are a reversible phenomenon[9], and that alone they are not capable of causing gross alterations of the ducts (mucoviscidosis is instructive in this connection[10,11]). In addition, the existence of congenital lithostatin biosynthesis and secretion defects has still to be reliably confirmed. These latter observations emerge from clinicomorphological studies on the natural history of chronic pancreatitis in man, from anatomical and histological investigations into the presence and persistence of intraductal plugs in subjects without pancreatitis and their reversibility, as well as from immunohistochemical studies on the tissue expression of mRNA encoding for lithostatin.

What should be stressed, however, is that, quite apart from the likely error as to the pathophysiological sequence of events, credit is due to the Marseilles hypothesis for identifying the specific factors (lithostatin) and the non-specific factors (all the other physicochemical alterations of the pancreatic juice) involved in pancreatic lithogenesis; these are, or will be, of basic importance also in the interpretation of the intermediate stages described in the other hypotheses outlined below.

The necrosis–fibrosis hypothesis

Klöppel and Maillet, in a series of studies based on retrospective anatomopathological and histological observations[12–14], have suggested that chronic pancreatitis is the result of repeated attacks of acute pancreatitis, thus resuscitating a theory proposed by Comfort and Gambill almost 50 years ago[15].

In their working hypothesis, based on macro- and microscopic findings in surgical and/or autopsy specimens of pancreases from patients with acute and chronic pancreatitis mainly associated with alcohol, Klöppel and Maillet have suggested that the peri- and intrapancreatic fatty necrosis, which is a constant feature of acute pancreatitis, may in the later stages of the disease rapidly evolve into fibrosis and/or the formation of pseudocysts, both of which are capable of involving the interlobular ducts, creating stenosis and sacculation. The flow of juice would thus be obstructed and this would facilitate the precipitation of proteins and consequent calcifications. Eventually the acinar lobules would be replaced by fibrotic tissue, which would aggravate the pancreatic fibrosis, involving ducts as yet unaffected.

Support for this hypothesis was provided very recently by a morphoclinical and functional study conducted by the Zurich team[16] in a large patient sample with alcoholic pancreatitis, in which it was confirmed that the possible progression from acute to chronic pancreatitis is strictly related to two factors, one being the presence and severity of the attacks of acute pancreatitis, which are always clinically severe and morphologically of the necrotizing type, and the other being the site of the necrosis, which is mainly in the head of the pancreas with development of pseudocysts.

Apart from the fact that fibrotic scarring following acute pancreatitis is more often than not resolved (since, experimentally at least, it has been shown that this type of fibrosis involves short-lived collagen type III and procollagen type III and not the long-lasting collagen types I and IV[17–20]), from the clinical standpoint most cases of chronic pancreatitis are diagnosed at an advanced stage, i.e. with full-blown ductal lesions and, generally speaking, with a negative long-term medical history of repeated and severe acute episodes of a necrotizing type, which would be expected to characterize the natural history of chronic pancreatitis if the sequence postulated in this hypothesis were effectively the right one. In saying this, it is not our intention to rule out the possibility that severe acute necrotizing pancreatitis of any cause or origin may not lead to stenotic scarring, but such scarring, if anything, gives rise – and only when the main duct is involved – to chronic pancreatitis of the obstructive type[21–23] and not to primary-type chronic pancreatitis.

On the other hand, we feel one can hardly postulate that widespread small foci of steatonecrosis alone, which are also common in the course of clinically mild or relatively symptom-free oedematous pancreatitis, are capable of causing the scattering of major lesions so typical of primary chronic pancreatitis. This is because we have to admit that any focus of steatonecrosis, however limited, is capable of forming permanent connective tissue. This idea clashes blatantly with the available experimental data and the clinical findings and follow-up data for patients suffering from recurrent acute pancreatitis.

What, to our mind, should nevertheless be appreciated in this hypothesis is that it represents the first serious attempt to interpret the pathogenesis of chronic pancreatitis in something other than the usual manner, i.e. seeking the primary factors responsible for the disease not in biochemical and physicochemical changes in the pancreatic juice, which are of basic importance, but only at a later stage in the pathogenesis, but in pathomorphological events capable of triggering the most important form of primary damage, namely the ductal stenoses responsible for the stasis of the pancreatic juice.

The toxic–metabolic hypothesis

Several years ago now, on the basis of anatomohistological investigations, Bordalo's team in Portugal[24] had suggested that a chronic alcohol intake caused accumulation of intracellular lipids and periacinar fibrosis in the pancreas (as it was already known to do in the liver) and that the cellular necrosis resulting from fatty degeneration might trigger more widespread fibrosis phenomena, even at a subclinical level, with impairment of the pancreatic microcirculation.

The result of a sequence of this type might be interpreted, by analogy with cirrhosis of the liver, as a fully fledged form of macro–micronodular chronic pancreatitis[25].

This hypothesis, which has been seriously challenged, particularly by the Marseilles School, was later taken up by the advocates of *oxidative stress* as the main factor responsible for the earliest lesions in chronic pancreatitis[26,27]. It has been suggested that, via direct and indirect mechanisms, alcohol may lead, at the level of the liver and pancreas, to a depletion of antioxidants, the so-called scavengers (such as selenium, vitamin E, riboflavin, vitamin C, beta-carotene and the S amino acids) and an accumulation of toxic oxidant substances (such as free radicals), capable of acting with a cytotoxic mechanism. The substances are thought to reach the pancreas both via the systemic circulation and via episodes of bile duct/Wirsung's duct reflux. The death of the cells is thought to come about in a progressive yet surreptitious manner, with the result that the process, though of the destructive type, would never be capable of causing clinical episodes of acute pancreatitis. However, the pancreatic juice in the course of time would be altered, possibly even impairing the actual secretion of lithostatin and thereby facilitating the intraductal precipitation of proteins, obstruction of the ducts, fibrosis, etc. More severe damage as occasioned by particularly severe relapses is thought to aggravate both the parenchymal and the vascular lesions, giving rise to a deterioration of the circulation and of the state of oxidative stress, and increasing tissue necrosis, thus facilitating the formation of fibrosis and consequently stasis of the pancreatic juice.

There are therefore many points of contact between this hypothesis and the necrosis–fibrosis hypothesis discussed previously, since, in both of them, the ductal impairment (stenosis) appears to be secondary to a periductal fibrosis and the latter appears to be the result of more or less extensive cell death phenomena. Nevertheless, if acinar necrosis, induced by factors such as alcohol and cigarette smoking, and the resulting fibrosis were really the first lesions to occur in chronic pancreatitis, we would expect that most, if not all, the subjects subjected to a chronic load of xenobiotics (alcohol, smoking, nutritional errors) would develop pancreatitis. It is, however, well known that a minority of subjects among those exposed, for instance, to alcohol, present chronic pancreatitis. What is more, this hypothesis can hardly be adduced to explain the occurrence of chronic pancreatitis in children and adolescents (so-called hereditary chronic pancreatitis) in Western countries, where chronic xenobiotic intoxication or some form of intrauterine damage due to nutritional deficiencies is hard to postulate. To these objections we should add those relating to the impossibility of reproducing lesions typical of human chronic pancreatitis in experimental animals by means of chronic alcohol intoxication alone, even when produced by extremely high doses for lengthy time periods[28].

This hypothesis, however, is important in that it has emphasized the finding that chronic alcohol intoxication can give rise directly or indirectly to steatosis with acinar cell degeneration and consequent intrapancreatic fibrosis, this latter form of damage probably being common to excessive drinkers, as occurring, for instance, in steatofibrosis of the liver. This type of widespread damage may, in fact, be an aggravating factor in the course of chronic pancreatitis, inasmuch as the cellular secretory abnormalities deriving from it all have a lithogenesis-promoting effect, as already stressed in the protein plug hypothesis.

The primary duct hypothesis

The three previous hypotheses all provide convincing information on what mechanisms intervene during the pathogenetic evolution of the lesions of chronic primary pancreatitis, but they do not help us to understand the initial stages of the disease, i.e. those without which the lesions described would continue to be of the non-specific type, common to all subjects engaging in habitual alcohol consumption and cigarette smoking or on the wrong diet. In other words, where may the genetic error lie that modulates and marshals the various aspects so far described and enables them to present the classic picture of primary chronic pancreatitis?

Indications in this connection are provided by studies in experimental animals and also by clinical trials in man. In experimental studies reviewed critically not long ago by Boros and Singer[28], it was suggested that alcohol, both alone and in association with various nutritional deficiencies, is incapable of reproducing the histological lesions typical of chronic pancreatitis in man and only in some cases causes the formation of plugs; these plugs are, however, also present in control animals. The observation of actual intraductal calcifications was a very sporadic event and one which was not confirmed by other similar studies. The only animal model capable of causing irreversible pancreatic alterations compatible with those of chronic pancreatitis in man is the one employing partial obstruction of the pancreatic ducts in the dog and rat[29–31]. Disturbance of flow alone was capable of causing the formation of ductal stones and pancreatic lesions, mainly of an obstructive type, with a histological picture similar to that described in human COP. When, however, chronic administration of alcohol was added to the partial obstruction – even only temporary – of the ducts, the lesions took on the appearance of human chronic calcific pancreatitis, in both the rat and the dog, with stenotic ductal alterations producing dilatation upstream of the stenoses, preceding the formation of plugs and stones and associated with irreversible parenchymal damage at both the microscopic and ultramicroscropic levels. From these experiments we deduce that outflow obstruction, obtained by manipulation at the ductal level, is the key initial factor in experimental chronic pancreatitis and that some such defect must also be sought in human pathology.

While the hypothesis of periductal postnecrotic secondary fibrosis as a cause of outflow obstruction may be convincing as the pathogenetic trigger factor only in the case of COP secondary to acute necrotizing pancreatitis, but is unsatisfactory when we seek to interpret the multiplicity of the lesions of primary chronic pancreatitis, it is only logical to wonder whether periductal fibrotic phenomena at the pancreatic level should not be regarded as being of a primary type, as considered in the liver in the course of primary sclerosing cholangitis.

The close analogies between primary sclerosing pancreatitis in morphological, epidemiological and clinical terms, as well as a number of observations of the immunohistochemical type[2,32], suggest that primary chronic pancreatitis may depend upon a mechanism of the immune type operating via two channels, one of which relates to the aberrant expression of major histocompatibility antigens by the ductal epithelium and the other to an infiltration of activated lymphocytes capable of mediating a periductal cytotoxic reaction. The various lymphocyte products may also act in a fibroblastic way and may trigger processes of periductal inflammatory fibrosis with stenosis and distortion of the affected segments. From this point on, the pathogenetic chain of events is the one with which we are familiar: ductal stasis promotes protein precipitation, plug formation, acinar damage, and so on. Exogenous toxic factors such as alcohol and cigarette smoking are thought to act not merely by boosting the lithogenic capability of the pancreatic juice (thus amplifying the effects of the obstructive phenomenon), but also possibly by enhancing the ductal epithelial defect, increasing its aberrant HLA expression[2,32].

This theory, like every new hypothesis, needs to be confirmed by more appropriate studies, since, while it is true that two reports have now confirmed a ductal epithelial defect of aberrant expression in patients with chronic pancreatitis and the activation of lymphocyte populations infiltrating the periductal spaces[33–35], what is equally certain is that aberrant HLA expression is a very common phenomenon in the vicinity of inflammatory foci, and is not always indicative of a primary immune reaction. The recent finding that HLA expression and ductal infiltration have also been described in areas of completely healthy pancreatic parenchyma lends support more to the primary than to the secondary nature of the process[35,36].

A pathogenetic interpretation such as the one proposed here might explain the onset of primary chronic pancreatitis in the various age brackets in line with the expression of the genetic defect and also offer new and as yet unexplored avenues in the field of medical treatment.

Figure 2.1 Classification of chronic pancreatitis.

1. Primary chronic pancreatitis (PCP)
    Calcific or Non-calcific
        Juvenile form
        Adult form

2. Secondary (obstructive) chronic pancreatitis
    Calcific or Non-calcific
        Due to sphincter of Oddi's disease
            Inflammatory (Odditis)
            Neoplastic (ampulloma)
        Due to stenosis of the main pancreatic duct, as a result of
            Pseudocysts (aftermath)
            Acute necrotizing pancreatitis (scars)
            Trauma (aftermath)
            Ductal tumours, intraductal mucinous tumours, endocrine tumours
        Due to alterations of the duodenal wall
            Cystic dystrophy
            Congenital malformations
            Neoplasms

3. Inflammatory
    In the course of autoimmune diseases

4. Pancreatic fibrosis
    Due to chronic alcohol abuse
    In the course of inflammatory bowel diseases or coeliac disease

5. Pancreatic lithiasis
    Of old age
    In the course of chronic hypercalcaemia or dyslipidaemia
    Drug-induced

N.B. Fibrosis (4) and lithiasis (5) are not to be regarded as chronic pancreatitis

CONCLUSION

The chapter on the pathogenesis of primary chronic pancreatitis undoubtedly needs rewriting without, however, discarding *en bloc* the pathogenetic hypotheses advocated to date. The pathophysiological events described in the various sequences proposed are, in fact, essential stages in the histogenesis of the disease and must be regarded as such. What remains unknown is the initial event, which can hardly be of a biochemical nature and is unlikely to be of the postnecrotic scarring or cellular atrophy type. Perhaps true cases of primary chronic pancreatitis are actually far less frequent than has been reported and may have a fully fledged immune aetiopathogenesis. Many of the forms of chronic pancreatitis regarded as primary, because they are calcific, might actually be cases of COP, overhastily labelled as primary owing to the mistaken belief that ductal lithiasis is exclusively a feature of this form of the disease. On the strength of these observations, it is, as we see it, advisable to abandon the more or less outdated classification proposed so far and adopt, at least provisionally, the nosographic scheme illustrated in Figure 2.1; though subject to extensive review and laying no claim to being definitive, to our mind this offers the advantage of true flexibility and manageability.

SECONDARY CHRONIC (OBSTRUCTIVE) PANCREATITIS

This form of pancreatitis now needs to be reviewed, particularly the epidemiology and aetiology. For years it has been claimed that COP accounts for only a minority of all cases of chronic pancreatitis observed, though specific studies on the incidence and prevalence of the disease have never been completed.

In a multicentre survey of a few years ago, conducted to more clearly define the anatomopathological characteristics of chronic pancreatitis, more than 87% of cases analysed were labelled as CCP, as against only 13% for chronic obstruction[37]. The latter were regarded as such if there was evidence of ampullary or ductal neoplastic occlusion, whereas other possible causes of COP were not reported, which would undoubtedly have raised the percentage total of patients with this particular form of disease.

The aetiological picture thus appears to be closely related to the epidemiological pattern and only a knowledge of all the possible causes of the disease can enhance the identification rate for this disease. From this standpoint we should explain that, alongside the better known causative factors reported since the Marseilles Symposium in 1984, such as tumours or scars occluding the pancreatic duct[21], several other pathological conditions – more often than not overlooked or disregarded – are capable of causing calcific or non-calcific COP (see Figure 2.1).

In particular, over the past few years it has emerged that COP may follow in the wake of alterations of the duodenal wall such as cystic dysplasia or slow-growth neoplasms such as neuroendocrine tumours to an extent as yet not fully defined, as in the case of an intraductal mucinous tumour (personal data). More often, however, the key event, in our opinion, can be identified as benign stenosis of Oddi's sphincter secondary to previous or concomitant lithiasic disease.

Unfortunately, precisely because of the relatively brief experience in this field, it is not possible as yet to define the real frequency of the phenomenon, but it would appear absolutely mandatory to know all the possible causes of COP so as not to make overhasty alternative diagnoses.

The pathogenesis of secondary chronic (obstructive) pancreatitis is very simple and can easily be inferred: partial yet chronic obstruction of outflow facilitates the thickening of the pancreatic juice and ductal dilatation. The addition of exogenous factors such as alcohol or cigarette smoking (and apparently also dietary factors) contribute towards aggravation of the phenomenon and formation of stones. The poorly drained parenchyma undergoes progressive atrophic degeneration with consequent exocrine and endocrine anatomical and functional impoverishment.

The (surgical or endoscopic) removal of the obstruction is, theoretically at least, capable not only of restoring the normal clinical picture but also of arresting the morphological and functional damage and perhaps even allows a certain degree of recovery. This latter possibility is probably related to the stage at which the diagnosis is made and therapeutic measures are implemented.

References

1. Sarles H. Definition and classification of pancreatitis. *Pancreas*; 1991; 6(4):470-4.
2. Cavallini G, Di Francesco V, Bovo P et al. Do chronic pancreatitis patients all have the same disease? In *Facing the Pancreatic Dilemma*. Edited by P Pederzoli et al. Springer-Verlag, Berlin; 1993: 110-21.
3. Sarles H, Payan M-J, Choux R. Morphology and classification of chronic pancreatitis geographical differences. In *Pancreatitis*. Edited by H Sarles et al. Arnette-Blackwell, Paris; 991: 3-18.
4. Sarles H. Etiopathogenesis and definition of chronic pancreatitis. *Dig Dis Sci*, 1986; 31(S9):91-107.
5. Sarles H, Bernard JP. Lithostatin and pancreatic lithogenesis. *Gastroenterol Int*, 1991; 4:30-4.
6. Scuro LA, Cavallini G. La patologia inflammatoria del pancreas. Nosografia clinica e contributo di gruppo. In *Atti del XCI Congresso della Societa Italiana di Medicina Interna*. Luigi Pozzi, Rome; 1990: 483-634.
7. Bernades P. Belghiti J, Athouel M et al. Histoire naturelle de la pancréatite chronique: étude en 120 cas. *Gastroentérol Clin Biol* 1983; 7:8-13.
8. Amman RW, Akovbiantz A, Largiader F et al. Course and outcome of chronic pancreatitis. Longitudinal study of a mixed medical-surgical series of 245 patients. *Gastroenterology* 1984; 86:820-8.
9. Sarles H, Bernard JP, Johnson C. Pathogenesis and epidemiology of chronic pancreatitis. *Ann Rev Med* 1989; 40:453-68.
10. Lebenthal L. Lerner A, Heitlinger L. The pancreas in cystic fibrosis. In *The Exocrine Pancreas: Biology, Pathobiology and Disease*. Edited by WLV Go et al. Raven Press, New York; 1986: 783-817.
11. Allen R, Baggenstoss A. The pathogenesis of fibrocystic disease of the pancreas. Study of the ducts by serial section. *Am J Pathol* 1955; 31:337-51.
12. Klöppel G. Pathomorphology of chronic pancreatitis. In *Diagnostic Procedures in Pancreatic Disease*. Edited by P Malfertheiner, H Dischuneit. Springer-Verlag, Berlin; 1986: 135-9.
13. Klöppel G, Maillet B. Chronic pancreatitis. Evolution of the disease. *Hepatogastroenterology* 1991; 38:408-12.
14. Klöppel G, Maillet B. The morphological basis for the evolution of acute pancreatitis into chronic pancreatitis. *Virchows Arch A* 1992; 420:1-4.
15. Comfort MW, Gambill EE, Baggenstoss AH. Chronic relapsing pancreatitis. *Gastroenterology* 1946; 6:376-408.
16. Amman RW, Muellhaupt B, Meyenberger C, Heitz PU. Alcoholic non-progressive chronic pancreatitis. Pre-operative long-term study of a large cohort with alcoholic acute pancreatitis (1976-1992). *Pancreas* 1994; 9(3):365-73.
17. Odaira G, Iovanna JL, Berger Z, Sarles H. Localized necrotic-hemorrhagic pancreatitis in rats after trypsin injection in pancreatic interstitium. *Digestion* 1984; 30:97.
18. Uscagna L, Kennedy RH, Grimaud JA, Sarles H. Immunolocalisation des colonnes de la lamine (LM) dans la matrice connective (MC) du pancréas normal et dans la pancréatite obstructive du rat. *Gastroentérol Clin Biol* 1984; 8(ii):20.
19. Uscagna L, Kennedy RH, Choux R et al. The evolution of connective matrix changes in experimental acute pancreatitis. *Dig Dis Sci* 1984; 29:970.
20. Uscagna L, Kennedy RH, Stocker S et al. Immunolocalisation of collagen types, laminin and fibronectin in the normal human pancreas. *Digestion* 1984; 30:158-64.
21. Gyr K, Singer MV, Sarles H (Eds) *Pancreatitis: Concepts and Classification*. Excerpta Medica, Amsterdam. 1984; xxiii-xxiv.

22. Angelini G Pederzoli P, Caliari S *et al.* Long-term outcome of acute necrohemorrhagic pancreatitis. A 4 year follow-up. *Digestion* 1984; 30:131-7.

23. Angelini G, Cavallini G, Pedrazoli P *et al.* Long-term outcome of acute pancreatitis: a prospective study of 118 patients. *Digestion* 1993; 54:143-7.

24. Bordalo O, Goncalves D, Noronha M *et al.* Newer concept for the pathogenesis of chronic alcoholic pancreatitis. *Am J Gastroenterol* 1977; 68:278-85.

25. Noronha M, Baptista A, Bordalo O. Sequential aspects of pathology in chronic alcoholic disease of the pancreas. *In Pancreatitis: Concepts and Classification.* Edited by K Gyr *et al.* Excerpta Medica, Amsterdam; 1984: 61-5.

26. Braganza JM. Pancreatic disease: a casualty of hepatic 'detoxification'? *Lancet* 1983; ii:1000-3.

27. Braganza JM, Wickens FG, Cawood P, Dordmandy TL. Lipid peroxidation (free-radical oxidation) products in bile from patients with pancreatic disease. *Lancet* 1983; ii: 375-9.

28. Boros LG, Singer MV. Animal models of chronic pancreatitis. A critical review of experimental studies. In *Pancreatitis: Concepts and Classification.* Edited by K Gyr *et al.* Excerpta Medica, Amsterdam; 1984: 67-82.

29. Konishi K, Ryohei I, Kato O *et al.* Experimental pancreolithiasis in the dog. *Surgery* 1981; 6:687-91.

30. Sakakibara A, Okumura N, Hayakawa T, Kanazaki M. Ultra-structural changes in the exocrine pancreas of experimental pancreolithiasis in the dog. *Am J Gastroenterol* 1982; 77:498-503.

31. Tanaka T, Ichiba Y, Miura Y et al. Pathogenesis of chronic alcoholic pancreatitis. *Am J Gastroenterol* 1990; 85:1536-7.

32. Cavallini G. Is chronic pancreatitis a primary disease of the pancreatic ducts? A new pathogenetic hypothesis. *Ital J Gastroenterol* 1993; 25(7):391-6.

33. Bovo P, Mirachian R, Merigo F *et al.* HLA molecule expression on chronic pancreatitis specimens: is there any role for autoimmunity? A preliminary study. *Pancreas* 1987; 2:350-6.

34. Bedossa P, Bacci J, Lemaigre G, Martin E. Lymphocyte subset and HLA-DR expression in normal pancreas and in chronic pancreatitis. *Pancreas* 1990; 5:415-20.

35. Jalleh RP, Gilbertson JA, Williamson RCN *et al.* Expression of major histocompatibility antigens in human chronic pancreatitis. *Gut* 1993; 34:1452-7.

36. Cavallini G, Frulloni L, Di Francesco V *et al.* Autoimmunity and chronic pancreatitis. *Gut* 1995; 36(5):799 (letter).

37. Sahel J, Cros RC, Durbec JP *et al.* Multicenter pathological study of chronic pancreatitis: morphological regional variations and differences between chronic calcifying pancreatitis and obstructive pancreatitis. *Pancreas* 1986; 6:471-7.

Diagnosis:
Endoscopy-related techniques

2

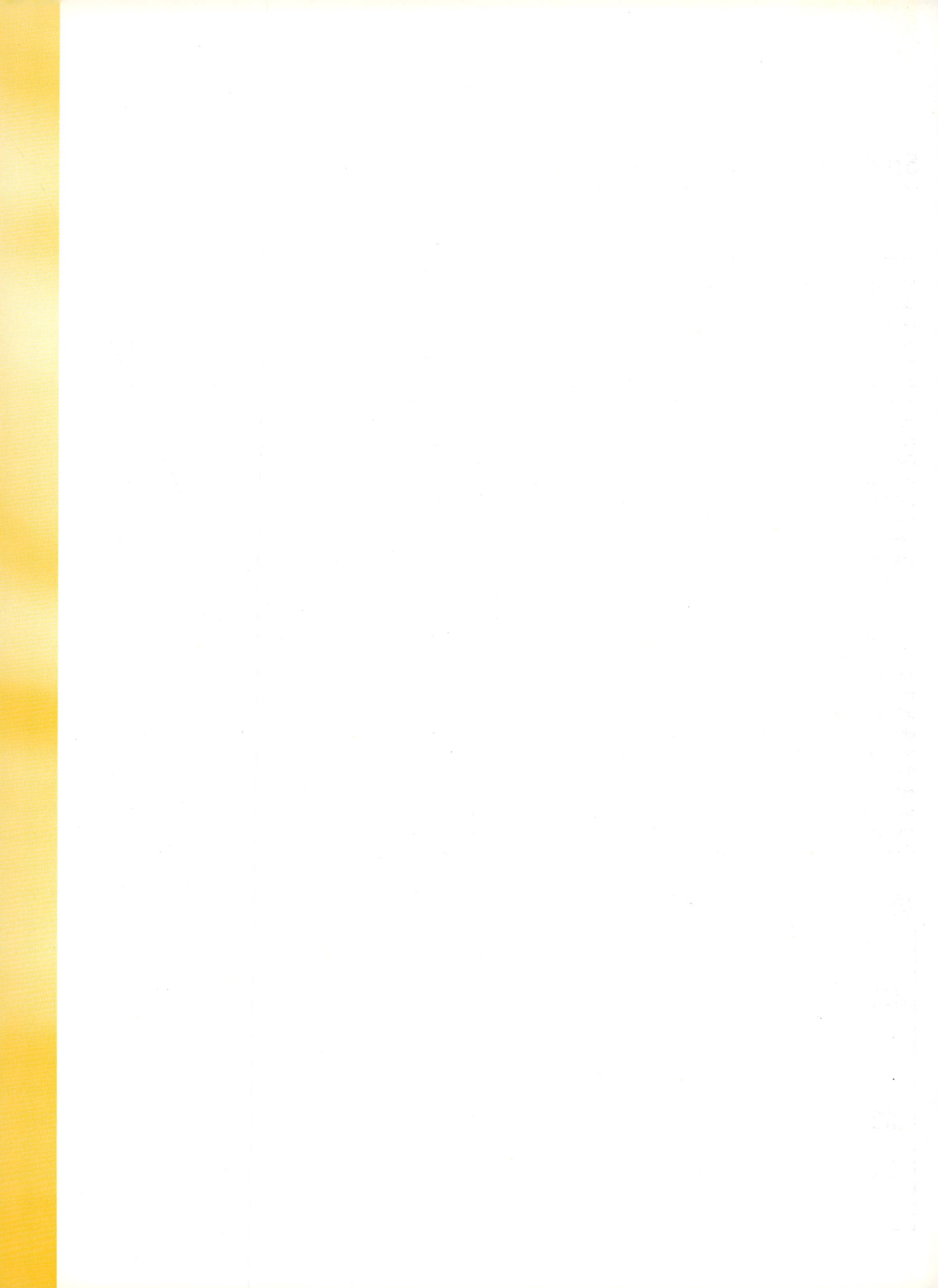

3

Sphincter of Oddi manometry

Walter J. Hogan

INTRODUCTION

Manometric pressure measurements of the sphincter of Oddi (SO) have been performed at the time of endoscopic retrograde cholangiopancreatography (ERCP) for more than two decades. SO manometry has been an aid in defining dysfunction of the SO (albeit of structural or muscular aetiology); it has been especially helpful in evaluating patients with suspected biliary tract disorders[1]. The use of manometry in defining potential dysfunction of the pancreatic portion of the SO has received far less clinical application. Only recently has attention been directed to the use of SO manometry in helping define potential SO dysfunction in patients with acute and chronic pancreatitis[2]. To appreciate the use of this diagnostic modality in helping define disorders such as recurrent pancreatitis, one has to appreciate the relationship of the pancreatic duct portion of the SO to adjacent structures.

SO MANOMETRY: CBD AND PD SEGMENTS

The SO is a muscular bundle that encircles the confluence of the distal common bile duct (CBD) and the pancreatic duct (PD) as it penetrates the wall of the duodenum; a common channel or ampulla is usually found to be present 80% of the time on endoscopic retrograde cholangiopancreatography (ERCP)[3]. The American anatomist Boyden described a sphincteric arrangement that primarily encompasses the biliary duct and described 'vestiges' of SO muscle that involved the distal PD in less than 10% of the human cadaver dissections[4]. Little, if any, physiological importance was

attributed to this sphincteric 'remnant' (Figure 3.1). However, these anatomical observations have not been substantiated by SO manometric pressure recordings. The SO manometric pressure measurements and clinical experience indicate that there is an equivalent amount of sphincteric musculature that involves the terminal PD structure over a 6–8mm length. During ERCP manometric pressure recordings from the PD portion of the SO, a basal pressure and phasic wave contractions similar to those found in the CBD segment are recorded routinely[5]. The concept of SO dysfunction involving pancreatic drainage is based on the belief that dysfunction can occur predominantly in the CBD, exclusively in the PD segment of the SO, or in the entire sphincteric apparatus, influencing pancreatic secretory flow (Figure 3.2).

INDICATIONS FOR SO MANOMETRY

Indications for SO manometry in pancreatic disease have been confined almost exclusively to patients with acute recurrent pancreatitis without a demonstrable structural aetiology[6]. This suggests the possibility of a 'papillary stenosis' *versus* a primary muscular dysfunction as the potential cause for recurrent pancreatitis. In an attempt to more clearly define structural from functional causes for SO disorders, the following classification of three types of patients with recurrent pancreatitis has been proposed[7].

Classification of SO dysfunction

This classification of three types of patient with recurrent pancreatitis who may have SO dysfunction has its counterpart in the biliary tract. A similar classification has been very

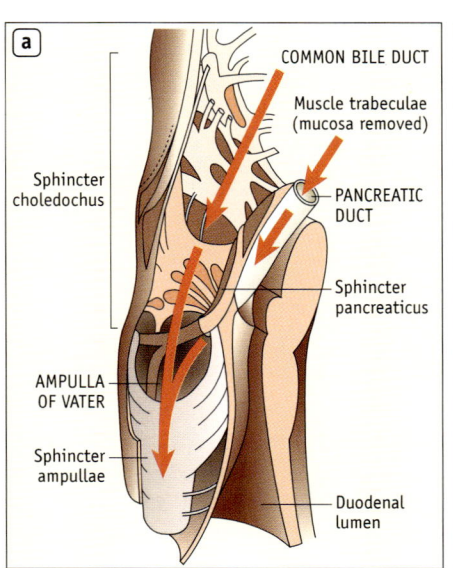

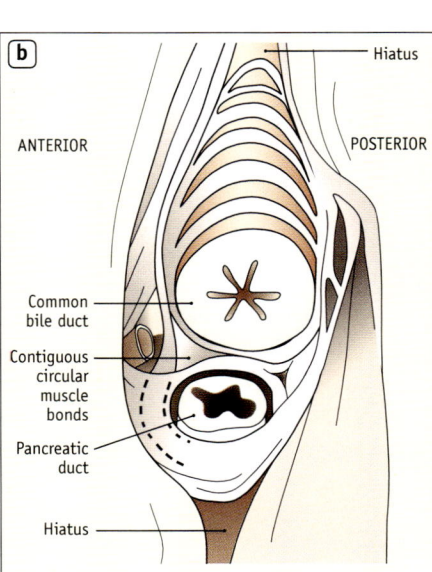

Figure 3.1 Boyden's anatomy of the sphincter of Oddi.
(a) SO zone demonstrating discrete areas of smooth muscle (mini-sphincters) and a relatively 'negligible' sphincter pancreatitis.
(b) Cross-section of the distal confluence of the CBD and PD showing contiguous intertwining of circular muscle around both ducts. (After Boyden.)

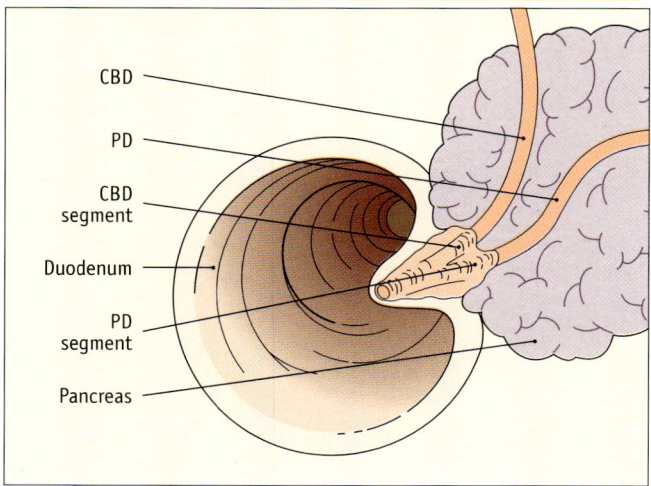

Figure 3.2 Distal pancreaticobiliary junction: ERCP schema. Based on diagnostic ERCP study and manometric pressure recordings, the SO is a contiguous 8–10cm zone of motor activity that involves both the distal choledochus and pancreatic ducts.

CBD

PD

CBD segment

Duodenum

PD segment

Pancreas

Figure 3.3 The ERCP manometric recording system. The SO manometric catheter (internal) is shown exiting the biopsy channel of the duodenoscope. The circumferential rings and three pressure recording ports are detailed. An external catheter, attached to the shaft of the endoscope by parafilm, records duodenal pressure transients. Pressure recordings are transmitted to transducers and subsequently displayed on a graphical direct writing recorder or computer screen. The use of a hydraulic capillary pump assures a low perfusion pressure and non-compliant pressure recording.

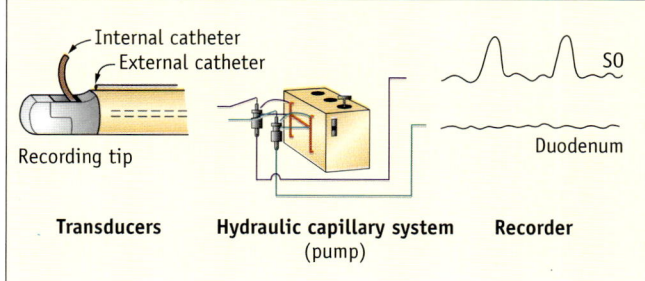

Internal catheter
External catheter

Recording tip

Transducers | Hydraulic capillary system (pump) | Recorder

SO

Duodenum

useful in helping define patients with biliary dyskinesia[8].

Type I: These patients have pancreatic-type pain (mid-epigastrium radiating into the back, lasting for hours to days) associated with a dilated PD (> 7mm) and delayed secretory drainage from the PD (> 10 min) and an elevated serum amylase. These patients most likely have a structural abnormality of the SO.

Type II: These patients have pancreatic-type pain, but only two of the additional features described above. In this patient group there is probably an even distribution of patients with functional or structural disorder of the SO.

Type III: These patients have only the pancreatic-type pain. They do not have enzymatic abnormalities or demonstrable PD drainage problems. Documentation of this patient group is extremely rare and the diagnosis is based solely on the parameter of SO pressure abnormality.

It should be pointed out that a recent report demonstrated SO dysfunction associated with chronic pancreatitis in 37% (18/49) of patients with mild to moderate chronic pancreatitis and interestingly 44% (8/18) had this dysfunction isolated to the PD segment of the SO[9].

TECHNIQUE

Manometric catheter pressure recording from the SO is accomplished using a triple-lumen polyvinyl catheter with an outer diameter of 1.7mm, an individual luminal diameter of 0.5mm and a length of 200mm. A pressure recording port is fashioned in each lumen; the most distal orifice is 5mm from the end of the catheter and the three orifices are each 2mm apart. The catheter is tattooed with circumferential black marks beginning at the most distal orifice and spaced 2mm apart to enable the endoscopist to observe the depth of penetration of the catheter into the SO zone during manometric pressure recording. Each catheter lumen is infused with bubble-free saline at a rate of 0.25ml/min by a mini-

mally compliant hydraulic capillary infusion system using a reservoir pressure of 350mmHg (Arndorfer Industries; Greendale, WI)[10] (Figure 3.3).

For recording pressures from the PD, a catheter has been developed which aspirates fluid from one of the three tips during the manometric pressure recording from the PD. Utilization of this catheter has been reported to decrease the incidence of post-ERCP pancreatitis in patients who undergo concurrent SO manometry[11].

Manometric catheters with miniature solid-state intraluminal transducers located at the distal tip have been used to measure pancreaticobiliary duct pressure. This system also avoids infusion of fluid and enables the recording of intraductal pressures over a long period[12].

Continuous recording of intraluminal duodenal pressure is obtained by a single lumen Teflon catheter that is affixed to the endoscope by parafilm tape and records concurrent intraluminal duodenal pressure transients. This tube is perfused similarly during recording periods.

SO PRESSURE RECORDING

Prior to endoscopy, the patients are administered conscious sedation with incremental IV doses of diazepam or midazolam. Following the diagnostic ERCP examination, intraductal contrast medium is allowed to escape into the duodenum. (Diagnostic ERCP preceding SO manometry does not alter the validity of the subsequent recording and is cost-effective[13].)

The diagnostic ERCP cannula is removed over a guide wire and subsequently replaced by the manometry catheter. The Arndorfer manometry catheter incorporates a small distal sheath that slides over the guide wire. This guide wire is removed prior to SO recording because it tends to cause trace artefact. Following the completion of the manometric recording, a small amount of contrast medium can be intro-

Figure 3.4 SO pressure recording technique from the SO zone. The manometry catheter is freely inserted into the CBD segment of the SO. A stationed pullthrough into the duodenum is performed at least twice.

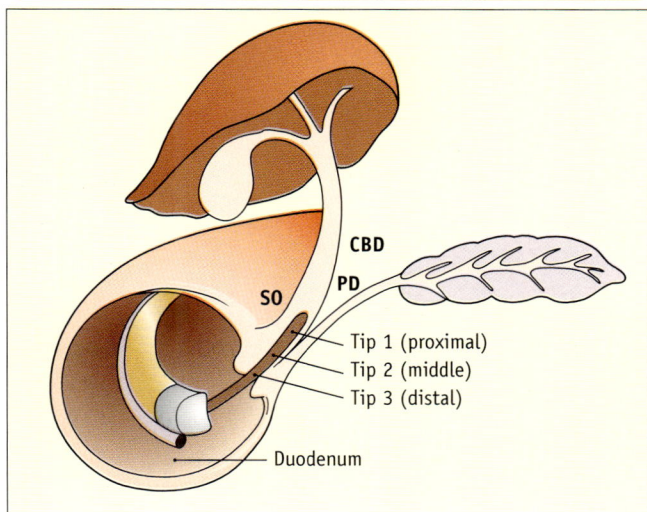

Figure 3.5 SO pressure profile obtained during catheter pullthrough of the CBD, showing the CBD/duodenal pressure gradient, the basal SO pressure and superimposed phasic SO waves.

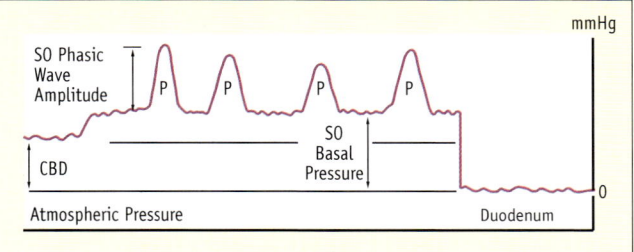

Figure 3.6 Phasic SO waves are recorded in all three orifices of the manometric catheter. Pressures are indicated on the vertical axis and time on the horizontal. In this triple sequence, the wave propagation is antegrade, i.e. towards the duodenum.

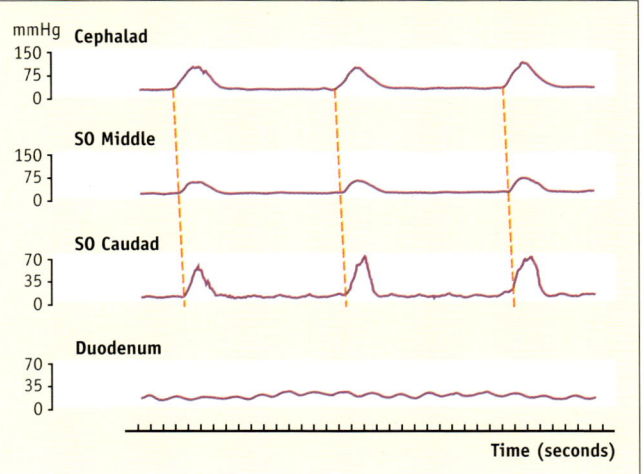

duced through the manometric catheter to verify which segment of the SO has been measured. Assessment of the ductal orientation of the SO manometric catheter is often based on the colour of the aspirated fluid, although the accuracy of this method has never been validated.

The manometry catheter is passed through the biopsy channel of the duodenoscope and inserted through the papilla and into the PD (Figure 3.4). The catheter should be freely inserted into the ductal system without kinking or bowing. The recording orifices are stationed initially for 2 or 3 min within the duct to record pressure and to permit a 'stabilization' of the SO mechanism[14]. Subsequently, the manometry catheter is withdrawn across the SO segment in 2mm incremental 'stations' using the circumferential rings as reference points for depth determination. The SO pressure is recorded during two relatively rapid pullthroughs. Finally, the catheter is stationed in the SO zone to record basal SO pressure and/or phasic SO contractions for a 3–5 min period from all three ports with the polygraph speed increased to 5cm/s. Paper speed is increased so that the temporal relationship of the phasic wave recorded in the three orifices can be determined much more accurately.

Because of the increased incidence of pancreatitis following SO manometry[15], especially when the PD is involved in the recording procedure, recording time is carefully monitored and compacted to 5 min of interpretable recording. As mentioned, the aspiration catheter has been used more successfully, with a significantly lower incidence of post-ERCP pancreatitis. However, determination of basal SO pressure may be influenced when pressures are averaged from two rather than three recording ports and, for that reason, there has not been universal adoption of the aspirating catheter.

During pullthrough of the SO zone, PD pressure is obtained initially. As the catheter is withdrawn into the zone of the SO, there is an elevated basal SO pressure created that is an intermittently sustained or plateaued pressure (Figure 3.5). The basal pressure is often 8–10mm above the

intraductal pressure and 20–25mmHg above duodenal pressure. We record 'actual' duodenal pressures because atmospheric pressure is used as our zero point. A basal SO pressure is obtained for at least 2 min from each recording port; the average of these three values determines the mean basal SO pressure[16].

Phasic SO waves can be recorded from each recording orifice. The frequency, amplitude and duration of phasic waves are calculated over the same recording period and the mean value is determined for each minute. Amplitude of the phasic waves is determined by subtracting the basal SO pressure from the peak wave pressure, and the direction of propagation of wave sequences is determined by drawing a line from the onset point of the major upstroke of the proximal phasic wave to the onset point of the corresponding distal phasic wave (Figure 3.6). In this manner, the phasic wave sequences over a 4m recording span are classified as: antegrade, i.e. towards the duodenum; retrograde, away from the duodenum; or simultaneous. Analysis of SO pressure has shown no difference in values recorded from 'control' patients or volunteer subjects with or without a gall bladder[17].

Figure 3.7 CCK-OP administration. (a) The normal response to an intravenous bolus of CCK-OP (20ng/kg) is shown in this trace. Rapid SO phasic wave activity (tachyoddia) is ablated almost immediately following CCK injection (arrow). (b) Paradoxical response to CCK-OP. There is a sequential contraction response recorded in all three tips within the SO zone. (Note the duodenal contraction is delayed relative to the SO.)

Figure 3.8 Portions of manometric pressure recordings from the CBD and the PD segments of the SO. Basal SO pressures are similar in the CBD and PD, and phasic SO waves are also comparable.

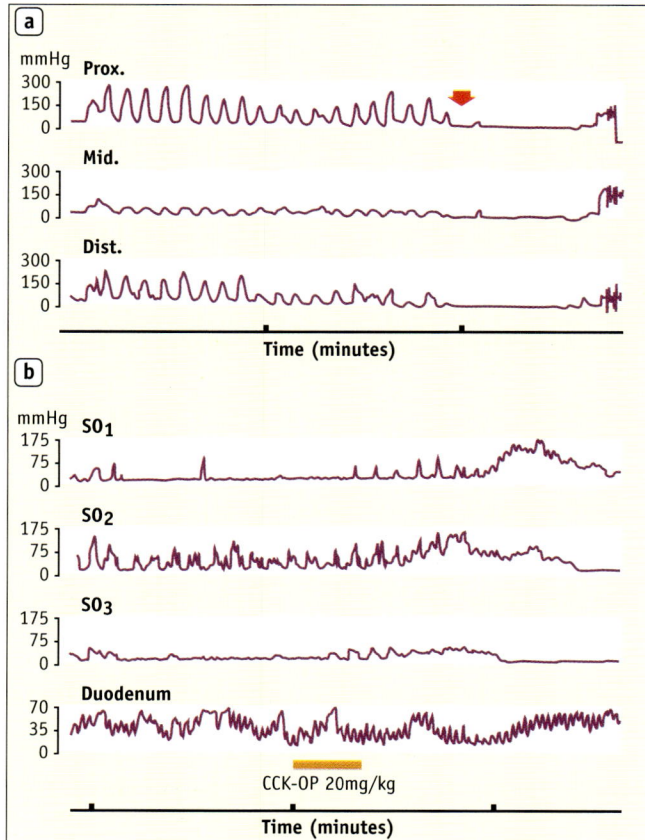

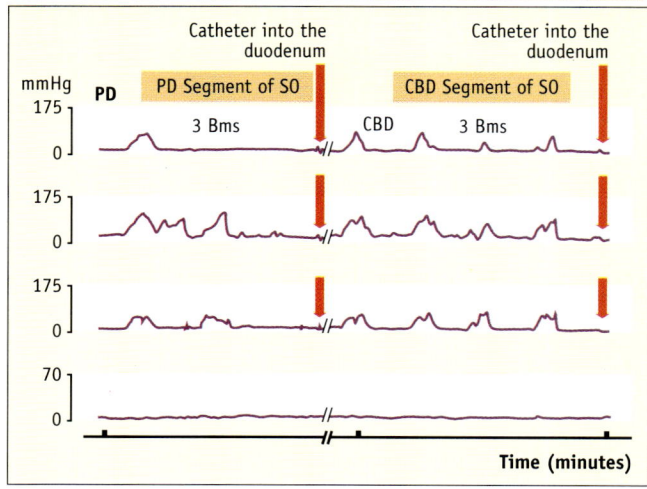

Duodenal pressure, ductal pressure and basal SO pressure are each averaged from all three recording tips. Basal SO pressure must be reproducible in at least two of the three recording tips on at least two pullthroughs. During the recording of SO pressure, certain provocative tests can be performed. Cholecystokinin (CCK-OP), 20ng/kg IV, can be administered as a pulse bolus and phasic SO activity observed for 3–5 min following administration. Normally, phasic SO activity and basal SO pressure markedly decrease at this dosage (Figure 3.7a). In some patients there is a paradoxical pressure increase in the basal SO pressure and this 'paradoxical response' is felt to represent a denervated sphincter[18] (Figure 3.7b). In another test, an ampoule of amyl nitrate is broken and the patient is instructed to take four deep 'sniffs'. The patient's pulse is monitored during this time and both basal and phasic SO activity is observed for 2–3 min. Normally, there is a profound decrease in both SO features[19].

There are caveats for recording SO manometry, ranging from the need for an experienced manometrist and endoscopist to appropriate supervised training in SO manometric pressure recording. The reproducibility of SO manometric pressure recording in the same groups of patients has been demonstrated by a number of investigators throughout the world[20]. In a group of 47 patients studied on two occasions over a 12-month period, there was significant correlation in reproducibility of basal SO pressure[21].

SO manometric pressure values have been standardized throughout the world. A basal SO pressure of 40mm Hg has been determined to be 2–3 standard deviations above the mean[22]. A study of 50 healthy volunteers showed the average basal pressure was 35mmHg[23]. The average amplitude of phasic SO contractions ranges from 350 to 400mmHg. The upper limits for the frequency of phasic SO contractions ranges from 7 to 10/min. The sequence of phasic contractions, i.e. antegrade or retrograde, varies. Retrograde sequence is abnormal if it occurs in more than 50% of total waveforms, based on two studies in patients; however, studies in normal subjects indicate that the majority of phasic waves are simultaneous in propagation sequence.

SO manometry has been used in an attempt to separate SO dysfunction into the categories of stenosis and dyskinesia[24]. The recording of rapid SO phasic waves or paradoxical response to CCK-OP would suggest dyskinesia. An elevated basal SO pressure does not differentiate a stenosis from dyskinesia. However, the administration of a smooth muscle relaxant such as CCK, amyl nitrate or glucagon and subsequent SO relaxation is highly suggestive of a muscular rather than a structural disorder.

CLINICAL SIGNIFICANCE

Evidence on the clinical significance of SO manometry in relation to pancreatic disorders has been accruing at a relatively rapid pace over the last few years. A recent study reported SO manometric pressures recorded from both the CBD and the PD segments in a group of 58 patients could be divided into three groups: functional abdominal pain, partial biliary obstruction and idiopathic recurrent pancreat-

Figure 3.9 Basal SO pressure is markedly elevated during manometric catheter pull-through of the pancreatic duct. Evidence of phasic SO pressure is seen in the proximal recording port.

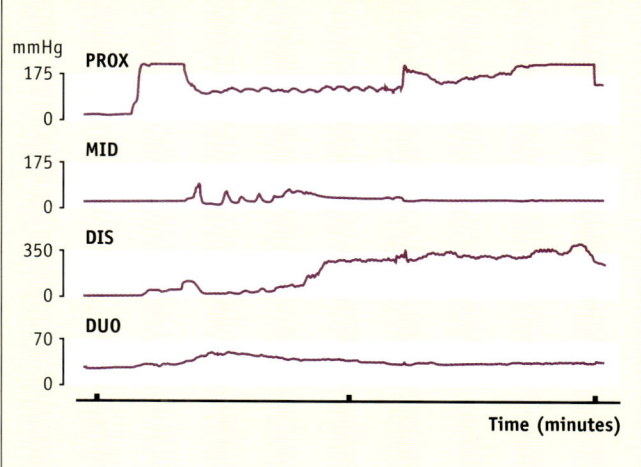

Figure 3.10 The SO pressure recorded from the PD portion of the SO is preserved following conventional sphincterotomy. However, the group of patients with recurrent episodes of pancreatitis (right) demonstrate an abnormal elevation of their basal SO pressure.

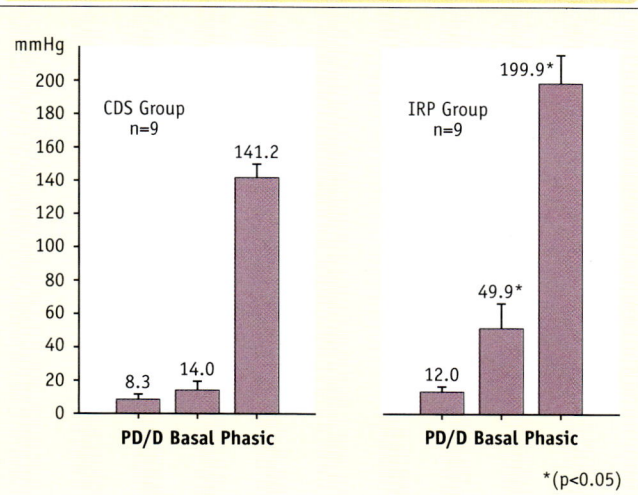

*(p<0.05)

itis[5]. Resting ductal pressures in either the CBD or the PD were equivalent in all three patient groups. Basal SO pressure in the patient group with functional abdominal pain, was comparable whether it was recorded from the CBD or PD segment (Figure 3.8). In the patient group with partial biliary obstruction, mean basal SO pressure was comparable from either ductal source but it was significantly higher than basal pressures in the group of patients with functional pain. Additionally, five of eight patients in the partial biliary obstruction group had the elevated basal SO pressure confined to the CBD segment. Three of the patients also had elevated basal pressures in both SO segments. The patients with acute recurrent pancreatitis, however, had basal SO pressure significantly greater in the PD segment (mean 37.7mmHg) compared to their CBD segment (mean 21.0mmHg). In this group, five of seven patients demonstrated the abnormal pressure exclusively in the PD segment (Figure 3.9). These study results suggested that select cannulation of the CBD or the PD segment should be considered when one wishes to diagnose or exclude SO dysfunction as a cause for a specific clinical condition suggesting a biliary or pancreatic disorder.

Most recently, a specific aetiology was identified in the majority of patients (76%) with an unexplained pancreatitis, using advanced endoscopic techniques including SO manometry. SO dysfunction was found in 24 of 68 patients (35%) with unexplained pancreatitis. SO manometry was considered an 'essential tool' when evaluating unexplained acute pancreatitis[25].

In another study, SO manometry was obtained from both ducts in 100 of 122 (82%) patients with pancreaticobiliary disorders. The overall concordance for biliary and pancreatic SO manometry results was 73%. Of the patients with abnormal SO manometry studies, 27 (42%) had abnormalities confined to only one duct. For instance, 17 patients had

abnormalities in the PD segment of the SO. Ten patients had abnormalities in the CBD portion of the SO while 37 patients (37%) had abnormalities in both ducts. It was felt that diagnostic information is increased by studying both ducts and if SO manometry is normal in one duct, study of the other duct should be attempted[26]. In another study that supports these findings, discordance between biliary and pancreatic basal SO pressure on dual sphincter manometry was observed in 47% of patients. SO manometry of both sphincters is urged when a suspected sphincter of dysfunction problem exists[27].

THERAPEUTIC INDICATIONS

Recently a number of studies have pointed more and more to the importance of SO manometry in patients with recurrent unexplained pancreatitis[28]. We have had the opportunity of following, for periods ranging from 27 to 81 months, a group of patients with acute recurrent pancreatitis who have had endoscopic or operative sphincterotomy for recurrent pancreatitis[29]. Clinical outcome was scored as 'good' only if no further attacks of pancreatitis occurred during the follow-up period. Otherwise, the patients were rated as 'poor'. Fifteen of 18 patients with elevated SO pressure have had long-term good outcome from either endoscopic or operative sphincteroplasty. In contrast, only 4 of 12 patients with normal basal SO pressure fared well after sphincterotomy. These results have been supported in a recent report that looked at the effectiveness of SO manometry and bile crystal analysis in detecting the aetiology of idiopathic pancreatitis. An abnormality found in one or other test identified an endoscopically treatable condition in these patients[30].

Conventional sphincterotomy does not always guarantee that patients with recurrent acute pancreatitis will respond[31]. A group of patients has been reported who continued to have 'attacks' of acute pancreatitis after the failure of endoscopic or conventional operative sphincteroplasty. Nine patients had two or more attacks of pancreatitis after sphincterotomy (five conventional operative sphincteroplasties; four endoscopic sphincteroplasties). SO manometry was performed with pressures recorded from both the CBD and PD. Pancreaticobiliary anatomy and secretin-stimulated pancreatic secretory test were normal. For comparison, nine patients who had endoscopic sphincterotomy for CBD were evaluated concurrently.

SO manometry pressures obtained from the CBD segment in all 18 patients were virtually identical to duodenal pressures, reflecting ablation of the CBD portion of the SO. Conversely, pressures within the PD were preserved. There was a normal PD-to-duodenal pressure gradient and preservation of basal and phasic SO contraction. However, eight of nine patients with acute recurrent pancreatitis had a significant elevation of basal and phasic SO contraction within the PD segment (Figure 3.10). This finding demonstrated persistence of an abnormally elevated PD SO pressure that did not respond to therapy. Subsequently, seven of the patients with elevated basal SO pressure in their PD segment had endoscopic sphincterotomy. Follow-up over a 5-year period has shown them to be without recurrence of pancreatitis.

References

1. Hogan WJ, Geenen JE. Biliary dyskinesia. *Endoscopy* 1988; 20:179–83.
2. Venu RP, Geenen JE, Hogan WJ *et al.* Idiopathic recurrent pancreatitis. An approach to diagnosis and treatment. *Dig Dis Sci* 1989; 34:56–60.
3. Komorowski RA, Beggs BL, Geenen JE *et al.* Assessment of ampulla of Vater pathology: an endoscopic approach. *Am J Surg Path* 1991; 15:1188–96.
4. Boyden EA. The anatomy of the choledochoduodenal junction in man. *Surg Gynecol Obstet* 1957; 104:641–52.
5. Raddawi H, Geenen JE, Hogan WJ, Dodds WJ, Venu RP, Johnson GK. Pressure measurement from the biliary and pancreatic segments of the sphincter of Oddi: comparison between patients with functional biliary and pancreatic disease. *Dig Dis Sci* 1991; 36(1):71–4.
6. Toouli J, Roberts-Thomson IC, Dent J *et al.* Sphincter of Oddi motility disorders in patients with idiopathic recurrent pancreatitis. *Br J Surg* 1985; 72:859–63.
7. Geenen JE, Hogan WJ, Dodds WJ *et al.* Intraluminal pressure recording from the human sphincter of Oddi. *Gastroenterology* 1980; 78:317–24.
8. Hogan WJ, Geenen JE. Dysmotility disturbances of the biliary tract; classification, diagnosis and treatment. *Semin Liver Dis* 1987; 7:302–10.
9. Tamasky P, Knapple W, Coyle W *et al.* Does sphincter of Oddi dysfunction cause chronic pancreatitis? *Gastrointest Endosc* 1996; 43(4):398.
10. Hogan WJ. Gallbladder and biliary tract. In *Atlas of Gastrointestinal Motility in Health and Disease*. Edited by MM Schuster. Williams & Wilkins; 1993: 250–67.
11. Sherman S, Troiano FP, Hawes RH *et al.* Sphincter of Oddi manometry: decreased risk of clinical pancreatitis with use of a modified aspirating catheter. *Gastrointest Endosc* 1990; 36:462–6.
12. Tanaka M, Ikeda S. Sphincter of Oddi manometry: comparison of microtransducer and perfusion methods. *Endoscopy* 1988; 20:184–8.
13. Sherman S, Hawes RH, Madura JA *et al.* Comparison of intraoperative and endoscopic manometry of the sphincter of Oddi. *Surg Gynecol Obstet* 1992; 175:410–8.
14. Funch-Jensen P, Kruse A, Ravnsbaek J. Endoscopic sphincter of Oddi manometry in healthy volunteers. *Scand J Gastroenterol* 1987; 22:243–9.
15. Sherman S, Lehman GA. ERCP and endoscopic sphincterotomy-induced pancreatitis. *Pancreas* 1991; 6:350–67.
16. Toouli J. Clinical relevance of sphincter of Oddi dysfunction. *Br J Surg* 1990; 77:723–4.
17. Guelrud M. Results of sphincter of Oddi manometry studies in healthy humans. *Gastrointest Endosc Clin N Am* 1993; 3:93–105.
18. Rolny P, Arleback A, Funch-Jensen P *et al.* Paradoxical response of sphincter of Oddi to intravenous injection of cholecystokinin or ceruletide. Manometric findings and results of treatment in biliary dyskinesia. *Gut* 1986; 27:1507–11.
19. Dodds WJ. Biliary tract motility and its relationship to clinical disorders. *Am J Radiol* 1990; 155:247–58.
20. Smithline A, Hawes R, Lehman G. Sphincter of Oddi manometry: interobserver variability. *Gastrointest Endosc* 1993; 39:486–91.
21. Geenen JE, Hogan WJ, Dodds WJ *et al.* The efficacy of endoscopic sphincterotomy after cholecystectomy in patients with sphincter of Oddi dysfunction. *New Engl J Med* 1989; 320:82–7.
22. Toouli J. What is sphincter of Oddi dysfunction? *Gut* 1989; 30:753–61.
23. Guelrud M, Mendoza S, Rossiter G *et al.* Sphincter of Oddi manometry in healthy volunteers. *Dig Dis Sci* 1990; 35:38–46.
24. Hogan WJ. Sphincter of Oddi physiology and pathophysiology. *Regul Pept Let III* 1991; 2:23–8.
25. Coyle W, Tamasky P, Knapple W *et al.* Evaluation of unexplained acute pancreatitis using ERCP, sphincter of Oddi manometry (SOM) and endoscopic ultrasound (EUS). *Gastrointest Endosc* 1996; 43(4):378.
26. Knapple W, Tarnasky P, Coyle W *et al.* Sphincter of Oddi manometry (SOM) of both ducts after conscious sedation with meperidine. *Gastrointest Endosc* 1996; 43(4):385.
27. Kaw M, Verma R, Brodmerkel GJ. Biliary and/or pancreatic sphincter of Oddi dysfunction (SOD). Response to endoscopic sphincterotomy (ES). *Gastrointest Endosc* 1996; 43(4):384.
28. Gregg JW, Carr-Locke DL. Endoscopic pancreatic and biliary manometry in pancreatic, biliary and papillary disease and after endoscopic sphincterotomy and surgical sphincteroplasty. *Gut* 1984; 25:1247.
29. Stone JE, Hogan WJ, Geenen JE *et al.* Acute recurrent pancreatitis: the role of sphincter of Oddi (SO) manometry in predicting long-term benefit of therapy. *Gastroenterol* 1988; 94(5):A446.
30. Kaw M, Verma R, Brodmerkel GJ. ERCP, biliary analysis, sphincter of Oddi manometry (SOM) in idiopathic pancreatitis (IP) and response to endoscopic sphincterotomy (ES). *Gastrointest Endosc* 1996; 43(4):408.
31. Geenen DJ, Hogan WJ, Geenen JE *et al.* The importance of the pancreatic duct segment of the sphincter of Oddi (SO): why conventional sphincteroplasty may fail in recurrent pancreatitis. *Gastroenterology* 1995; 108:A356.

4

Main pancreatic duct manometry

Niels Ebbehøj & Peter Funch-Jensen

INTRODUCTION

The pressure in the pancreas has been addressed throughout more than a hundred years as part of the physiology of pancreatic exocrine secretion and as part of the pain mechanism in chronic pancreatitis. The first reports were observations on the secretory pressures in the main pancreatic duct (MPD) in rabbits[1], dogs, cats and monkeys[2]. In man, measurements have been performed of: pressure after insertion of water or contrast medium in the pancreatic duct[3,4]; pseudocyst needle pressure[5]; endoscopically measured intraductal pressure[6-8]; and, most recently, tissue fluid pressure[9,10].

Until recently, the methods applied for measuring pancreatic pressure have been limited to direct measurement of intraductal pressure by cannulation via fistulas by direct intraoperative needle puncture. The introduction of pressure measurements by endoscopic transampullary cannulation[6,11] and by transcutaneous sonographically guided fine-needle puncture[10,12] has increased the understanding of fluid transport in the pancreatic duct and ampulla.

METHODS OF MEASURING PANCREATIC PRESSURE

Theoretically, the areas of interest for pressure investigations within the pancreas are: (a) intravascular pressure related to haemodynamics; (b) pressure in the duct system related to the production and drainage of pancreatic juice; and (c) fluid pressure in the interstitial space related to Starling forces (i.e. capillary pressure, capillary permeability, osmotic pressure in plasma and interstitial fluid, and properties and structures of the tissue).

Experimental evidence excluded portal haemodynamics from playing a major part in the regulation of pancreatic pressures and the interstitial pressure is not in itself able to create the relatively high pressures measured, regarding the possibility of continuous flow in the pancreatic duct[13, 14].

In 1958 it was demonstrated that the pancreatic part of the sphincter of Oddi is a distinct sphincter zone with influence on the flow of pancreatic juice into the duodenum[15]. Peripheral contractions in the duct system have also been described[16],but today it is generally accepted that no active contractility is present in the duct system[6].

Various manometric techniques have been applied in the pancreatic duct system, but the most widely used system today incorporates a catheter with side-holes, combined with external transducers, with perfusion effected by a capillary infusion pump[11]. This system has a high frequency response even at low perfusion rates. For ductal manometry the frequency response is of minor- importance. However, employing such a system allows endo-

Author (ref)	n	Pressure (mmHg)
Du Val (3)	9	21
White and Bourde (17)	1	14
Christoffersen *et al.* (19)	3	29
Madsen and Winkler (20)	7	26
Bradley (5)	19	26
Ebbehøj *et al.* (9)	6	24
Anderson *et al.* (21)	1	18
Rolny *et al.* (8)	13	12 * $
Sato *et al.* (22)	5	16
Okazaki *et al.* (23)	19	50 * $
Ebbehøj *et al.* (24)	39	17 *
Total/Mean	**122**	**25**

Figure 4.1 Some pancreatic pressure measurements in patients with chronic pancreatitis since 1958. Adapted from Ebbehøj 1992[18].

* denotes inclusion of patients with and without pain.
$ denotes endoscopic measurements.

scopic registration of ductal pressures as well as sphincter of Oddi manometry during the same investigation. Employing a triple-lumen catheter with side-holes spaced 2mm apart allows the recording of baseline pressure, phasic contractions and the direction of the contractions[11].

In the MPD pressure is measured by direct fine-needle puncture intraoperatively[9] or by sonographically guided puncture[10] but this can only be done when the MPD is dilated. For long-term measurements the introduction of narrow catheters through the puncture has been tried but so far without any particular success. Figure 4.1 shows some pancreatic pressure measurements taken in patients with chronic pancreatitis.

Pancreatic pressure and physiology

Normal MPD pressure is around 7–10mmHg, slightly higher than the common bile duct (CBD) pressure[9,25]. This pressure is determined by the production of pancreatic juice and the flow into the duodenum as regulated by the sphincter of Oddi or, as described later, by obstructions distally in the MPD. Sphincter of Oddi motility is described elsewhere in this book.

This formation of pressure is one of the pathophysiological considerations in various diseases of the pancreas. Pancreatitis, acute and chronic, in the dorsal part of a pancreas divisum is suggested to be associated with elevated pressure[26]. Variuos surgical and endoscopic drainage procedures for pain in chronic pancreatitis have as a prerequisite an impeded drainage of pancreatic juice as part of the pathophysiology of the disease.

Pancreatic pressure and morphology

Okazaki found higher intraductal pressures in mild and moderate chronic pancreatitis than in severely diseased glands, but did not relate the pressure differences to pain[27,28]. As for the morphology as seen by endoscopic retrograde pancreatography (ERP), there is apparently no overall relation between pressure and MPD diameter[29]. Patients with small cavities on ERP or ultrasonography (US) have significantly higher pressures and more pronounced pain[24]. This had not been reported before, but the existence of small cavities is one of the signs of severe chronic pancreatitis included in the Marseilles classification of 1984[30,31]. Thus, the higher pressure and pain score probably represent a more severe stage of disease.

Regional pressure differences are significantly but not uniformly related to ERP morphology[29]: obstruction of the MPD by stone, total obstruction or stenosis may be associated with pressure gradients; in the individual patient the pressure is usually highest in the region with the largest duct diameter. Regional pressure differences are found in many patients with chronic pancreatitis[29], the highest pressure usually being in the upstream region (Figure 4.2). The regional pressure differences may explain in part some of the contradictions in the literature[8,28] and may also be one of the reasons for the operative failures. In one study, the regional pressure differences were found to be larger in four patients with previous pancreatic surgery[29]. These patients underwent reoperation (drainage or resection) because of recurrent or persistent pain, and it seems likely that local pressure barriers being exceeded might explain their pathology. This is in agreement with Prinz, who found redrainage and extended drainage to be quite successful in a similar group of patients[32].

No clear relation between pancreatic morphology and pain in chronic pancreatitis has been established[33–41], although pancreatic calcifications were more frequent among patients without pain in some series[42,43].

Pancreatic pressure and exocrine function

A significant relation between pancreatic (tissue fluid) pressure and function has never been described. In a study of percutaneous pressure measurements the pressure was not found to be related to the results of a Lundh's meal-stimulated test[24]. No significant relation between pressure and exocrine secretory capacity was found in groups of patients with or without previous surgery, or with or without pain[24].

Amman[44,45] suggested that residual pancreatic exocrine function is an important element in the pain mechanism of chronic pancreatitis, since they found that pain ceased when exocrine function deteriorated. Girdwood[33] found more pronounced exocrine insufficiency in patients without abdominal pain. Others have not been able to confirm the relation between deteriorating exocrine function and subsequent pain relief[46–50] and the theory of the 'burning out pancreas' as the principal pain-relieving mechanism in chronic pancreatitis is debatable[51].

Pancreatic pressure and pain

The first evidence of a causal relation between pressure and pain was the observation that raising the pressure to above 25cm of water in an intubated MPD in a patient with chronic pancreatitis caused pain[17]. Later it was found that an intraoperative pressure decrease was associated with at least short-term pain relief[52]. Endoscopic pancreatic duct manometry with a microtransducer technique revealed elevated pancreatic pressures in patients with

Figure 4.2 Regional pancreatic tissue fluid pressure (mmHg) compared with duct morphology in 16 patients with chronic pancreatitis. A vertical line denotes a stone, total stop or major stenosis in the pancreatic duct at the approximate location, demonstrated by ERCP. Adapted from Ebbehøj et al. 1990[29].

Figure 4.3 Median values and maximum values of pancreatic tissue fluid pressure (obtained by percutaneous sonographically guided puncture by the needle method) and pain in 39 patients with chronic pancreatitis. $p = 0.00001$ and $p = 0.000001$, respectively. Data from Ebbehøj et al. 1990[13]

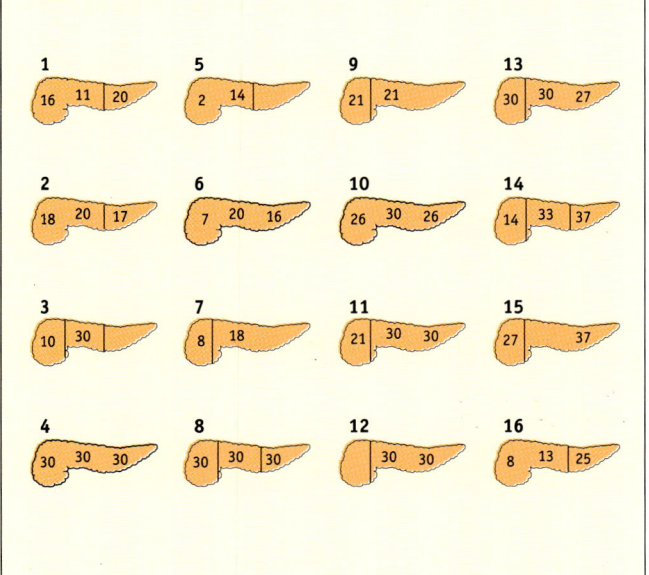

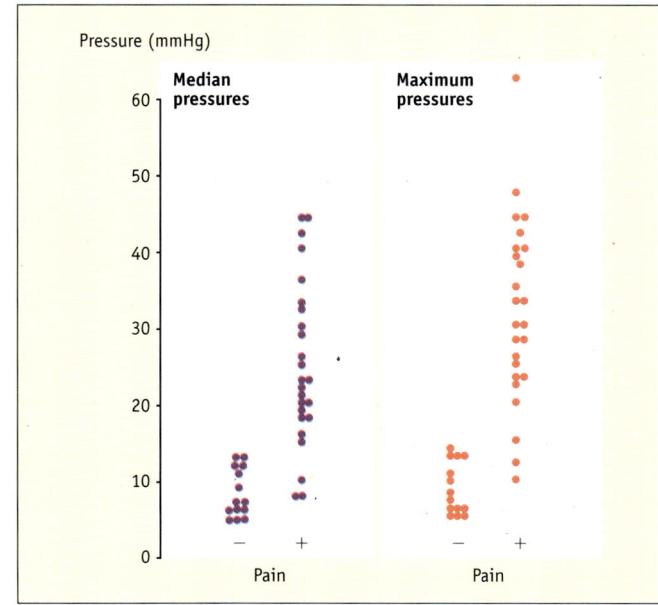

chronic pancreatitis with pain, whereas patients free of pain had normal pressures[23]. These results were in contrast to a previous study using an endoscopic perfusion manometry technique[8].

These two studies included patients with and without pain, but lacked any specific description of the criteria applied. In studies with well defined pain assessments, pancreatic tissue fluid pressures obtained by the needle method related well to pain (Figure 4.3)[24]. Thus, significantly higher pressures were found in patients with pain than without it, and a significant correlation was found between pressure and pain score when all patients were considered[24]. However, when the group of patients with pain was considered alone, the correlation was not significant[24]. This may be considered to be a reminder of the differences in pain perception in individual patients, and of the existence of mechanisms modulating the perception of a given peripheral nociceptive stimulus[53].

The apparent pain threshold in this study was a pancreatic tissue fluid pressure of 15mmHg[24], in agreement with previous results[17], and slightly above normal values[9]. However, this pressure is probably not high enough to initiate a compartment syndrome with tissue ischaemia[54]. Patients with previous pancreatic surgery were not distinctive in revealing the pressure-and-pain relation[24].

In a longitudinal study, drainage operations for pain in chronic pancreatitis led to pressure decreases and subsequent pain relief[24,52]. A decisive factor for a postoperative pain-free period, which in some studies was achieved in up to 90% of the patients (Figure 4.4), was an intraoperative pressure decrease of at least 10mmHg. The duration of the postoperative pain-free period was significantly related to the magnitude of the intraoperative pressure decrease[65].

Future studies

Despite increasing evidence that MPD pressure plays a part in the pathophysiology of pancreatic disease, four main issues still need intensive research. First, the cause of increased pressure in various diseases should be investigated, and anatomical and physiological obstructions to the flow of pancreatic juice should be taken into consideration. Secondly, the effects of the numerous drainage procedures need evaluation with respect to defectiveness in drainage of whole or part of the pancreas. Thirdly, the relation between MPD pressure and blood perfusion calls for research, as a possible reason for decreasing endocrine pancreatic function in chronic pancreatitis. Finally, in acute pancreatitis the possibility that impeded drainage plays a role in the early pathophysiological mechanisms could lead to new early therapies, either pharmaceutical or endoscopic. For this purpose, the safety of the different pressure measurement techniques in acute pancreatitis must be evaluated.

Figure 4.4 Short-term (<1 year) and long-term (>1 year) pain relief after drainage operations for chronic pancreatitis. Adapted from Ebbehøj 1992 [18].

Author (ref)	Drainage procedure	n	Pain relief (%) Short-term	Long-term
White (55)	PJ	55		63
Amman (56)	PJ + resect	47		40
Warshaw (57)	PJ	10		80
Prinz (58)	PJ	87		37
Taylor (59)	PJ	16	87	50
Scuro (60)	PJ	93		63
Amman (44)	PJ	69		48
Sato (22)	PJ	43		90
Holmberg (61)	PJ	51		60
Ebbehøj (10)	PG	13	46	
Bradley (62)	PJ	64		58
Pain (63)	PG	53	80	60
Ebbehøj (64)	PG	45		56
Total/Mean		**646**	**81**	**55**

PJ = pancreaticojejunostomy
PG = pancreaticogastrostomy

References

1. Henry, Wollheim: Einige Beobachtungen über das Pankreassecret pflanzenfressender Tiere. *Arch Physiol* 1877; xiv:465.

2. Herring PT, Simpson S. The pressure of pancreatic secretion and the mode of absorption of pancreatic juice after obstruction of the main ducts of the pancreas. *J Q Physiol Rev* 1909; 2:99–108.

3. Du Val MK. The effect of chronic pancreatitis on pressure tolerance in the human pancreatic duct. *Surgery* 1958; 43:798–801.

4. White TT, Elmslie RG, Magee DF. Observations on the human intraductal pancreatic pressure. *Surg Gynecol Obstet* 1964; 118:1043–5.

5. Bradley EL. Pancreatic duct pressure in chronic pancreatitis. *Am J Surg* 1982; 144:313–16.

6. Csendes A, Kruse A, Funch-Jensen P et al. Pressure measurements in the biliary and pancreatic duct systems in controls and in patients with gallstones, previous cholecystectomy, or common bile duct stones. *Gastroenterology* 1979; 77:1203–10.

7. Gregg JA, Carr-Locke DL. Endoscopic pancreatic and biliary manometry in pancreatic, biliary and papillary disease and after endoscopic sphincterotomy. *Gut* 1984; 25:1247–54.

8. Rolny P, Ärlebäck A, Järnerot G, Andersson T. Endoscopic manometry of the sphincter of Oddi and pancreatic duct in chronic pancreatitis. *Scand J Gastroenterol* 1986; 21:415–20.

9. Ebbehøj N, Svendsen LB, Madsen P. Pancreatic tissue pressure. Techniques and pathophysiological aspects. *Scand J Gastroenterol* 1984; 19:1066–8.

10. Ebbehøj N, Bülow J, Madsen P. Tissue pressure in the pancreas measured via sonographically-guided fine needle puncture. *Ugeskr Læger* 1987; 149:2786–8.

11. Geenen JE, Hogan WJ, Dodds WJ et al. Intraluminal pressure recording from the human sphincter of Oddi. *Gastroenterology* 1980; 78:317–24.

12. Ebbehøj N, Borly L, Bülow J, Henriksen JH, Heyeraas KJ, Rasmussen SG. Evaluation of pancreatic pressure measurements intraoperatively and by sonographically guided fine-needle puncture. *Scand J Gastroenterol* 1990; 25:1097–102.

13. Ebbehøj N, Borly L, Heyeraas KJ, Henriksen JH. The effect of portal hypertension and duct ligature on pancreatic tissue fluid pressures in cats. *Scand J Gastroenterol* 1990; 25:609–12.

14. Karanjia ND, Singh SM, Widdison AL, Lutrin FJ, Reber HA. Pancreatic ductal and interstitial pressures in cats with chronic pancreatitis. *Dig Dis Sci* 1992; 37:268–73.

15. Menguy RB, Hallenbeck GA, Bollman JL, Grindley JH. Intraductal pressures and sphincteric resistance in canine pancreatic and biliary ducts after various stimuli. *Surg Gynecol Obstet* 1958; 106(3):306–20.

16. Korovitsky LK. The part played by the ducts in the pancreatic secretion. *J Physiol* 1923; 57:215–23.

17. White TT, Bourde J. A new observation on human intraductal pancreatic pressure. *Surg Gynecol Obstet* 1970; 124:275–8.

18. Ebbehøj N. *Pancreatic Tissue Fluid Pressure and Pain*. Lægeforeningens Forlag, Copenhagen; 1992.

19. Christoffersen I, Madsen P, Philbert A, Smith K. Chronic obstructive pancreatitis treated by pancreatogastrostomy. *Gastroenterology* 1981; 80:1124.

20. Madsen P, Winkler K. The intraductal pancreatic pressure in chronic pancreatitis. *Scand J Gastroenterol* 1982; 17:553–4.

21. Anderson TM, Pitt HA, Longmire WP. Experience with sphincteroplasty and sphincterotomy in pancreaticobiliary surgery. *Ann Surg* 1985; 201:399–401.

22. Sato T, Miyashita E, Matsuno S, Yamauchi H. The role of surgical treatment for chronic pancreatitis. *Ann Surg* 1986; 203:266–71.

23. Okazaki K, Yamamoto Y, Kagiyama S et al. Pressure of papillary sphincter zone and pancreatic main duct in patients with alcoholic and idiopathic chronic pancreatitis. *Int J Pancreatol* 1988; 3:457–68.

24. Ebbehøj N, Borly L, Bülow J, et al. Pancreatic tissue fluid pressure in chronic pancreatitis. Relation to pain, morphology and function. *Scand J Gastroenterol* 1990; 25:1046–51.

25. Tanaka M, Ikeda S, Nakayama F. Nonoperative measurements of pancreatic and common bile duct pressures with a microtransducer catheter and effects of duodenoscopic sphincterotomy. *Dig Dis Sci* 1981; 26:545–52.

26. Staritz M, Meyer zum Buschenfelde KH. Elevated pressure in the dorsal part of pancreas divisum: the cause of chronic pancreatitis? *Pancreas* 1988; 3(1):108–10.

27. Okazaki K, Yamamoto Y, Ito K et al. Endoscopic measurement of papilla sphincter zone and pancreatic main duct pressure in patients with chronic pancreatitis. *Gastroenterology* 1986; 91:409–18.

28. Okazaki K, Yamamoto Y, Kagiyama S et al. Pressure of papillary sphincter zone and pancreatic main duct in patients with chronic pancreatitis in the early stage. *Scand J Gastroenterol* 1988; 23:501–7.

29. Ebbehøj N, Borly L, Madsen P, Matzen P. Comparison of regional pancreatic tissue fluid pressures and ERP-morphology in chronic pancreatitis. *Scand J Gastroenterol* 1990; 25:756–60.

30. Sarner M, Cotton P. Classification of pancreatitis. *Gut* 1984; 25:756–9.

31. Sarner M, Cotton PB. Definitions of acute and chronic pancreatitis. *Clin Gastroenterol* 1984; 13:865–71.

32. Prinz RA, Aranha GV, Greenlee HB. Redrainage of the pancreatic duct in chronic pancreatitis. *Am J Surg* 1986; 151:150–6.

33. Girdwood AH, Merks IN, Bornman PC, Kottler RE, Cohen M. Does progressive pancreatic insufficiency limit pain in calcific pancreatitis with duct stricture or continued alcohol insult? *J Clin Gastroenterol* 1981; 3:241–5.

34. Braganza JM, Hunt L, Warwick F. Relationship between pancreatic exocrine function and ductal morphology in chronic pancreatitis. *Gastroenterology* 1982; 62:1341–7.

35. Lauridsen KN, Raahede J, Kruse A, Thommesen P. ERP in chronic pancreatitis - ductal morphology, relation to exocrine function and pain - clinical value. *Röntgenblatter* 1985; 38:258–60.

36. Kugelberg C, Wehlin L, Arnesjö B, Tylén U. Endoscopic pancreaticography in evaluating results of pancreatico-jejunostomy. *Gut* 1976; 17:167–72.

37. Bornman PC, Girdwood AH, Marks IN, Hatfield ARW, Kottler RE. The influence of continued alcohol intake, pancreatic duct hold-up, and pancreatic insufficiency on the pain pattern in chronic noncalcific and calcific pancreatitis: a comparative study. *Surg Gastroenterol* 1982; 1:5-9.

38. Girdwood AH, Hatfield ARW, Bornman PC, Denyer ME, Kottler RE, Marks IN. Structure and function in non-calcific pancreatitis. *Dig Dis Sci* 1984; 29:721–6.

39. Jensen AR, Matzen P, Malchow-Møller A, Christoffersen I et al. Pattern of pain, duct morphology, and pancreatic function in chronic pancreatitis. *Scand J Gastroenterol* 1984; 19:334–8.

40. Malfertheiner P, Büchler M, Stanescu A, Ditschuneit H. Pancreatic morphology and function in relation to pain in chronic pancreatitis. *Int J Pancreatol* 1987; 1:59–66.

41. Bornman PC, Marks IN, Girdwood AH et al. Is pancreatic duct obstruction or stricture a major cause of pain in calcific pancreatitis? *Br J Surg* 1980; 67:425–8.

42. Bornman PC, Marks IN, Girdwood AH. Mechanism of pain in chronic alcohol-induced pancreatitis. In *Pancreatitis – Concepts and Classification*. Edited by Gyr K, Singer MV, Sarles H. Elsevier, Amsterdam; 1984.

43. Keith RG, Keshavjee SH, Kerenyi NR. Neuropathology of chronic pancreatitis in humans. *Can J Surg* 1985; 28:207–11.

44. Amman RW, Akovbiantz A, Largiader F. Pain relief in chronic pancreatitis with and without surgery. *Gastroenterology* 1984; 87:746–7.

45. Amman RW, Akovbiantz A, Largiader F, Schueler G. Course and outcome of chronic pancreatitis. Longitudinal study of a mixed medical-surgical series of 245 patients. *Gastroenterology* 1984; 86:820–8.

46. Warshaw AL. Conservation of pancreatic tissue by combined gastric, biliary, and pancreatic duct drainage for pain from chronic pancreatitis. *Am J Surg* 1985; 149:563–9.

47. Moossa AR. Surgical treatment of chronic pancreatitis: an overview. *Br J Surg* 1987; 74:661–7.

48. Ink O, Labayle D, Buffet C, Chaput JC, Étienne JP. Pancreatite chronique alcoolique: relations de la doleur avec le sevrage et la chirurgie pancréatique. *Gastroenterol Clin Biol* 1984; 8:419–25.

49. Ink O, Attali P, Pelletier G, Buffet C, Etienne JP. Pain in chronic pancreatitis. *Gastroenterology* 1985; 88:603–4.

50. Pedersen NT, Andersen BN, Pedersen G, Worning H. Chronic pancreatitis in Copenhagen. A retrospective study of 64 consecutive cases. *Scand J Gastroenterol* 1982; 17:925–31.

51. Warshaw AL. Pain in chronic pancreatitis. Patients, patience and the impatient surgeon. *Gastroenterology* 1984; 86:987–9.

52. Ebbehøj N, Borly L, Madsen P, Svendsen LB. Pancreatic tissue pressure and pain in chronic pancreatitis. *Pancreas* 1986; 1:556–8.

53. Cervero F. Neurophysiology of gastrointestinal pain. *Baillières Clin Gastroenterol* 1988; 2:183–99.

54. Perry MO. Compartment syndromes and reperfusion injury. *Surg Clin North Am* 1988; 68:853–64.

55. White TT, Slavotinek AH. Results of surgical treatment of chronic pancreatitis. Report of 142 cases. *Ann Surg* 1979; 189:217–24.

56. Amman RW, Largiader F, Akovbiantz A. Pain relief by surgery in chronic pancreatitis? Relationship between pain relief, pancreatic dysfunction and alcohol withdrawal. *Scand J Gastroenterol* 1979; 14:209–14.

57. Warshaw AL, Popp JW, Schapiro RH. Long term patency, pancreatic function, and pain relief after lateral pancreaticojejunostomy for chronic pancreatitis. *Gastroenterology* 1980; 79:289–93.

58. Prinz RA, Herbert MD, Greenlee B. Pancreatic duct drainage in 100 patients with chronic pancreatitis. *Ann Surg* 1981; 194:313–20.

59. Taylor RH, Bagley FH, Braasch JW, Warren KW. Ductal drainage or resection for chronic pancreatitis. *Am J Surg* 1981; 141:28–33.

60. Scuro LA, Vantini I, Piubello W et al. Evolution of pain in chronic relapsing pancreatitis: a study of operated and nonoperated patients. *Am J Gastroenterol* 1983; 78:495–500.

61. Holmberg JT, Isaksson G, Ihse I. Long term results of pancreaticojejunostomy in chronic pancreatitis. *Surg Gynecol Obstet* 1985; 160:339–46.

62. Bradley EL. Long term results of pancreaticojejunostomy in patients with chronic pancreatitis. *Am J Surg* 1987; 153:207–13.

63. Pain JA, Knight MJ. Pancreaticogastrostomy: the preferred operation for pain relief in chronic pancreatitis. *Br J Surg* 1988; 75:220–2.

64. Ebbehøj N, Klaaborg KE, Kronborg O, Madsen P. Pancreaticogastrostomy for chronic pancreatitis. *Am J Surg* 1989; 157:315–17.

65. Ebbehøj N, Borly L, Bülow J, Rasmussen SG, Madsen P. Evaluation of pancreatic tissue fluid pressure and pain in chronic pancreatitis - a longitudinal study. *Scand J Gastroenterol* 1990; 25:462–6.

5

Endoscopic ultrasonography

T. Lok Tio

INTRODUCTION

In Europe and Japan abdominal ultrasonography (US) is widely used as the primary diagnostic imaging modality in diagnosing pancreatic diseases because it is non-invasive, relatively mobile and particularly user-friendly. In daily clinical practice, however, abdominal adipose tissue, low-standing ribs in patients with lung emphysema, and previous abdominal surgery, may lead to unsuccessful investigation. Endoscopic retrograde cholangiopancreatography (ERCP) has become the standard diagnostic procedure in patients with pancreaticobiliary diseases. Since the late 1970s, there has been a trend towards the development of a combination of US and endoscopy in a single instrument, in which an echoprobe is attached to the tip of the endoscope[1-3]. Recently, endoscopic ultrasonography (EUS) has been increasingly performed in Europe, Japan and the United States[2-7]. The direct approach to the target of interest with high-frequency US enables clear, detailed imaging of the pancreas, the ampulla of Vater and the extrahepatic bile duct that cannot be obtained by conventional abdominal US[11-19]. Intraductal US, performed transhepatically during antegrade cholangiography, or transpapillary during ERCP, or during laparoscopy or laparascopic cholecystectomy, has been introduced for clinical evaluation. The preliminary results of such intraductal US (IDUS) are promising, and it is likely that this will become the future trend.

INSTRUMENTS

The state-of-the-art instrument is either a radial scanning or a curve-array scanning echoendoscope, in which a small ultrasound transducer is mounted on the tip of a lateral-viewing endoscope. The choice of a lateral-viewing echoendoscope is based on experience gathered from ERCP that such an endoscope enables the operator to visualize the papilla accurately and to cannulate the bile duct and the pancreatic duct. The transducer can be readily inserted into the duodenum and placed accurately at the target, using the endoscopic control system. At present, the most widely used instrument is an Olympus radial-scanning echoendoscope because of its rather easy anatomical orientation on US. The biopsy channel equipped with an elevator can be used for EUS-guided aspiration cytology. The maximum length of needle that can be inserted through the biopsy channel is 16mm. The length of the needle protruding from the Teflon overtube is only 7–8mm and the outer diameter is approximately 2mm. Only lesions with close proximity to the transducer, such as submucosal abnormalities, can be punctured and aspirated. Recently, a Pentax curve-array echoendoscope equipped with colour Doppler has become available. Such an instrument is

suitable for aspiration cytology, as a modified transbronchial needle can be used and imaged continuously on EUS during the puncture procedure. Since 1988 a catheter echoprobe, which can be inserted through the large biopsy channel of the endoscope has also been available. Recently, such a catheter echoprobe has also been employed in evaluating biliary and pancreatic duct abnormalities by direct insertion into the duct system via a duodenoscope. A 'Microvasive' catheter echoprobe can be inserted via a guide wire previously inserted during routine ERCP or percutaneous cholangiography (PTC). Such a procedure requires fluoroscopy for controlling the position of the transducer.

INVESTIGATIVE TECHNIQUE

The method of investigation resembles the endoscopic manoeuvre during ERCP. Intravenous sedation and topical oropharyngeal anaesthesia are necessary for smooth and successful investigation. The transducer should be positioned adequately for insertion into the duodenal bulb. Thereafter, the transducer must be further inserted into the second part of the duodenum. In pancreatic EUS the tip of the echoendoscope must be placed distally from the papilla in order to visualize the entire head of the pancreas and particularly to image the uncinate process. In the case of an ampullary lesion the papilla of Vater must be found endoscopically. Thereafter, the transducer is placed as closely as possible to the papilla. For biliary EUS the common bile duct and the portal vein should be imaged side by side by placing the echoprobe along the medial wall of the periampullary duodenum. After successful imaging of the target the echoprobe must be gradually withdrawn into the duodenal bulb and the stomach for complete examination. In IDUS the catheter echoprobe must be inserted into the bile duct or the pancreatic duct under fluoroscopic control. The detailed description of these investigative techniques will be further explained below. The body and tail of the pancreas should be examined from the stomach during the withdrawal of the instrument at the final stage of the examination.

ANATOMICAL ORIENTATION

In the duodenum, cross-sectional images resembling those obtained by computed tomography (CT) should be obtained for purposes of standardization. Abdominal US using cross-sectional, longitudinal and oblique orientations is very helpful for anatomical orientation and essential for complete examination. For practical reasons, the anatomy will be discussed according to the target of interest, either the pancreas or the ampulla of Vater.

Pancreas

The pancreas is imaged by placing the transducer in the descending duodenum, the duodenal bulb and the stomach. In order to minimize the duration of examination and to improve patient tolerance, the transducer should initially be inserted into the descending duodenum for the complete evaluation of the head of the pancreas.

Transduodenal approach: In the duodenum, cross-sectional images resembling those of CT or abdominal US are very helpful for standardization. The aorta and the inferior vena cava (IVC) are the most important landmarks and should be positioned at 5 and 7 o'clock, respectively. The spinal body, seen as a bright acoustic shadow, should be placed between the aorta and IVC at 6 o'clock. Occasionally the gall bladder can be found adjacent to the IVC. With these landmarks held in position, the transducer is gradually withdrawn proximally. The right lobe of the liver is seen at the right lateral or lateroventral quadrant. The mesenteric vessels are seen adjacent to the aorta at the left lateral quadrant; the superior mesenteric vein is seen at the ventral portion and the corresponding artery at the dorsal portion at about 3 to 4 o'clock. These blood vessels are crucial for imaging the uncinate process of the pancreas, which is visualized as a fine granulated parenchyma between the aorta, the vena cava and the mesenteric vessels (Figure 5.1). With further withdrawal of the transducer, the confluence between the portal vein, the superior mesenteric vein and the splenic vein should be clearly seen. The common bile duct (CBD) is found adjacent and parallel to the portal vein. In an oblique section the CBD, portal vein and IVC can be seen simultaneously (Figure 5.2). The gastroduodenal artery originating from the main hepat-

ic artery is seen running almost tangentially to the pancreas. The junction between the head and the body of the pancreas, the so-called neck of the pancreas, can be visualized from the proximal portion of the descending duodenum or the duodenal bulb. This area is of paramount interest in the evaluation of patients with endocrine tumours of the pancreas, particularly insulinoma. The body and the tail of the pancreas can be accurately assessed by placing the echoprobe along the posterior wall of the antrum and the body of the stomach. The splenic vein is the key to complete imaging as it runs along the dorsal portion of the entire distal pancreas into the splenic hilum. The left renal artery runs parallel to the splenic vein, originating from the IVC (Figure 5.3). In cases where imaging the splenic vein is difficult, the left renal vein is very helpful for identifying the splenic vein.

Imaging the regional lymph nodes of the pancreas requires a sound knowledge of their anatomical location. In the pancreatic head, regional lymph nodes are located adjacent to the aorta and IVC and adjacent to the splenic vessels. The so-called retropancreatic lymph nodes are found adjacent to the gastroduodenal artery or the pancreaticoduodenal artery, along the distal common bile duct and the portal vein. The pyloric lymph nodes are found at the proximal end of the gastroduodenal artery adjacent to the hepatic artery. The coeliac nodes are located at the coeliac axis – the bifurcation between the hepatic artery and the splenic artery. The lymph nodes at the distal part of the pancreas – the body and the tail of the pancreas – are located along the splenic artery and at the splenic hilum. The most proximal lymph nodes to be investigated are the lymph nodes along the left gastric artery, which can be visualized along the lesser curvature of the proximal body of the stomach.

Figure 5.1 EUS cross-sectional image from the middle part of the descending duodenum showing the aorta (AO) at 6 o'clock, the left renal vein (RV) running ventrally to the aorta, the superior mesenteric vein (MSV) at 3 o'clock, the superior mesenteric artery (MSA) at 4 o'clock. Note that the parenchyma of the uncinate process of the pancreas and the pancreatic duct (PD) are located between the aorta and the mesenteric vessels.

Figure 5.2 EUS oblique image from the level adjacent to the papilla of Vater showing the common bile duct (CBD), portal vein (PV) and inferior vena cava (IVC). The PV and IVC veins run parallel to each other. Note the clear image and fine texture of the head of the pancreas (P).

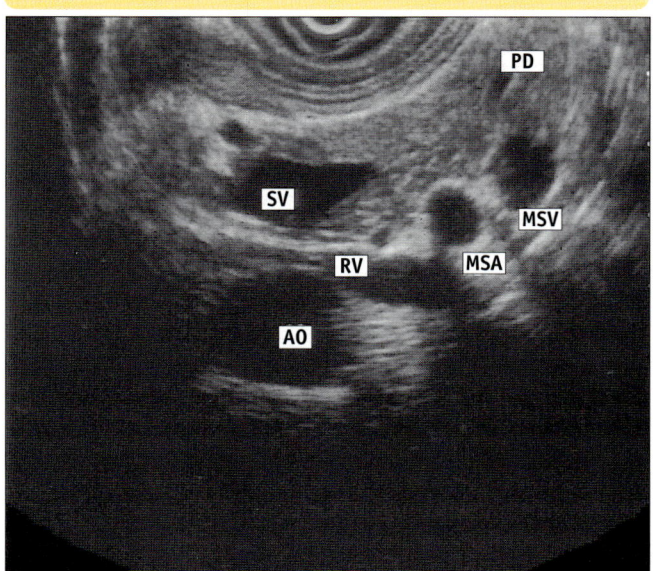

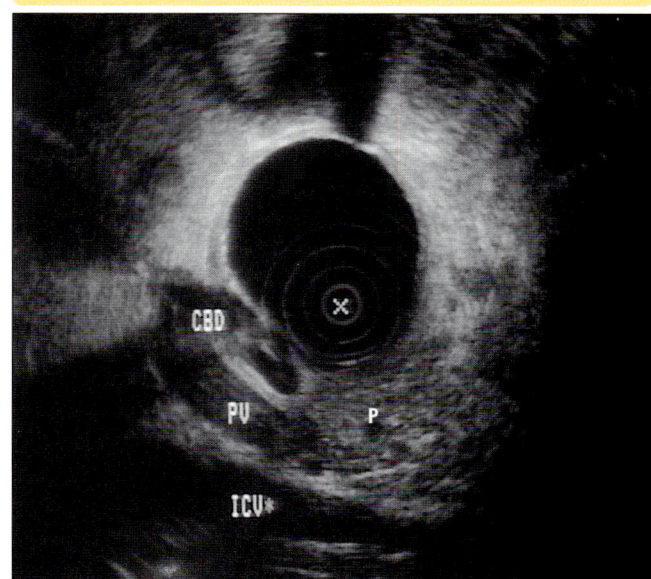

Figure 5.3 Cross-sectional EUS from the body of the stomach showing the body of the pancreas (PB) and the tail (PT), with normal texture and contours. Note that the splenic vein (SV) runs along the posterior borders of the pancreas. The left renal vein (RV) is parallel to the splenic vein. LK = left kidney.

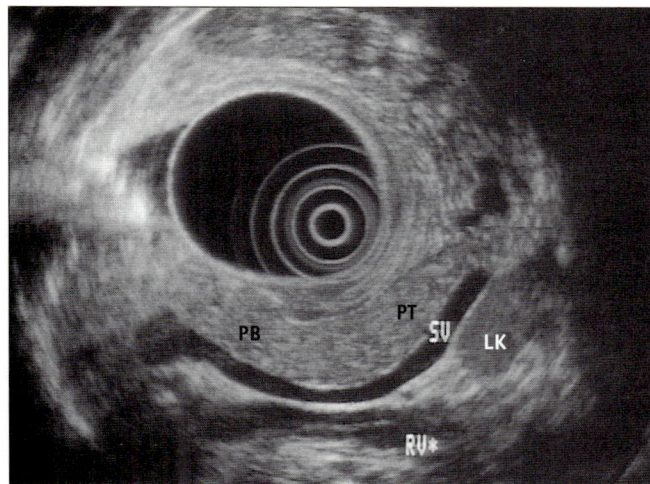

Ampulla of Vater

Imaging the ampulla of Vater requires accurate positioning of the transducer to the papilla of Vater endoscopically and sono-graphically. On EUS the papilla is seen as a nodule containing the common channel or the bile duct and the pancreatic duct. On cross-sectional images the sphincter of Oddi – the sphinc-ter ampullae – appears as a circular muscle bundle surround-ing the common channel. The sphincter of the ampulla of the

bile duct is seen as a muscle bundle encircling the bile duct, often seen as local thickening of the muscle layer of the common bile duct wall. The sphincter of the pancreatic duct resembles a muscle layer surrounding the pancreatic duct. The ampulla is located in the submucosa of the duodenum. Imaging of the major blood vessels and the regional lymph nodes resembles that for the pancreas. The lymph nodes at the splenic hilum, however, are classified as distant lymph nodes.

EUS RESULTS AND INTERPRETATION

The most important roles for EUS are in the diagnosis and staging of malignant disease of the pancreas, ampulla of Vater and bile duct, and in the localization and diagnosis of endocrine tumour of the pancreas.

Pancreatic cancer

A diagnosis of pancreatic cancer is made when a hypoechoic pancreatic tumour is seen obstructing the pancreatic duct (Figures 5.4 and 5.5). In the case of cancer of the head of the pancreas, prestenotic dilatation of the pancreatic duct and the common bile duct is often found; this is generally known as the 'double duct' sign (Figures 5.6 and 5.7). In cancer of the body or the tail of the pancreas, only dilatation of the corre-sponding pancreatic duct is seen because the common bile duct (CBD) is usually not involved unless the tumour invades the head of the pancreas (Figure 5.8). A biliary stent, either plastic or metal, is visualized as a hypoechoic pattern within the CBD (Figure 5.10). In staging pancreatic cancers the TNM classification appears to be clinically important because the depth of cancer invasion is the main criterion, replacing

Figure 5.4 EUS reveals a limited intrapancreatic tumour (T) of 2cm diameter that is located adjacent to the biliary stent (seen as two hyperechoic white lines, arrowed) without invasion of the parapancreatic tissue. From its size alone the tumour would be classified as a T1 cancer. However, due to involvement of the CBD the tumour is defined as a T2 cancer. This was confirmed by histology of a resected specimen. SV = splenic vein; SMA = superior mesenteric artery.

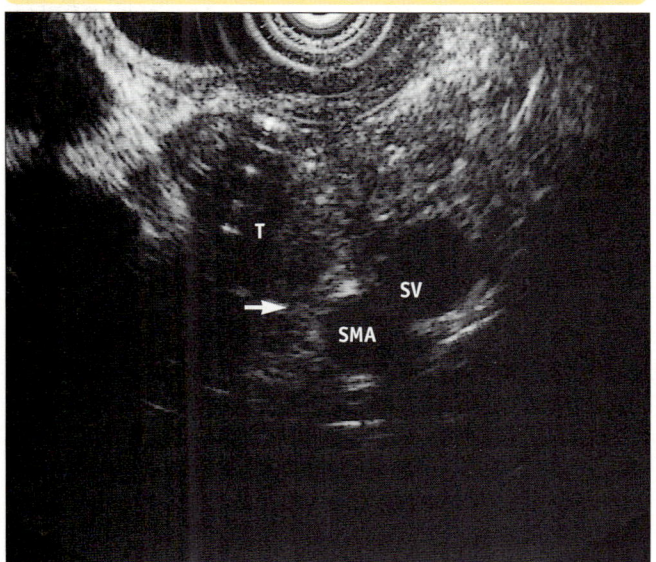

Figure 5.5 EUS reveals an intrapancreatic hypoechoic tumour (T) obstructing the common bile duct (CBD) and pancreatic duct (PD). The dilated CBD and PD are clearly seen immediately adjacent to the tumour. The splenic vein (SV), the splenoportal confluence (CF) and the superior mesenteric artery (MSA) are normal. Note the difference in echogenicity between the normal pancreas and the tumour. P = pancreas.

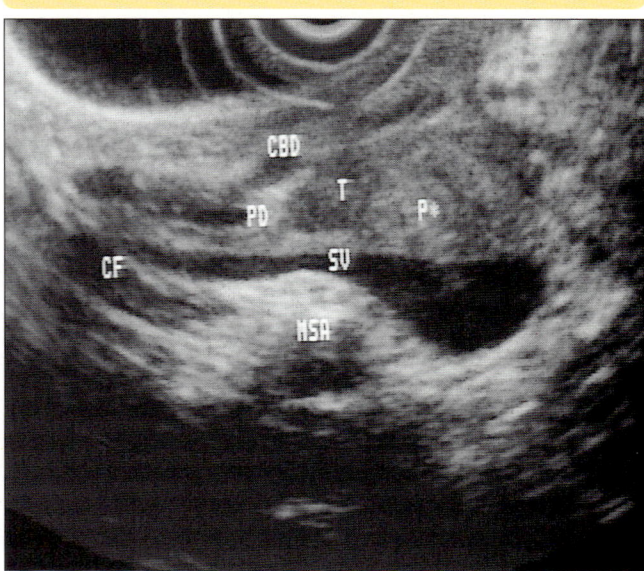

resectability of tumour as the gold standard. The definition of regional lymph nodes has been simplified. The size and extent of pancreatic carcinoma have been shown to have a close correlation with long-term prognosis of the disease[8–10b]. The TNM classification adopted for EUS is shown in Figure 5.11.

In our initial series involving 43 patients who had undergone surgery for pancreatic cancer, the histology revealed T1 cancer in 5 cases (c.11 %) (Figure 5.3). The accuracy of EUS was 100%. T2 cancer was diagnosed correctly in 88% of 17 cases. Tumour invasion was seen in the duodenum (n = 3), in

Figure 5.6 EUS reveals a limited intrapancreatic tumour (T) obstructing the pancreatic duct (PD) and common bile duct (CBD). The adjacent splenic vein (SV) appears to be of normal calibre. The tumour is classified as a T2 cancer because of the invasion into parapancreatic tissue and the CBD.

Figure 5.7 EUS reveals a hypoechoic tumour mass (T) resulting in dilatation of the common bile duct (CBD) and pancreatic duct (PD). The tumour shows direct penetration into the adjacent splenic vein (SV) (arrowed) and is classified as T3.

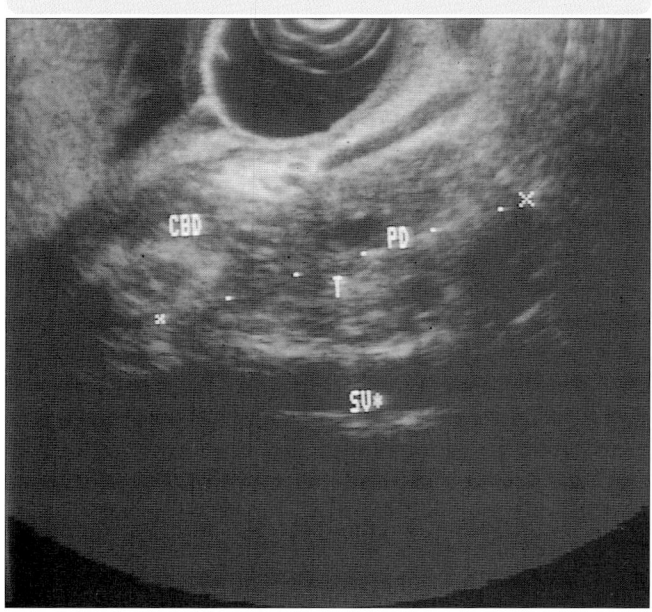

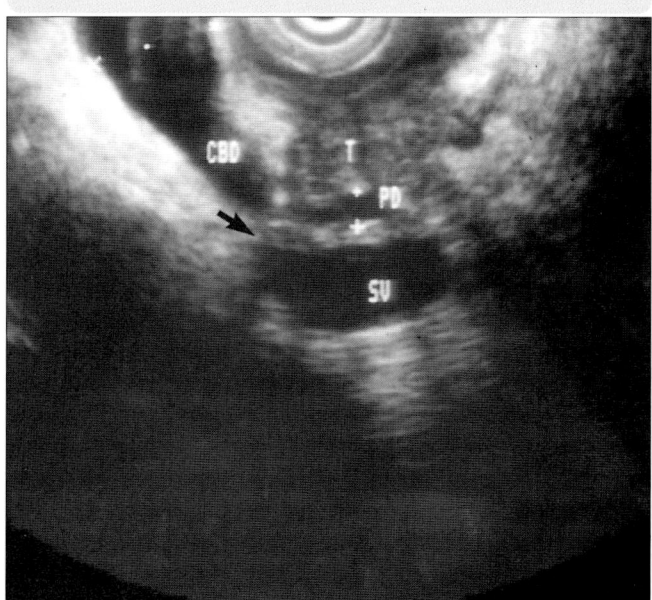

Figure 5.8 EUS reveals a hypoechoic tumour mass (T) in the head of the pancreas, with limited invasion into the adjacent wall of the splenoportal confluence (arrowed). The portal vein (PV) and the splenic vein (SV) are clearly seen, starting in the hilum of the liver (LH) and ending up in the hilum of the spleen (SH).

Figure 5.9 EUS reveals an extremely large hypoechoic tumour mass (T) in the tail of the pancreas that is invading the adjacent submucosa of the gastric wall. Note the junction (arrowed) between the pancreatic mass and the gastric submucosal invasion. Note the tumour is penetrating adjacent to the jejunal loop, which is seen as an anechoic pattern with some hyperechoic pattern representing air (J). The findings were confirmed by surgical exploration for ileus.

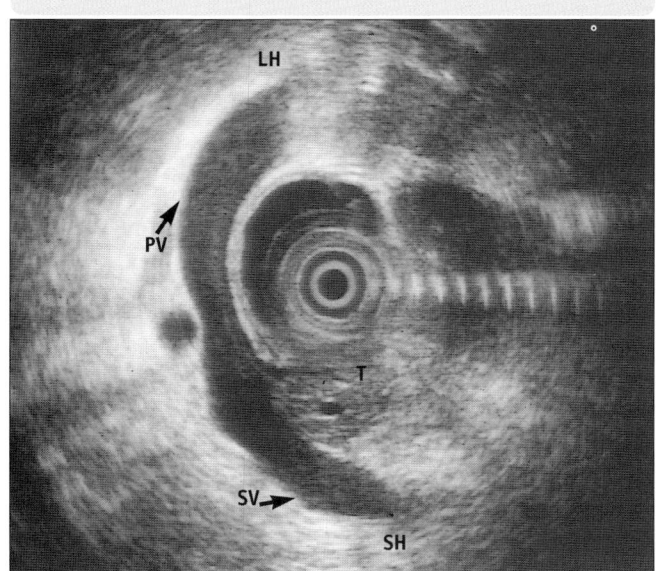

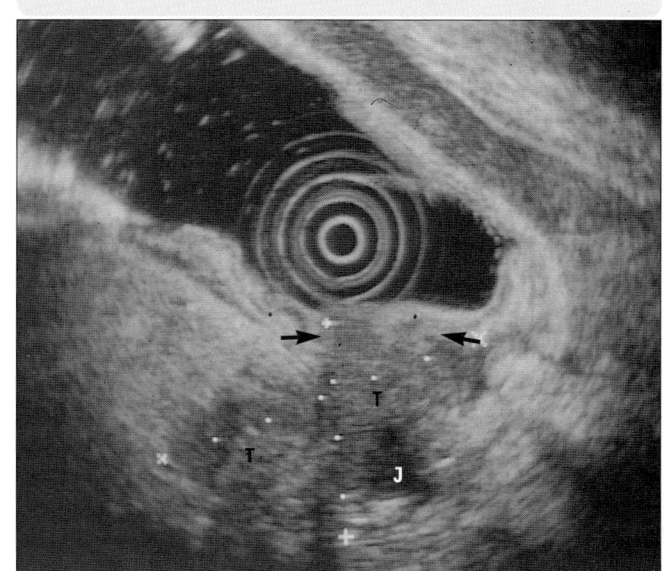

Figure 5.10 EUS shows a biliary metallic stent as a hyperechoic tube-like structure with anechoic bile content (arrowed). The mass in the pancreatic head is visualized as a hypoechoic pattern (T) adjacent to the stent.

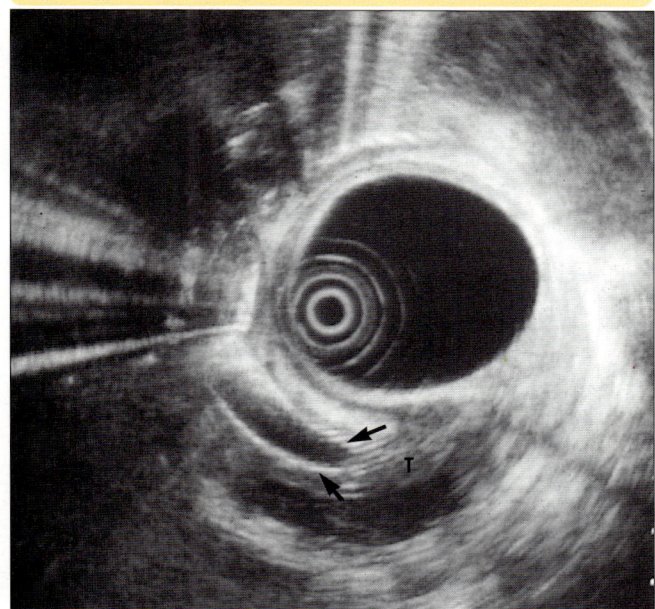

Figure 5.11 The TNM classification for pancreatic cancer adopted for EUS.

T:	**Primary tumour**
T1:	Primary hypoechoic tumour limited to the pancreas
	T1a: Hypoechoic tumour 2cm or less in the greatest dimension
	T1b: Tumour > 2cm in the greatest dimension
T2:	Primary hypoechoic tumour extending directly into the duodenum, CBD or peripancreatic tissue
T3:	Primary hypoechoic tumour extending to the stomach, colon, spleen or adjacent blood vessels, e.g. portal vein, splenic vein, mesenteric vessels, aorta, IVC
N:	**Regional lymph nodes**
N0:	No regional lymph node metastasis
N1:	Regional lymph node metastasis
Nx:	. Regional lymph node cannot be assessed
M:	**Distant metastasis**
M0:	No distant metastasis
M1:	Distant metastasis, e.g. liver metastases or peritoneal dissemination
	Stage grouping
Stage I:	T1 N0 M0
Stage II:	T2 N0 M0 or T3 N0 M0
Stage III:	T1 N1 M0 or T2 N1 M0 or T3 N1 M0
Stage IV:	T4, any N, M0 or any T, any N, M1

M classification of distant metastases resembles that for pancreatic cancer except that lymph node metastases at the splenic hilum are considered to be distant metastases.

the CBD (n = 3) and in the peripancreatic tissue (n = 9). In diagnosing non-resectability, EUS was accurate based on imaging tumour invasion of the splenoportal confluence in 13 of 14 cases. In the remaining case, EUS overdiagnosed T3 cancer – tumour-associated compression of the splenoportal confluence gave a false impression of invasion. The overall accuracy of EUS in diagnosing non-resectability was 92%[11].

In a comparative study Rosch *et al.* reported that EUS was superior to angiography, CT and abdominal US in assessing the involvement of the portal vein in pancreatic carcinoma. The accuracy of EUS, angiography, CT and abdominal US was 95%, 85%, 75% and 55%, respectively[12]. Snady *et al.* reported that EUS was significantly more accurate than combined CT and ERCP in predicting the resectability of cancer regarding periduodenal, periportal, mesenteric vessel and coeliac axis involvement[13]. In our updated study involving 70 cases of pancreatic cancer, EUS was inaccurate in assessing mesocolon involvement because the junction between the pancreas and the corresponding colonic segment could not be visualized[13a]. The diagnosis of distal pancreatic cancer involving the gastric wall was confirmed by EUS aspiration cytology using a radial-scanning echoendoscope[14] (Figure 5.9). Vilman *et al.* reported the use of a curve-array echoendoscope in diagnosing pancreatic mass[15]. Recently Yasuda has described the use of a miniature radial scanning catheter echoprobe during ERCP[16]. The very limited penetration depth of the miniature echoprobe and the lack of adequate contact with the duct wall may create difficulties for obtaining clear images. Moreover, the durability of such an instrument should be improved before routine use can be advocated.

Multifocal intraductal cancer: In rare cases multifocal ductal cancer can be found, characterized by the presence of multiple intraductal growing tumours and an extremely dilat-

ed pancreatic duct. On ERCP the tumours are visualized as multiple filling defects within an extremely dilated pancreatic duct. On EUS the tumours are imaged as polypoid lesions within the dilated duct. Multifocality and intraductal spread are the characteristic features of such tumours. The prognosis is unfavourable even if total pancreatectomy is performed. The highly malignant nature of the disease was illustrated in the first *Atlas of Transintestinal Ultrasonography*, which was published and distributed during the World Congress of Gastroenterology in Sao Paolo, Brazil[16a]. In a patient with multiductal pancreatic cancer, total pancreatectomy with radical resection of the tumours did not improve survival.

Tissue diagnosis with EUS-guided FNA cytology: Where tissue diagnosis is needed, EUS-guided fine-needle aspiration (FNA) can be useful. A radial scanning echoprobe may be helpful in diagnosing submucosal invasion by pancreatic cancer[14]. The target can be reached endoscopically and the tip of the needle visualized by EUS. It is important to control the position of the needle endoscopically and sonographically. In the case of pancreatic tumours, which are usually located some distance from the gastroduodenal wall, a radial scanning echoprobe may not be sufficient to achieve the tissue diagnosis. The use of a long needle may not be helpful because the tip of the needle cannot be seen by EUS. Moreover, the manoeuvre of such a needle through the biopsy channel of the instrument is usually very difficult because of the almost 90-degree angle of the biopsy channel.

Cystic pancreatic mass versus ***pancreatic cancer:*** A cystic mass in the pancreas and periampullary region may represent cystadenoma or cystadenocarcinoma. The distinction between benign lesions and malignant tumours is difficult to make based solely on imaging morphology. The architecture of the lesion can be imaged in detail: the wall structure; the content regarding fluid *versus* cystic or mixed; the topographical relationship with the adjacent pancreatic duct; and the effect on adjacent major blood vessels such as the portal or splenic vein and the splenic or mesenteric artery. On ERCP, segmental dilatation of the pancreatic duct, particularly the side branches, may suggest cystic lesions or cystic tumours – cystadenoma or cystadenocarcinoma. Differentiation of cystic lesions from chronic pancreatitis by CT is difficult. EUS is often helpful because of its clear imaging of the pancreas.

The following case report may illustrate the usefulness of EUS. A 35-year-old male had episodes of discomfort and pain in the abdomen, with radiation to the back. CT revealed a small hypodense lesion in the region of the uncinate process without evidence of calcification. ERCP showed a normal main pancreatic duct with slightly dilated side branch at the level of the uncinate process. The distinction between pancreatitis and cystic tumours could not be made. EUS revealed diffuse small hyperechoic spots in the head of the pancreas with some extension into the body and tail of the pancreas. Cystic lesions were not visualized. There were some acoustic shadows seen in the uncinate process. FNA was not attempted because no mass was found. The findings were consistent with a diagnosis of idiopathic chronic pancreatitis. Follow-up CT, ERCP and EUS over 3 months revealed no change in the previous findings.

Ampullary cancer

The definition of tumour categories for ampullary cancer (Figure 5.12) is substantially different from that for pancreatic cancer. The demarcation between early stage and advanced stage disease is involvement of the muscularis propria of the duodenum, which in advanced stages of ampullary cancer resembles that in oesophagogastric cancer.

In a series of 24 consecutive cases of ampullary cancer, EUS correctly diagnosed two of three cases of T1 cancer. Overstaging occurred due to peritumoural inflammation. T2 cancer was correctly diagnosed in 11 of 12 cases (Figure 5.13). In one case EUS led to overstaging again because of peritumoural pancreatitis. T3 cancer was correctly diagnosed in seven of eight cases (Figure 5.14). Interestingly, EUS-guided aspiration cytology was positive in one case in which the endoscopic biopsy was negative. Understaging occurred in one case because very small tumour penetration was not seen on EUS. T4 cancer was found in only one case and correctly diagnosed by EUS based on a tumour extension with diameter > 2cm. The accuracy of EUS was 67% in T1 cancers, 92% in T2, 87% in T3 and 100% in T4. The overall accuracy was 87% [11].

In a case report we described the role of EUS in diagnosing and in determining local tumour resection on a mucosal type of early ampullary cancer[17a]. This is important because an extended Whipple procedure may be unsuitable in the treatment of early ampullary cancer of mucosal type. In the case of submucosal T1 cancer, however, Whipple resection is needed because of the approximately 25% chance of lymph nodes being affected. EUS has also been reported to be more accurate than other imaging techniques in staging ampullary cancers. The use of a miniature catheter echoprobe with ERCP is promising, particularly in cancer staging and in distinguishing villous adenomas from advanced cancers. EUS-guided FNA may be helpful in achieving the tissue diagnosis of malignancy in the case of focal malignant degeneration,

---

Figure 5.12 Classification of ampullary cancer for EUS.

T:	Primary tumour
T1:	Tumour limited to the ampulla of Vater
T2:	Tumour invading the duodenal wall
T3:	Tumour invading 2cm into the pancreatic parenchyma
T4:	Tumour invading > 2cm into the pancreas and/or adjacent organs

N:	Regional lymph nodes
N0:	No regional lymph node metastasis
N1:	Regional lymph node metastasis
Nx:	Regional lymph node cannot be assessed

	Stage grouping
Stage I:	T1 N0 M0
Stage II:	T2 N0 M0 or T3 N0 M0
Stage III:	T1 N1 M0 or T2 N1 M0 or T3 N1 M0
Stage IV:	T4, any N, M0 or any T, any N, M1

M classification of distant metastases resembles that for pancreatic cancer except that lymph node metastases at the splenic hilum are considered to be distant metastases.

Figure 5.13 EUS reveals a hypoechoic tumour (T) in the ampulla of Vater, with close proximity to the pancreas. The pancreatic duct (PD) is normal in calibre. No invasion into the pancreas is seen, consistent with T2 ampullary cancer. There is a small periduodenal lymph node (LN) of approximately 3mm in diameter, considered to be non-metastatic (N0). SV = splenic vein; SMA = superior mesentric artery.

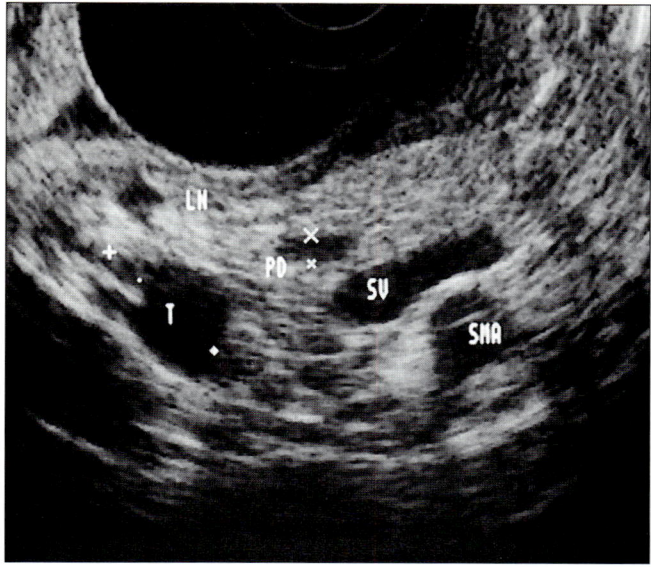

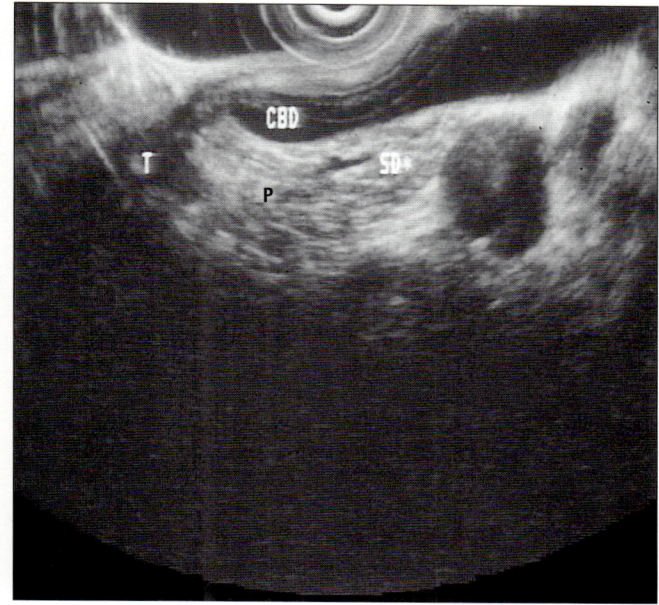

Figure 5.14 EUS reveals a hypoechoic tumour (T) in the ampulla of Vater invading the extremely dilated common bile duct (CBD) and the pancreas (P). The pancreatic duct adjacent to the tumour is minimally dilated. The finding is consistent with T3 ampullary cancer. There is no evidence of metastasis to the lymph node. SD = Santorini duct.

which may not be diagnosed by endoscopic biopsy. A combination of ERCP, cholangioscopy and catheter EUS may become very helpful in ascertaining the diagnosis of malignancy by endoscopic biopsy and FNA.

The use of an intraoperative intravasal miniature probe has been reported to be helpful to the surgeon in diagnosing portal vein invasion because tumour compression can be differentiated from tumour invasion.

Advanced duodenal cancer* versus *advanced pancreatic cancer: Primary duodenal carcinoma is extremely rare. In advanced stage duodenal carcinoma the distinction between primary duodenal carcinomas and pancreatic cancers is difficult to make. Duodenal obstruction is usually the common symptom of such advanced diseases. Endoscopic biopsy may reveal adenocarcinoma, which may represent 'the tip of the iceberg' where the primary tumour is located in the pancreas. The best method for final diagnosis is EUS, since the transducer can be placed adjacent to the target lesion. Where a stenosis cannot be passed with an echoendoscope, a catheter echoprobe can be inserted. The major tumour mass may be located primarily in the pancreas, with penetration into the duodenal wall. The diagnosis should be ascertained prior to surgery to help the surgeon plan the treatment strategy. Whipple resection with extended resection, probably with portal vein reconstruction, may become necessary where the splenoportal confluence is infiltrated. In primary ampullary carcinoma with advanced invasion, the distinction between primary pancreatic carcinomas and pancreatic cancers is difficult to make. The prognosis may not be significantly different, however, because of the advanced stage.

The following case report may illustrate the power of EUS in helping clinicians in decision making. A 54-year-old male patient had a history of dyspepsia for about 6 months. Endoscopy was normal but tests for *Helicobacter pylori* were positive. Follow-up endoscopy over 3 months revealed a stenosis at the junction between the duodenal bulb and the descending duodenum. Biopsy was inconclusive. A barium swallow did not show other abnormalities. Endoscopic biopsy prior to hospital admission revealed adenocarcinoma consistent with duodenal carcinoma. A CT scan revealed slight thickening of the duodenum without evidence of pancreatic mass. The patient was referred for further evaluation. EUS was performed for staging. The stenosis was impassable for the standard echoendoscope with an outer diameter of 13mm. The transducer was placed proximally to the stenosis. EUS revealed a hypoechoic tumour mass in the pancreas with direct invasion into the duodenal wall. The connection between the pancreatic tumour mass and the duodenal wall abnormality was seen as a path-like structure. There were some adjacent lymph nodes giving rise to the suspicion of metastasis (Figure 5.15). To evaluate the maximal tumour extension a small catheter echoprobe was inserted via the biopsy channel into the stenotic area. The tumour was seen invading the splenic vein, with prestenotic dilatation of the pancreatic duct. ERCP was not attempted because of the duodenal stenosis. Whipple resection was performed and the histology confirmed the diagnosis of adenocarcinoma consistent with pancreatic cancer.

Chronic pancreatitis

The diagnosis of chronic pancreatitis is based on findings such as disintegration of glands (psuedolobuli architecture with increased fibrosis within the organ), a diffuse hyperechoic pattern with or without calcification, irregular changes in calibre of the pancreatic duct and its side branches, the presence or absence of pseudocysts within or adjacent to the pancreas, and enlargement or atrophy of the organ (Figure 5.16). It is interesting to note that a pancreatic pseudocyst may migrate to structures within the parapancreatic space such as the perigastroduodenal wall, the hepatoduodenal ligament or even the hilum of the liver. The wall of a pancreatic pseudocyst is usually the surrounding tissue, since by definition a pancreatic pseudocyst does not have a covering wall structure. A true pancreatic cyst, however, has a wall structure. In clinical practice, the role of EUS in diagnosing pancreatic pseudocyst is important not only to localize the lesion but also to determine the anatomical relationship between the pseudocyst and the duodenal wall, the presence of any connection between the pseudocyst and the pancreatic duct, the presence or absence of splenic vein or portal vein compression or thrombosis, and the presence or absence of splenic artery aneurysm or, in rare cases, portal vein aneurysm. The therapeutic use of EUS lies in the endoscopic drainage of pancreatic pseudocysts; the optimal indication would be a pancreatic pseudocyst with a close proximity to the duodenum and the stomach (Figure 5.17). It is crucial to know that no blood vessel lies between the pancreatic pseudocyst and the duodenal wall or the gastric wall when EUS-guided drainage is attempted (Figure 5.18).

Pancreatic pseudocyst* versus *cystic lesion of the pancreas: The differential diagnosis of pancreatic pseudocyst from a cystic lesion of the pancreas, such as cystadenoma or

Figure 5.15 (a) Endoscopy reveals a mass in the duodenal bulb proven to be adenocarcinoma by biopsy. (b) EUS reveals a hyperechoic tumour (T) in the pancreas invading the splenic vein (SV) and the duodenal wall (arrows). Note the dilated pancreatic duct (PD).

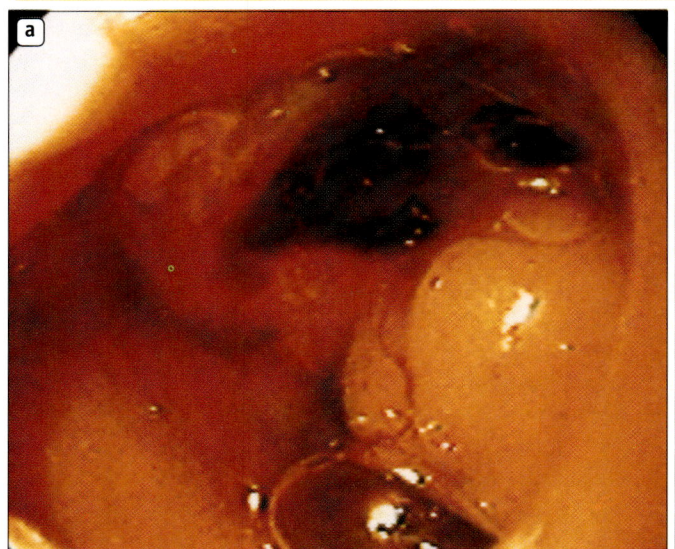

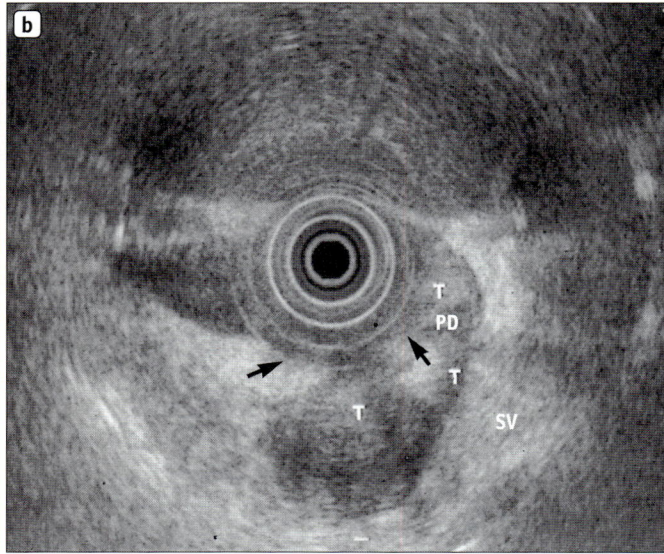

cystadenocarcinoma, is often difficult. Where no evidence of chronic pancreatitis is found, the presence of a cystic lesion in the pancreas is worrisome if the wall of the cyst is lobulated, if pseudopodia boundaries are present, and if narrowing of the splenic or portal vein or of their junction is visualized. Colour Doppler may become helpful in imaging the blood flow or the presence of a thrombus adjacent to the narrowed area. The use of EUS-guided puncture to obtain malignant cells may be controversial because of the risk of tumour spread. Some surgeons believe that adding to the risk of tumour spread is not acceptable because of the chance of curing the disease. Others believe that resection

should be attempted only in cases where there is a strong suspicion of malignancy. FNA should be attempted to achieve the final diagnosis. Imaging a connection between the cystic lesion and the pancreatic duct is sometimes difficult because it is not easy to place them in one plane.

Endocrine tumours

Endocrine tumours may be intrapancreatic, extrapancreatic, single or multiple. The main extrapancreatic site is the duodenum, in particular the second part of the duodenum.

The localization and the diagnosis of endocrine tumours may be very difficult because the size may be very small or

Figure 5.16 EUS reveals a heterogeneous pattern of the head of the pancreas with some calcification (arrows). Note the dorsal shadows beyond the calcification. The findings are consistent with chronic pancreatitis.

Figure 5.17 EUS reveals a large pancreatic pseudocyst (CY) in close proximity to the duodenal wall. There is no evidence of blood vessels between the duodenal wall and the pseudocyst. EUS-guided pseudocyst drainage was carried out successfully.

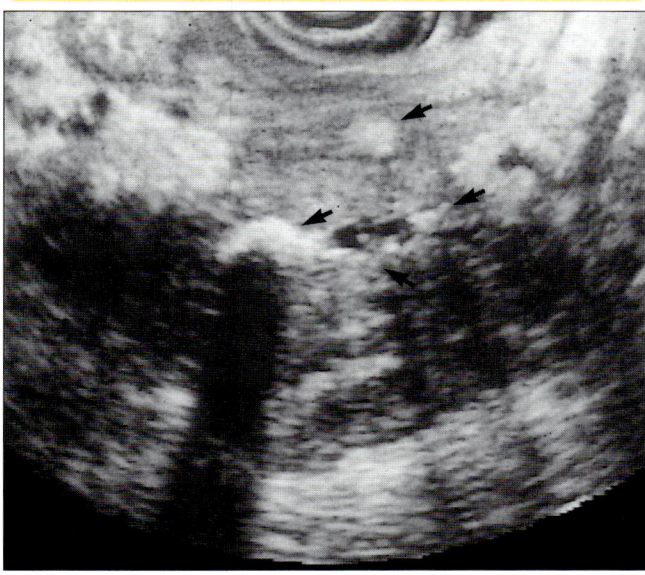

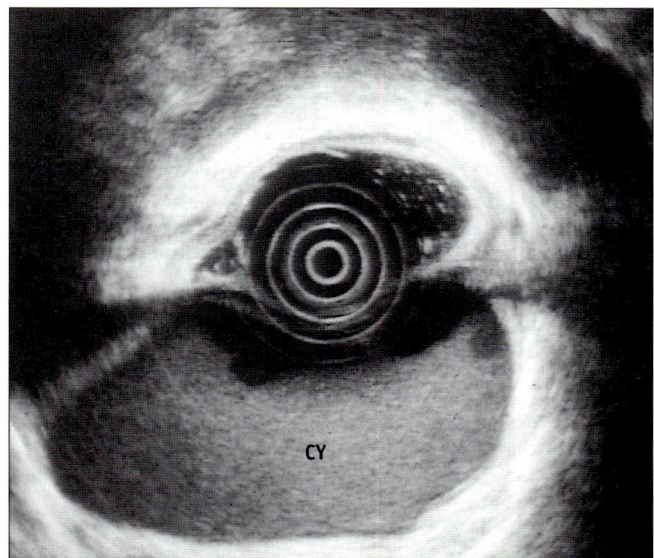

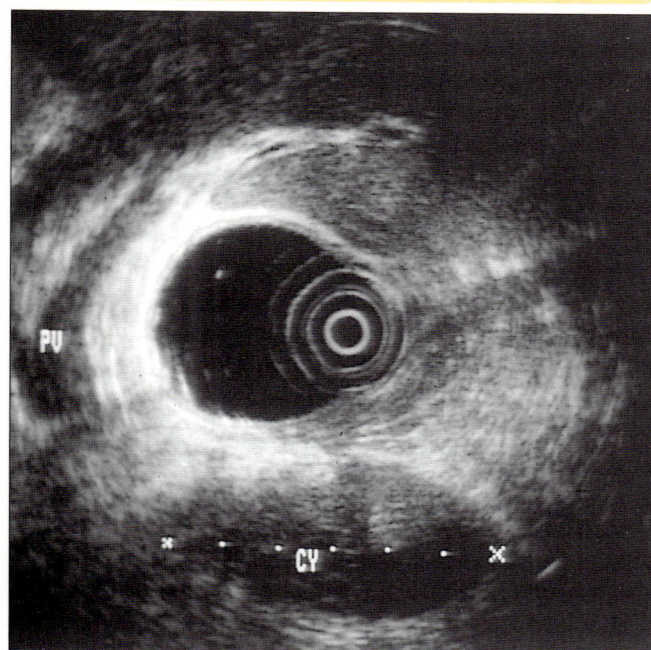

Figure 5.18 EUS reveals a pancreatic pseudocyst (CY) with heterogeneous pattern, which may represent debris within the cyst. Note the relatively long distance between the duodenal wall and the pseudocyst. The portal vein (PV) is clearly seen adjacent to the pseudocyst.

the tumour pattern may not be distinguishable from the surrounding normal tissue. Diagnosis and location of the tumours are essential since the disease can be cured surgically.

In the literature EUS has been reported to be the most accurate way of diagnosing and locating endocrine tumours of the pancreas because of its capability of imaging small lesions[24]. Moreover, the tumour pattern can be readily distinguished from the normal surrounding tissue (Figure 5.19). Where a small tumour is found and pinpointed, minimal surgery can be attempted. A small tumour found by EUS and visualized during laparoscopic US can be enucleated. Such surgery will become the trend in the future because of the minimally invasive nature of the procedure and the similar cure rate to that of standard surgery. Preoperative diagnosis can be integrated into routine patient care in planning the strategy for treatment.

In the case of extrapancreatic endocrine tumours, which are often localized in the second and third parts of the duodenum, it may be difficult to locate and visualise the tumour using EUS. Such tumours are usually small and nodular and may be compressed by the water-filled balloon attached to the transducer. The water-filled method used for the gastrointestinal lumen may not be appropriate because the water may just run away into the more distal part of the duodenum and jejunum. An initial step would be the identification of duodenal nodules by duodenoscopy. Thereafter, a catheter echoprobe could be inserted to identify the extent of the submucosal lesion, which is usually localized. In order to obtain clear EUS images the duodenal lumen needs to be filled with water. Where a catheter echoprobe with a balloon at its tip is used, simultaneous filling of the duodenal lumen and the balloon with water may lead to clear images of duodenal nodules without creating compression and artefacts. Subsequently, standard EUS with an echoen-

doscope should be carried out in imaging extrapancreatic and intrapancreatic lesions. EUS-guided FNA can be used in diagnosing an endocrine tumour using special tissue staining. If the duodenal lesion is of limited size it may be appropriate to remove it endoscopically, particularly if surgery is contraindicated or the patient refuses to undergo surgery.

Zollinger–Ellison syndrome: In cases where the tumour is found by other imaging techniques such as abdominal US, CT and angiography, EUS can deliver additional information regarding the anatomical relationship with the surrounding organs such as the duodenum, pancreas, bile duct and liver parenchyma. Clear delineation of the tumour is very helpful for the surgeon attempting radical resection with or without preservation of the surrounding organ.

There is an ongoing protocol at the National Institutes of Health in Bethesda comparing preoperative imaging diagnosis – US, EUS, CT, angiography, endoscopy and octreotide scanning – with surgery and histology of resected specimens. In the author's own experience EUS is helpful not only in identifying small lesions that may not be detected by other imaging techniques but also for visualizing large tumour masses in order to achieve additional information: is the tumour intrapancreatic or extrapancreatic; are there feeding blood vessels; what is the relationship between the tumour and the major blood vessels and the duodenum? (Whipple *versus* non-Whipple procedure). Interestingly an extrapancreatic tumour mass, even of excessive size, can be removed surgically if the major blood vessels are only compressed and not invaded by the tumour. In general such tumour masses represent metastatic disease such as a conglomerate of lymph nodes. In contrast, a small intrapancreatic tumour requires resection, though a tumour located at the surface of the pancreas may be removable by laparascopic surgery with tumour enucleation. The main sites of metastatic disease identified by EUS are the

Figure 5.19 EUS reveals a small hypoechoic tumour (stars) of approximately 2cm diameter adjacent to the splenic vein (SV). The tumour was shown to be an insulinoma by histology of the resected specimen.

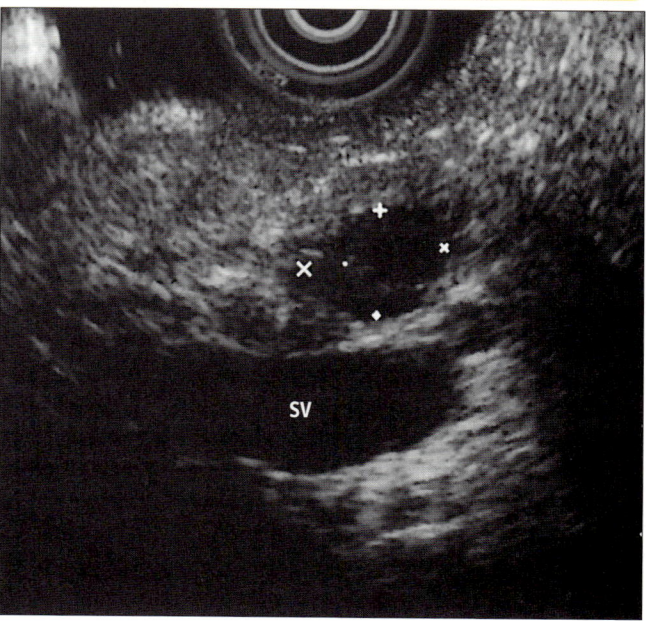

lymph nodes adjacent to the distal CBD, splenoportal confluence, vena cava or the left renal vein. In the literature the main site of intrapancreatic gastrinoma is the neck of the pancreas. Where intrapancreatic location of gastrinomas is excluded duodenal nodules are found in more than 50% of cases.

The following case report may illustrate the role of EUS with regard to the collaboration between gastroenterologists and surgeons. A 47-year-old man was treated for several months for diarrhoea. A traveller's disease was considered and giardiasis was confirmed. After antibiotic treatment the diarrhoea persisted. Gastrin testing revealed levels 10 times higher than normal, which has been found to be an indicator for Zollinger–Ellison syndrome (ZES). A CT scan revealed a mass adjacent to the pancreatic head, the duodenum and the liver. Duodenal involvement could not be excluded. Angiography revealed findings consistent with pancreatic tumour. Octreotide scanning was positive. The patient was referred for additional information regarding the exact location of the mass (extra-pancreatic *versus* intrapancreatic), relationship between the tumour and the duodenum, and whether blood vessels were present within the tumour. EUS revealed a large tumour mass located adjacent to the head of the pancreas, the second part of the duodenum and the CBD. Blood vessels were found within the tumour mass. Invasion into the duodenal wall was not found. The portal vein was dislocated dorsally but not invaded. After consultation with the surgeon, Whipple resection was performed because of the absence of pancreatic and duodenal invasion. Surgery and intraoperative US confirmed the EUS findings.

Diagnostic steps for patients with ZES are a blood gastrin test followed by imaging techniques such as octreotide scan for whole body check-up, followed by abdominal US, CT and angiography. EUS should be performed to precisely locate the tumour and duodenal nodules, and to rule out duodenal and pancreatic involvement. Endoscopy with side-viewing optics is necessary to visualize the duodenal abnormality. In some centres complete oesophagogastroduodenoscopy is integrated in diagnosing reflux oesophagitis and gastric and duodenal ulcers; this must be performed with a forward-viewing gastroscope. Thereafter, endoscopy with a lateral-viewing endoscope should be performed for diagnosing duodenal nodules. In the near future the use of small catheter echoprobes during standard endoscopy may become the choice for staging duodenal endocrine tumours. The tumours can be located endoscopically and the transducer placed accurately as close as possible to the target. In this way, compression of the water-filled balloon can be avoided.

References

1. Hisanaga K, Hisanaga A. A new real-time sector scanning system of ultra-wide angle and real-time recording to entire cardiac images: transesophagus and transchest method. *Ultrasound Med* 1978; 4:391–401.
2. Strohm WED, Philip F, Hagenmueller F, Classen M. Ultrasonic tomography by means of ultrasonic fiberendoscope. *Endoscopy* 1980; 12:241–4.
3. Di Magno EP, Buxton JL, Regan PT. The ultrasonic endoscope. *Lancet* 1980; 1:629–31.
4. Lux G, Heyder N, Demling L. Endoscopic ultrasonography: technique, orientation and diagnostic possibilities. *Endoscopy* 1982; 4:220–5.
5. Tio TL, Tytgat GNJ. Endoscopic ultrasonography in the assessment of intra- and transmural infiltration of tumours in the esophagus, stomach and papilla of Vater and in the detection of extra-esophageal lesions. *Endoscopy* 1984; 16:203–10.
6. Murata Y, Muroi M, Yoshida M. Endoscopic ultrasonography in the diagnosis of esophageal carcinoma. *Surg Endosc* 1987; 1:11–16.
7. Yasuda K, Kiyota K, Nakajima M. Fundamentals of endoscopic laser therapy (ELT) for GI-tumors – new aspects with endoscopic ultrasonography (EUS). *Endoscopy* 1987; 19(suppl 1):2–6.
8. Hermanek P, Sobin LH (Eds) *TNM Classification of Malignant Tumours, 4th ed.* Springer-Verlag, Berlin; 1987.
9. Sobin LH, Hermanek P, Hutter RP. TNM classification of malignant tumours. *Cancer* 1988; 61:2310–14.
10. Spiessl B, Beahrs OH, Hermanek P, *et al.* (Eds) *TNM Atlas, 3rd ed.* Springer-Verlag, Berlin; 1989.
10a.Cubilla AL, Fortner J, Fitzgerald J. Lymph node involvement in carcinoma of the head of the pancreas area. *Cancer* 1978; 41:880–7.
10b.Nagai H, Kuroda A, Moroika Y. Lymphatic and local spread of T1 and T2 pancreatic cancer: a study of autopsy material. *Ann Surg* 1986; 204:65–71.
11. Tio TL, Tytgat GNJ, Cikot RJLM, Houthoff HJ. Ampullopancreatic carcinoma preoperative TNM classification with endosonography. *Radiology* 1990; 175:455–61.
12. Rosch T, Braig C, Gain T, Classen M. Staging of pancreatic and ampullary carcinoma by endoscopic ultrasonography. *Gastroenterology* 1992; 102:188–99.
13. Snady H, Cooperman A, Siegel JH. Endoscopic ultrasonography compared with computed tomography and ERCP in patients with obstructive jaundice and small pancreatic mass. *Gastrointest Endosc* 1992; 38:27–34.
13a.Tio TL, Sie LH, Kallimanis G, *et al.* Staging of ampullary and pancreatic carcinoma: comparison between endosonography and surgery. *Gastrointest Endosc* 1996; 12:706–13.
14. Tio TL, Sie LH, Tytgat GNJ. Endosonography and cytology in diagnosing and staging pancreatic body and tail carcinoma. *Dig Dis Sci* 1993; 38:59–64.
15. Vilman P, Jacobsen JK, Henriksen FW. Endoscopic ultrasonography with guided fine needle aspiration biopsy in pancreatic disease. *Gastrointest Endosc* 1992; 38(2):172–3.
16. Yasuda K, Nukai H, Nakajima M. Clinical application of ultrasonic probes in biliary and pancreatic duct. *Endoscopy* 1992; 24(S1):370–5.
16a.Tio TL, Tytgat GNJ. *Atlas of Transintestinal Ultrasonography*. Mur-Kostverloren, Aalsmeer; 1986.
17. Tio TL, Wijers OB, Sars PRA, Tytgat GNJ. Preoperative TNM classification of proximal extrahepatic bile duct carcinoma by endosonography. *Semin Liver Dis* 1990;10:114–20.
17a.Tio Tl, Mulder, Eggink WF. Endosonography in staging early carcinoma of the ampulla of Vater. *Gastroenterology* 1992; 102:1392–5.
18. Tio TL, Cheng J, Sars PRA, Tytgat GNJ. Preoperative TNM classification of extrahepatic bile duct carcinoma by endosonography. *Gastroenterology* 1991; 10:1351–61.
19. Tio TL, Tytgat GNJ. Endoscopic ultrasonography in the preoperative staging of biliopancreatic carcinoma. In *Hepatobiliary and Pancreatic Malignancy*. Edited by NJ Lygidakis, GNJ Tytgat. Thieme, New York; 1989: 66–78.
20. Tio TL. *Endosonography in Gastroenterology*. Springer, Berlin, Heidelberg, New York; 1988.
21. Tio TL. *Atlas of Endosonography*. Interactive Video Laser Disc Program.Olympus, Lake Success, New York; 1993.
22. Tio TL. *TNM Cancer Staging by Endosonography*. Igaku-Shoin, New York; 1994.

Author (ref)	No. Patients	Source	Sensitivity (%)	Specificity (%)
Tada et al. (47)	9	Pancreatic juice	100	100
Van Laethem et al. (48)	45	Brushings	83	100
Urban et al. (46)	20	FNA	92	100
Trümper et al. (44)	27	Pancreatic juice	100	90
Berthélemy et al. (41)	75	Pancreatic juice and brushings	77	100
Watanabe et al. (42)	38	Pancreatic juice	55	100
Kondo et al. (50)	36	Pancreatic juice	67	100
Ihalainen et al. (49)	21	FNA	82	100
Villanueva et al. (50)	93	FNA	59	100
Shibata et al. (43)	47	FNA	56	100

FNA = fine needle aspirate

Figure 6.9 Reports of the detection of K-*ras* mutations.

Overexpression of the *erb*B-3 protein has also been associated with chronic pancreatitis, making this marker less attractive for the evaluation of suspected exocrine pancreatic cancer[37]. Over expression of the *erb*B-2 proto-oncogene has been found in approximately 20–40% of pancreatic malignancies[35,54]. Detection of this abnormality in pancreatic juice will only be useful in conjunction with other markers because of its low prevalence in pancreatic adenocarcinoma.

Mutations of the p53 tumour suppressor gene are common in many gastrointestinal malignancies. Alterations in the p53 gene have been found in 40–70% of pancreatic malignancies[39,40,46,55]. Mutations in the p53 gene have not been found in chronic pancreatitis specimens[39]. In addition, p53 gene mutations have been associated with a decreased survival in pancreatic duct malignancies[42]. This is not surprising, as p53 changes seem to be a late phenomenon in patients with pancreatic cancer[55]. Alone, detection of p53 expression in pancreatic juice specimens is of limited value, but it may be helpful in combination with other genetic markers for diagnosis and prognosis of pancreatic adenocarcinoma.

Mutations of the DCC tumour suppressor gene have been noted in up to 50% of pancreatic duct malignancies [36,38]. APC gene alterations are infrequently seen in exocrine tumours of the pancreas[41,56]. Neither the DCC suppressor gene nor the APC gene have been evaluated in cytology specimens in the current literature.

Conclusion

The detection of gene mutations appears to have great potential as an adjunctive diagnostic tool to standard cytology. Currently K-*ras* changes in pancreatic specimens are the most useful tool as these changes are highly sensitive and specific and seem to represent an early marker of pancreatic adenocarcinoma. The addition of other genetic markers may greatly add to the diagnostic sensitivity. Eventually, detection of these mutational changes could be obtained from serum or stool specimens, allowing for a non-invasive screening tool. Some early work on serum genetic markers has been done[48].

TUMOUR MARKERS

Pancreatic adenocarcinoma has been associated with a wide variety of tumour markers that can be detected in the serum or in pancreatic secretions (Figure 6.10). Unfortunately, tumour markers to date have lacked both organ and tumour specificity. Attempting to increase the sensitivity of tumour markers for pancreatic duct carcinoma by using multiple antigens leads to a decrease in specificity[57]. The most commonly studied marker is the glycoprotein antigen CA19-9. Other markers commonly investigated include CEA, CA95, CA242 and CA50.

CA19-9

Diagnosis: The tumour marker CA19-9 has been extensively studied in pancreatic disease. The sensitivity of this test for pancreatic cancer ranges from 50% to 95% and the specificity from 60% to 98%[58–70]. These wide ranges of sensitivity and specificity are reflective of the varied patient

Figure 6.10 Tumour markers assessed in pancreatic cancer: Review of recent literature.

Marker (ref)	Sensitivity(%)	Specificity (%)
PNA (57)	77	83
TPA (58,73,74)	52	85
CA195 (64,70)	76	53
CA242 (64,72,73)	57–81	80
CAM43 (64)	60	95
CA19-9 (55–60,62–65,67–70)	53–98	60–98
CA50 (58,65,72,73)	65–96	58–92
CEA (55,57–60,72,73)	38–92	47–87
DUPAN-2 (65)	48	85
Span-1 (65,75)	81	68–76
Elastase-1 (65)	51	76

populations studied, along with the different cut-off values for positive and negative tests. Most studies use a cut-off value of 37–40U/ml, which is quite sensitive for pancreatic cancer but is poorly specific. Some authors suggest a value of 100–200U/ml, but this reduces the sensitivity of the test to 55–65%[64,65,71]. Patients with other gastrointestinal malignancies and chronic or acute pancreatitis frequently have marked elevations in CA19-9. A CA19-9 level > 200U/ml in suspected pancreatic malignancy is almost diagnostic[66]. This test has no role in screening for pancreatic ductal malignancies because of its poor organ and disease specificity.

Staging: The level of CA19-9 has been evaluated to predict the stage of pancreatic adenocarcinoma with mixed results[66,71]. The sensitivity of the CA19-9 test does tend to increase with increasing stage of disease but there is significant overlap of CA19-9 levels between stages[64,66,68,71,72]. Highly anaplastic tumours may not have the ability to secrete CA19-9. In cases where the CA19-9 is > 1000U/ml the tumour is unlikely to be resectable[66].

CA19-9 in pancreatic juice: CA19-9 has also been evaluated in pancreatic secretions. A study by Malesci et al. showed that patients with pancreatic malignancies had significantly higher values of CA19-9 in pancreatic juice than normal controls and patients with chronic pancreatitis[72]. Two subsequent studies were not able to duplicate this early success and showed a great deal of overlap between pancreatic adenocarcinoma and patients with chronic pancreatitis and non-pancreatic processes[10,73]. Our own experience with CA19-9 levels in pancreatic juice has found a great deal of overlap between benign and malignant disease. Thus pancreatic juice CA19-9 level does not appear to be a useful discriminator of pancreatic processes.

CEA

Carcinoembryonic antigen (CEA) has frequently been evaluated as a tumour marker for pancreatic cancer. The sensitivity of the serum test has ranged from 40% to 80% and the specificity from 50% to 90%[62,63,68,74–76]. CEA has also been evaluated in pancreatic juice; it appears to be a more sensitive and specific marker than CA19-9 in pancreatic juice but there is still significant overlap between benign and malignant disease[10]. Currently, CEA levels in the serum do not appear to be as useful as CA19-9 in the evaluation of pancreatic malignancy. There does not appear to be a significant increase in the sensitivity and specificity in diagnosing a pancreatic malignancy if the tests are combined[64]. Further study is needed to determine whether measurement of pancreatic juice levels of CEA will prove worthwhile.

Other tumour markers

Other pancreatic tumour-associated markers studied include CA195, CAM43, CA242, CA50, DUPAN-2, Span-1, PNA (peanut agglutinin), elastase-1 and TPA (tissue polypeptide antigen).[58,60,61,67,68,75–78] None of the above tumour markers has consistently been shown to be superior to CA19-9. CA195 has also been assessed in pancreatic juice without success in differentiating benign from malignant pancreatic disease[73]. None of the above markers can currently be recommended as an adjunctive tool for the diagnosis or staging of pancreatic adenocarcinoma.

References

1. Keogan MT, Baker ME. Computed tomography and magnetic resonance imaging in the assessment of pancreatic disease. *Gastrointest Endosc Clin N Am* 1995; 5(1):31–59.
2. Yasuda K, Mukai H, Nakajima M. Endoscopic ultrasonography diagnosis of pancreatic cancer. *Gastrointest Endosc Clin N Am* 1995; 5(4):699–712.
3. Hawes RH, Zaidi S. Endoscopic ultrasonography of the pancreas. *Gastrointest Endosc Clin N Am* 1995; 5(1):61–80.
4. Pasanen PA, Eskelinen M, Partanen K et al. A prospective study of the value of imaging, serum markers and their combination in the diagnosis of pancreatic carcinoma in symptomatic patients. *Anticancer Res* 1992; 12(6B):2309–14.
5. Rösch T, Braig C, Gain T et al. Staging of pancreatic and ampullary carcinoma by endoscopic ultrasound. *Gastroenterology* 1992; 102:188–99.
6. Paksoy N, Lilleng R, Hagmar B et al. Diagnostic accuracy of fine needle aspiration cytology in pancreatic lesions. A review of 77 cases. *Acta Cytol* 1993; 37(6):889–93.
7. Niederau C, Grendell JH. Diagnosis of pancreatic carcinoma. Imaging techniques and tumour markers. *Pancreas* 1992; 7(1):66–86.
8. Layfield LJ, Wax TD, Lee JG et al. Accuracy and morphologic aspects of pancreatic and biliary brushings. *Acta Cytol* 1995; 39(1):8–11.
9. Giovannini M, Seitz JF, Monges G et al. Fine-needle aspiration cytology guided by endoscopic ultrasonography: results in 141 patients. *Endoscopy* 1995; 27(2):171–7.
10. Matsumoto S, Harada H, Tanaka J et al. Evaluation of cytology and tumor markers of pure pancreatic juice for the diagnosis of pancreatic cancer at early stages. *Pancreas* 1994; 9(6):741–7.
11. Ferrari AP, Lichtenstein DR, Slivka A et al. Brush cytology during ERCP for the diagnosis of biliary and pancreatic malignancies. *Gastrointest Endosc* 1994; 40:140–5.
12. Ryan ME. Cytologic brushings of ductal lesions during ERCP. *Gastrointest Endosc* 1991; 37(2):139–42.

13. Tao LC. Liver and pancreas: In *Comprehensive Cytopathology*. Edited by M Bibbo. WB Saunders, Philadelphia. 1991; 844.

14. Gupta RK, Wakefield SJ. Needle aspiration cytology, immunocytochemistry, and electron microscopic study of unusual pancreatic carcinoma with pleomorphic giant cells. *Diagn Cytopathol* 1992; 8(5):522–7.

15. Mikel UV, Becker RL Jr. A comparative study of quantitative stains for DNA in image cytometry. *Anal Quant Cytol Histol* 1991; 13(4):253–60.

16. Jorba R, Fernández-Cruz. Prognostic implications of DNA ploidy and cell-cycle analysis in pancreatic and periampullary carcinoma. *Hepato-Gastroenterol* 1994; 41:507–8.

17. Rickaert F, Gelin M, van Gansbeke D et al. Computerized morphonuclear characteristics and DNA content of adenocarcinoma of the pancreas, chronic pancreatitis, and normal tissues: relationship with histopathologic grading. *Hum Pathol* 1992; 23:1210–15.

18. Yeaton P, Kiss R, Deviere J et al. Use of cell image analysis in the detection of cancer from specimens obtained during endoscopic retrograde cholangiopancreatography. *Am J Clin Pathol* 1993; 100:497–501.

19. Linder S, Falkmer U, Hagmar T et al. Prognostic significance of DNA ploidy in pancreatic carcinoma. *Pancreas* 1994; 9(6):764–72.

20. Bui H, Ballouk F, del Rosario A et al. Nuclear DNA content and clinical follow-up in resected pancreatic adenocarcinoma. *Anal Quant Cytol Histol* 1993; 15(6):389–95.

21. Weger A, Glaser K, Schwab G et al. Quantitative nuclear DNA content in fine needle aspirates of pancreatic cancer. *Gut* 1991; 32:325–8.

22. Russack V. Image cytometry: current applications and future trends. *Crit Rev Clin Lab Sci* 1994; 31(1):1–34.

23. Gilman-Sachs A. Flow cytometry. *Anal Chem* 1994; 66(13): 700A–707A.

24. Ryan ME, Baldauf MC. Comparison of flow cytometry for DNA content and brush cytology for detection of malignancy in pancreatobiliary strictures. *Gastrointest Endosc* 1994; 40:133–9.

25. Schlichting E, Clausen OP, Hanssen AS et al. Ploidy and survival in resectable pancreatic cancers. A retrospective study over 9 years. *Eur J Surg* 1993; 159(4):229–33.

26. Eskelinen M, Lipponen P, Marin S et al. DNA ploidy, S-phase fraction, and G2 fraction as prognostic determinants in human pancreatic cancer. *Scand J Gastroenterol* 1992; 27(1):39–43.

27. Porschen R, Remy U, Bevers G et al. Prognostic significance of DNA ploidy in adenocarcinoma of the pancreas. A flow cytometric study of paraffin-embedded specimens. 1993; 71(12):3846–50.

28. Alanen KA, Joensuu H, Klemi PJ et al. Clinical significance of nuclear DNA content in pancreatic carcinoma. *J Pathol* 1990; 160:313–20.

29. Yoshimura T, Manabe T, Imamura T et al. Flow cytometric analysis of nuclear DNA content of duct cell carcinoma of the pancreas. *Cancer* 1992; 70:1069–74.

30. Hyoty M, Visakorpi T, Kallioniemi OP et al. Prognostic value of analysis of DNA in pancreatic adenocarcinoma by flow cytometry. *Eur J Surg* 1991; 157(10):595–600.

31. Herrera MF, van Heerden JA, Katzmann JA et al. Evaluation of DNA nuclear pattern as a prognostic determinant in resected pancreatic ductal adenocarcinoma. *Ann Surg* 1992; 215(2):120–4.

32. Dressler LG, Seamer LC. Controls, standards, and histogram interpretation in DNA flow cytometry. *Methods Cell Biol* 1994; 41:241–62.

33. Becker RL Jr. Standardization and quality control of quantitative microscopy in pathology. *J Cell Biochem* 1993; 17G:199–204.

34. Shibata D, Almoguera C, Forrester K et al. Detection of c-K-ras mutations in fine needle aspirates from human pancreatic adenocarcinomas. *Cancer Res* 1990; 50:1279–83.

35. Sakorafas GH, Tsiotou AG. Genetic basis of cancer of the pancreas: diagnostic and therapeutic applications. *Eur J Surg* 1994; 160:529–34.

36. Hohne MW, Halatsch ME, Kahl GF et al. Frequent loss of expression of the potential tumor suppresser gene DCC in ductal pancreatic adenocarcinoma. *Cancer Res* 1992; 52(9):2616–19.

37. Lemoine NR, Lobresco M, Leung H et al. The erbB-3 gene in human pancreatic cancer. *J Pathol* 1992; 168(3):269–73.

38. Simon B, Weinel R, Hohne M et al. Frequent alterations of the tumor suppressor genes p53 and DCC in human pancreatic carcinoma. *Gastroenterology* 1994; 106(6):1645–51.

39. Casey G, Yamanaka Y, Friess H et al. p53 mutations are common in pancreatic cancer and are absent in chronic pancreatitis. *Cancer Lett* 1993; 69(3):151–60.

40. Scarpa A, Capelli P, Mukai K et al. Pancreatic adenocarcinomas frequently show p53 gene mutations. *Am J Pathol* 1993; 142(5):1534–43.

41. Yashima K, Nakamori S, Murakami Y et al. Mutations of the adenomatous polyposis coli gene in the mutation cluster region: comparison of human pancreatic and colorectal cancers. *Int J Cancer* 1994; 59(1):43–7.

42. Nakamori S, Yashima K, Murakami Y et al. Association of p53 gene mutations with short survival in pancreatic adenocarcinoma. *Jpn J Cancer Res* 1995; 86(2):174–81.

43. Berthélemy P, Bouisson M, Escourrou J et al. Identification of K-ras mutations in pancreatic juice in the early diagnosis of pancreatic cancer. *Ann Intern Med* 1995; 123:188–91.

44. Watanabe H, Sawabu N, Ohta H et al. Identification of K-ras oncogene mutations in the pure pancreatic juice of patients with ductal pancreatic cancers. *Jpn J Cancer Res* 1993; 84:961–5.

45. Trümper LH, Bürger B, von Bonin F et al. Diagnosis of pancreatic adenocarcinoma by polymerase chain reaction from pancreatic secretions. *Br J Cancer* 1994; 70(2):278–84.

46. van Es JM, Polak MM, van den Berg FM et al. Molecular markers for diagnostic cytology of neoplasms in the head region of the pancreas: mutation of K-ras and overexpression of the p53 protein product. *J Clin Pathol* 1995; 48:218–22.

47. Urban T, Ricci S, Grange J-D et al. Detection of c-Ki-ras mutation by PCR/RFLP analysis and diagnosis of pancreatic adenocarcinomas. *J Natl Cancer Inst* 1993; 85:2008–12.

48. Tada M, Omata M, Ohto M. Clinical application of ras gene mutation for diagnosis of pancreatic adenocarcinoma. *Gastroenterology* 1991; 100:233–8.

49. Van Laethem J-L, Vertongen P, Deviere J et al. Detection of c-Ki-ras gene codon 12 mutations from pancreatic duct brushings in the diagnosis of pancreatic tumors. *Gut* 1995; 36:781–7.

50. Ihalainen J, Taavitsainen M, Salmivaara T et al. Diagnosis of pancreatic lesions using fine needle aspiration cytology: detection of K-ras point mutations using solid phase minisequencing. *J Clin Pathol* 1994; 47(12):1082–4.

51. Kondo H, Sugano K, Fukayama N et al. Detection of point mutations in the K-ras oncogene at codon 12 in pure pancreatic juice for diagnosis of pancreatic carcinoma. *Cancer* 1994; 73(6):1589–94.

52. Villanueva A, Reyes G, Cuatrecasas M et al. Diagnostic utility of K-ras mutations in fine-needle aspirates of pancreatic masses. *Gastroenterology* 1996; 110:1587–94.

53. Tada M, Ohashi M, Shiratori Y et al. Analysis of K-ras gene mutation in hyperplastic duct cells of the pancreas without pancreatic disease. *Gastroenterology* 1996; 110:227–31.

54. Jaskiewicz K, Krige JE, Thomson J. Expression of p53 tumor suppresser gene, oncoprotein c-erbB-2, cellular proliferation and differentiation in malignant and benign pancreatic lesions. *Anticancer Res* 1994; 14(5A):1919–22.

55. Pellegata NS, Sessa F, Renault B et al. K-ras and p53 gene mutations in pancreatic cancer: ductal and nonductal tumors progress through different genetic lesions. *Cancer Res* 1994; 54:1556–60.

56. Horii A, Nakatsuru S, Miyoshi Y et al. Frequent somatic mutations of the APC gene in human pancreatic cancer. *Cancer Res* 1992; 52(23):6696–8.

57. Metzgar RS, Asch HL. "Antigens of human pancreatic adenocarcinoma: their role in diagnosis and therapy". *Pancreas* 1988; 3(3):352–71.

58. Haglund C. Tumour marker antigen CA125 in pancreatic cancer: a comparison with CA19-9 and CEA. *Br J Cancer* 1986; 54(6):897–901.

59. Pleskow DK, Berger HJ, Gyves J et al. Evaluation of a serologic marker, CA19-9, in the diagnosis of pancreatic cancer. *Ann Intern Med* 1989; 110(9):704–9.

60. Ching CK, Rhodes JM. Enzyme-linked PNA lectin binding assay compared with CA19-9 and CEA radioimmunoassay as a diagnostic blood test for pancreatic cancer. *Br J Cancer* 1989; 59(6):949–53.

61. Benini L, Cavallini G, Zordan D et al. A clinical evaluation of monoclonal (CA19-9, CA50, CA12-5) and polyclonal (CEA, TPA) antibody-defined antigens for the diagnosis of pancreatic cancer. *Pancreas* 1988; 3(1):61–6.

62. Steinberg WM, Gelfand R, Anderson KK et al. Comparison of the sensitivity and specificity of the CA19-9 and carcinoembryonic antigen assays in detecting cancer of the pancreas. *Gastroenterology* 1986; 90(2):343–9.

63. Gupta MK, Arciaga R, Bocci L et al. Measurement of a monoclonal-antibody-defined antigen (CA19-9) in the sera of patients with malignant and nonmalignant diseases. Comparison with carcinoembryonic antigen. *Cancer* 1985; 56(2):277–83.

64. Gullo L. CA19-9: the Italian experience. *Pancreas* 1994; 9(6):717–19.

65. Malesci A, Montorsi M, Mariani A et al. Clinical utility of the serum CA19-9 test for diagnosing pancreatic carcinoma in symptomatic patients: a prospective study. *Pancreas* 1992; 7(4):497–502.

66. Forsmark CE, Lambiase L, Vogel SB. Diagnosis of pancreatic cancer and prediction of unresectability using the tumor-associated antigen CA19-9. *Pancreas* 1994; 9(6):731–4.

67. Banfi G, Zerbi A, Pastori S. Behavior of tumor markers CA19-9, CA195, CAM43, CA242, and TPS in the diagnosis and follow-up of pancreatic cancer. *Clin Chem* 1993; 39(3):420–3.

68. Satake K, Takeuchi T. Comparison of CA19-9 with other tumor markers in the diagnosis of cancer of the pancreas. *Pancreas* 1994; 9(6):720–4.

69. Richter JM, Christensen MR, Rustagi AK *et al*. The clinical utility of the Ca19-9 radioimmunoassay for the diagnosis of pancreatic cancer presenting as pain or weight loss. A cost-effectiveness analysis. *Arch Intern Med* 1989; 149(10):2292–7.

70. Fujii Y, Albers GH, Carre-Llopis A *et al*. The diagnostic value of the foetoacinar pancreatic (FAP) protein in cancer of the pancreas; a comparative study with CA19/9. *Br J Cancer* 1987; 56(4):495–500.

71. Ritts RE,Jr, Nagorney DM, Jacobsen VR *et al*. Comparison of preoperative serum CA19-9 levels with results of diagnostic imaging modalities in patients undergoing laparotomy for suspected pancreatic or gallbladder disease. *Pancreas* 1994; 9(6):707–16.

72. Malesci A, Tommasini MA, Bonata C *et al*. Determination of CA19-9 antigen in serum and pancreatic juice for differential diagnosis of pancreatic adenocarcinoma from chronic pancreatitis. *Gastroenterology* 1987; 92:60–7.

73. Hyöty M, Hyöty H, Ritva-Kaarina A *et al*. Tumour antigens CA195 and CA19-9 in pancreatic juice and serum for the diagnosis of pancreatic carcinoma. *Eur J Surg* 1992; 158:173–9.

74. Wang JY, Chen FZ, Yang YZ. Evaluation of non-invasive diagnostic tests in detecting cancer of the pancreas. *Chin Med J* 1990; 103(10):817–20.

75. Pasanen PA, Eskelinen M, Partanen K *et al*. Clinical evaluation of a new serum tumour marker CA 242 in pancreatic carcinoma. *Br J Cancer* 1992; 65:731–4.

76. Pasanen PA, Eskelinen M, Partanen K *et al*. A prospective study of serum tumour markers carcinoembryonic antigen, carbohydrate antigens 50 and 242, tissue polypeptide antigen and tissue polypeptide specific antigen in the diagnosis of pancreatic cancer with special reference to multivariate diagnostic score. *Br J Cancer* 1994; 69(3):562–5.

77. Pasanen PA, Eskelinen M, Partanen K *et al*. Clinical evaluation of tissue polypeptide antigen (TPA) in the diagnosis of pancreatic carcinoma. *Anticancer Res* 1993; 13:1883–8.

78. Kiriyama S, Hayakawa T, Kondo T, *et al*. Usefulness of a new tumor marker, Span-1, for the diagnosis of pancreatic cancer. *Cancer* 1990; 65(7):1557–61.

Diagnosis: ERCP **3**

7

Normal pancreatogram

Pier Alberto Testoni & Alberto Tittobello

INTRODUCTION

Endoscopic retrograde pancreatography (ERP) is still the most effective diagnostic tool for investigating the pancreatic duct system and studying the ampullary region. The endoscopic approach provides on one hand a complete examination of the descending duodenum and the papilla of Vater and, on the other hand, a well defined radiological documentation of the pancreatic ducts and, in selected cases, of the acinar tissue.

A correct evaluation of the normal pancreas must take into account: (a) the papillary region; (b) the confluence of the common bile duct (CBD) and pancreatic duct (PD); (c) the morphology of the main PD and of the duct of Santorini; and (d) the morphology of the side branches and of the acinar tissue.

Since anatomical variants are frequent, their recognition on pancreatography is also important for differential diagnosis between normal and pathological findings.

ENDOSCOPIC ANATOMY OF PAPILLA OF VATER

The major papilla is located on the mid-portion of the descending duodenum in most cases (more than 90%), closer to the posterior than to the anterior wall. On rare occasions it may be found in other sites, along a line extending from the duodenal bulb to the distal part of the descending duodenum. However, Classen *et al.* in a preliminary study[1], found it in the middle third of the descending duodenum in only 54% of cases, while it was in the lower third in 30% and in the upper third in 16% . In rare cases the major papilla is also found in the fourth duodenal portion.

Several structures are seen in the papillary area. A transverse semicircular mucosal fold, parallel to Kerkring's valvules, is located proximally to the orifice and sometimes hides it. The longitudinal mucosal protrusion that corresponds to the intramural segment of the CBD, properly called the papilla of Vater, varies in size and shape from person to person[2]; in some cases it may not project at all, making catheterization difficult. In our experience, the shape may vary over a period of time; in fact, a papilla that is flat at the beginning of catheterization may appear to project distinctly at the end of the procedure. The papillary orifice is generally punctiform and in a close view looks like a velvet area, darker than the surrounding mucosa. In most cases there is a single orifice and the catheter must be introduced obliquely upwards and to the right in the direction of the bile duct, more perpendicularly forward and to the right in the direction of the PD. Exceptionally there can be two separate orifices. Philip *et al.*[3] estimated that 2% of cases are of this type. The vertical mucosal relief, which extends caudally from the papillary region (the so-called frenulum of the caruncula), is the only vertical protrusion in the second part of the duodenum and, in practice, is identified endoscopically before the papilla proper. When the papilla is flat and difficult to identify, this mucosal relief is the main landmark for its identification.

Different aspects of the normal appearance of the papilla of Vater are shown in Figure 7.1. A periampullary duodenal

Figure 7.1   Different aspects of the normal papilla of Vater. The velvet appearance of the orifice at close view is shown in (c).

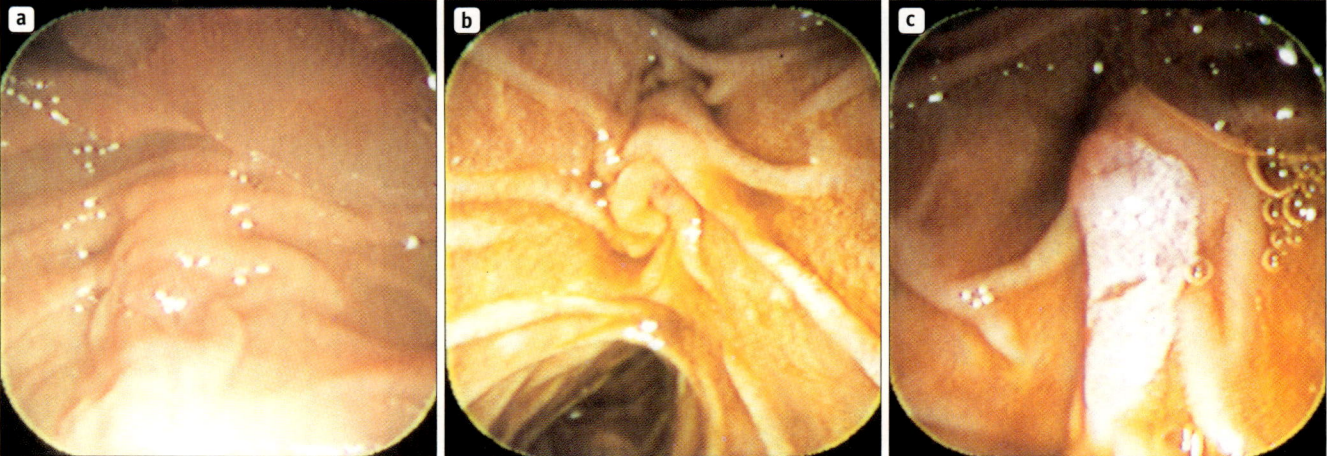

Figure 7.2 Different aspects of periampullary diverticula.

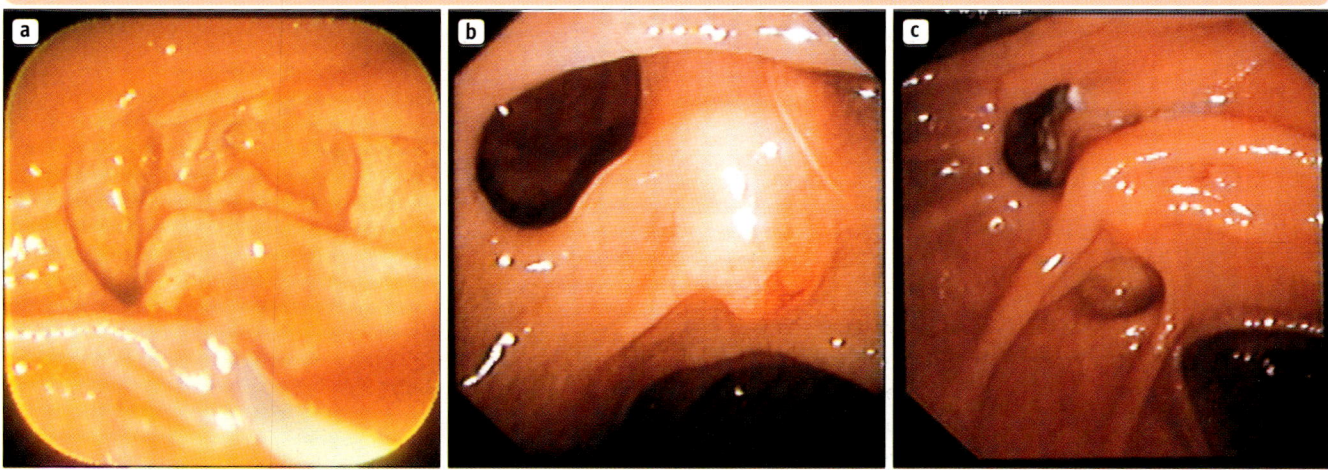

diverticulum or an intradiverticular papilla is seen in about 10% of cases. The frequency of this increases with advanced age (24% in our series) and it is found in as many as 20% of patients with CBD stones, suggesting a possible relationship between diverticula and biliary stone disease. The presence of periampullary diverticula may render it difficult to identify the papillary orifice and the proper orientation for cannulation. The difficulty is greater when the papilla is located within the diverticulum, especially if it lies on the inferior wall. In these cases, the longitudinal fold leading toward the diverticulum can be a useful landmark for identifying the papillary orifice. Several endoscopic views of periampullary diverticula are shown in Figures 7.2 and 7.3.

The minor papilla corresponds to the orifice of the duct of Santorini and is seen in about 80% of cases; it is usually located 2–3cm proximal, and slightly anterior, to the major papilla (Figure 7.4) and it can be used as a landmark for the identification of the major papilla when the latter is flat or hidden among large duodenal folds. There are several variations of position and also of size, permeability and functional prominence over the major papilla[3,4].

Figure 7.3 Endoscopic view of an intradiverticular papilla of Vater.

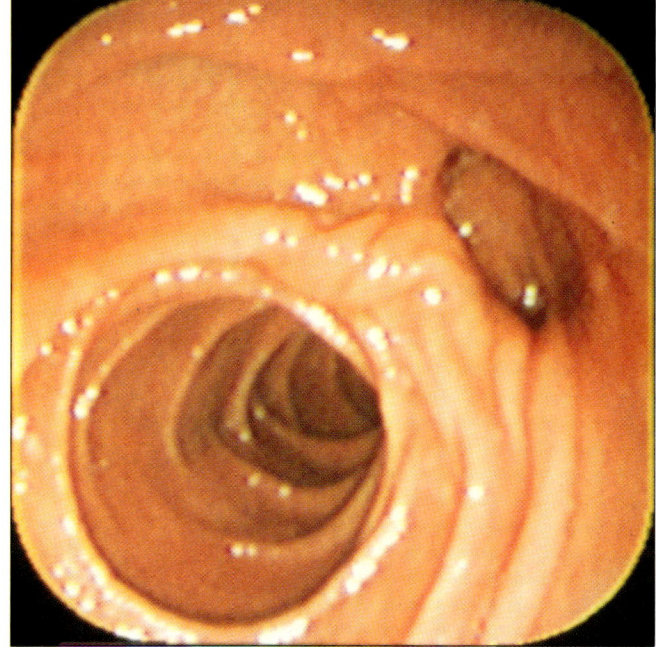

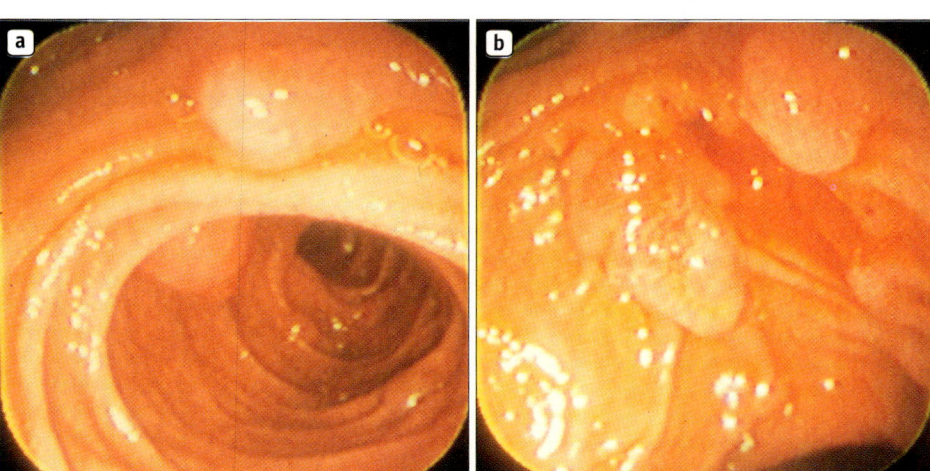

Figure 7.4 Endoscopic views of the minor papilla; it is usually located 2–3cm proximally and slightly anterior to the major papilla.

6

Pancreatic cancer: ancillary diagnostic techniques

Charles Duckworth, Robert Kiss & Paul Yeaton

INTRODUCTION

The diagnosis of pancreatic adenocarcinoma can often be difficult to establish. Computed tomography (CT), ultrasonography and magnetic resonance imaging detect neoplasms > 2cm with fair sensitivity, but small potentially curable lesions are frequently missed[1,2]. Endoscopic ultrasonography (EUS) is sensitive in detecting small lesions and improves staging accuracy[2,3]. Both endoscopic retrograde cholangiopancreatography (ERCP) and CT have 80–95% sensitivity in detecting pancreatic adenocarcinoma[2,4,5]. The specificity of CT ranges from 50% to 95%; ERCP is reported to be 90% specific[4,5]. Because images of chronic pancreatitis may closely resemble those of cancer, clinicians may be faced with inconclusive results. A confirmatory diagnosis is usually sought via light microscopy cytology or other supportive studies.

Currently endoscopic brush cytology and CT- or US-guided fine-needle aspiration (FNA) have a diagnostic sensitivity of only 40–75%[6–9]. Cytology has a specificity greater than 90%[6,8–12]. Brush cytology and FNA are both subject to sampling errors, either by missing the area of concern or obtaining insufficient material to establish a diagnosis (Figure 6.1). A small specimen may lack the architectural organization present in a resected specimen and the appearance of malignancy can resemble that of chronic pancreatitis[13]. These factors make cytological diagnosis a challenging endeavour, as much an art as a science, and help drive the quest for ancillary diagnostic techniques. Ideally, such examinations would be highly sensitive and specific and would have the potential to detect early, surgically curable disease.

The approaches to ancillary diagnostic techniques for pancreatic adenocarcinoma include adjuncts to light microscopic cytology (immunocytochemistry, electron microscopy, flow and image cytometry), biochemical tumour markers, and molecular biochemistry techniques designed to detect specific genetic aberrations[14]. While an exhaustive analysis of all such techniques is beyond the scope of this work, we will characterize the basic principles of these techniques and contrast their relative merits and current as well as future applications.

IMAGE CYTOMETRY

Image analysis is a computer-aided technique to quantify specific features of digitized images; image cytometry refers to the application of this technique to describe cellular morphology. The material to be examined is stained appropriately and examined with light microscopy. An appropriate image is identified by the operator for analysis and a video image is recorded (Figure 6.2). The recorded image can be displayed on a video monitor composed of pixels. Each pixel has a defined size and intensity that can be described numerically. Thus, the act of recording the image transfers the analogue microscopic image into a digital form and provides the basis for development of the mathematical algorithms describing the pixels and their relations with near neighbours.

The most well developed image cytometry applications describe nuclear material, but techniques are rapidly expand-

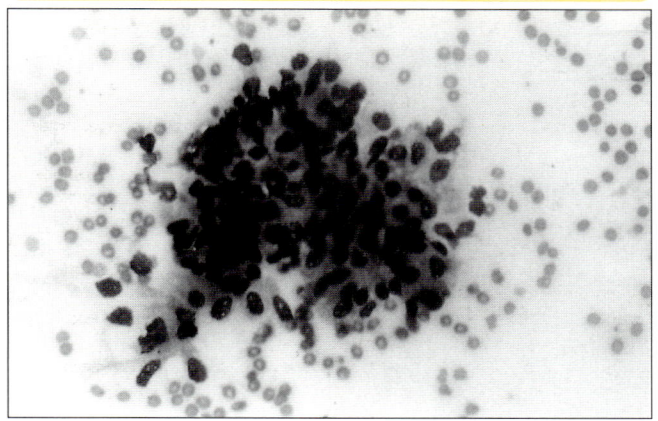

Figure 6.1 A pancreatic cytology specimen of malignant origin. Note the scant number of cells present and the lack of architecture; the basis of diagnosis is on cellular morphology alone.

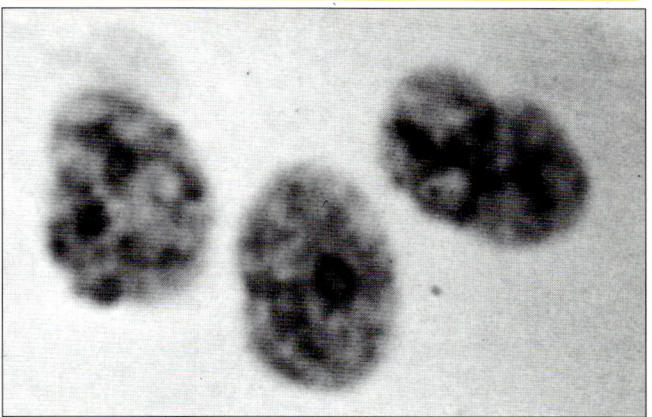

Figure 6.2 Photomicrograph of the video monitor image depicting three Feulgen-stained nuclei. Note the clear separation of the nuclei and the distribution of nuclear chromatin.

Figure 6.3 The cell cycle. G_0–G_1 represents the mature, differentiated cell. The S phase represents the synthesis of nuclear material. The end of the S-phase through to mitosis involves cells with twice the normal amount of DNA.

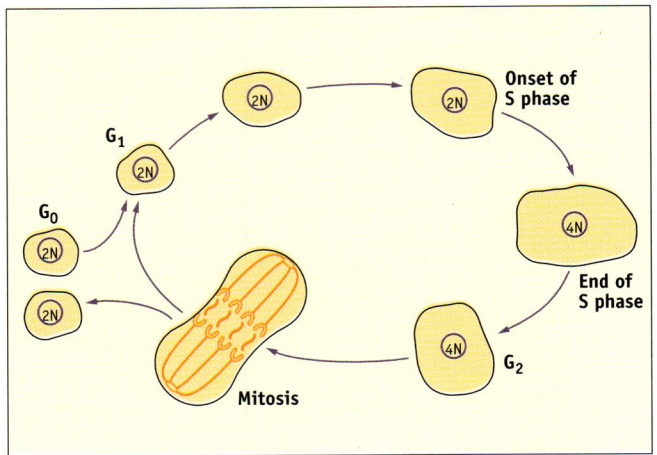

Figure 6.4 DNA histograms from normal and malignant pancreatic epithelia, derived by image cytometry.

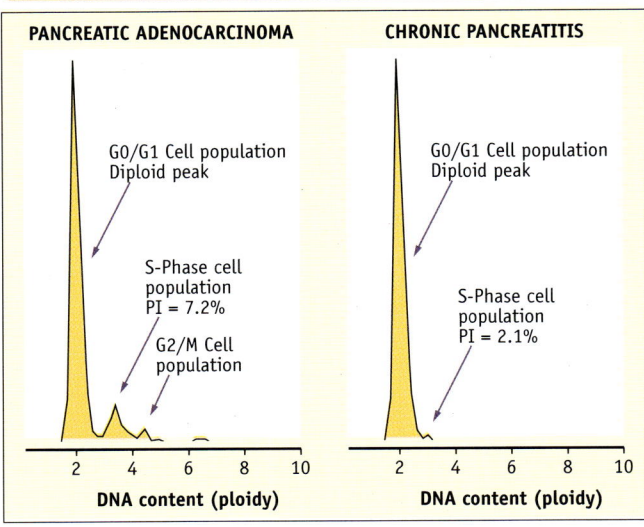

Figure 6.5 Examples of potential DNA histogram types. (Adapted from Deprez *et al. Am J Clin Pathol* 1993; 99:558–65).

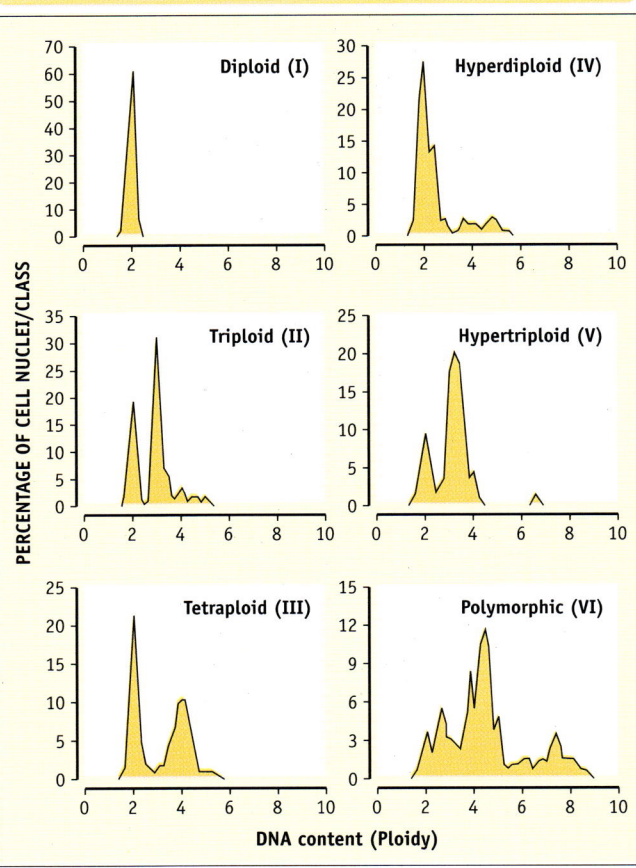

ing that encompass immunohistochemistry; in theory, anything that can be quantitatively stained can be quantitatively described with a high degree of accuracy employing image analysis. For the purposes of our discussion, we will concentrate on image analysis of nuclear material.

The Feulgen reaction is a quantitative staining method providing the basis for image cytometry of nuclear DNA. It is specific and stoichiometric and the intensity of the staining is directly proportional to the amount of nuclear material present[15]. Materials suitable for staining include cytological specimens, and therefore the method can be used in the diagnosis of pancreatic cancer.

Stained slides are examined microscopically for well separated, intact nuclei, and nuclear images are recorded with a CCD camera mounted on the microscope. Between 200 and 300 nuclear images are required to characterize accurately the population of cells included in the specimen. Three general types of information can be generated: morphometric, densitometric and textural.

Morphometric parameters describe the shape and/or size of the nuclei examined. The nuclear area is easily calculated by summation of the number of pixels representing the nuclear image. Nuclear shape may be quantified by other features, similar to those assessed during routine light microscopy. Quantification of the physical features describing nuclear distortion may be affected by the techniques used to transfer the specimen on to the slide for examination, some of which involve physical forces.

The density of individual pixels representing the stained nucleus is calculated on a 256 grey-scale index. This quantification is directly proportional to DNA content and from these data the total DNA content of individual nuclei can be calculated. By defining the nuclear content of the cell population examined, a DNA histogram can be generated, reflecting the ploidy status and characterizing the relative proportions of cell cycle components of the tissue examined (Figures 6.3, 6.4 and 6.5).

When viewing stained nuclear material with sufficient magnification, it is possible to discern variation in the distribution of DNA within the nucleus. This represents condensation of the nuclear material, or chromatin clumping. Textural parameters are mathematical descriptions of the topographical distribution of the nuclear DNA; a variety of constructs can be created describing the relationship of individual pixels, and their respective densities can be used to define their relationships. For example, 'pale' and 'dense' areas within the nucleus and descriptions of short and long lengths of chromatin can be defined.

APPLICATIONS

Diagnosis

Morphometric, densitometric and textural features can be used to differentiate benign from malignant pancreatic disease[16]. Rickaert et al., using archival paraffin-embedded specimens of pancreatic tissue, developed a scoring system based on nuclear area and chromatin density and distribution. Both the nuclear area and the total system score could be used to differentiate malignant from non-malignant pancreatic tissue[17]. Yeaton et al. performed image cytometry on brush cytology specimens obtained during ERCP, and created a scoring system based on the DNA index (determined from DNA content), histogram type and proliferative index. This scoring system was able to detect pancreatic malignancy with a 95% sensitivity and a 100% specificity[18]. 'Textural' features were reported by the authors to differentiate benign from malignant pancreatic disease but the data were not given.

Staging and survival: In addition to assisting diagnosis, the evaluation of cytology specimens using image analysis from pancreatic ductal carcinomas may provide useful information on survival and even stage or resectability. Rickaert et al. were able to distinguish grade I from grade III pancreatic duct malignancies utilizing a combination of morphometric, densitometric and textural parameters[17]. Linder et al. used image cytometry to assess the DNA content of cytology specimens from fine-needle aspirates. Patients with diploid tumours had a significant increase in survival time over those with non-diploid tumours[19]. These findings supported earlier work indicating a significant increase in survival among patients with diploid pancreatic tumours over tetraploid or aneuploid cases[20,21]. Survival data are useful in determining when to attempt resection and could assist the clinician in other decisions such as the type of stent to use in cases of palliation. Due to the high cost of expandable stents many clinicians recommend these stents only for those who will have a significant chance of extended survival.

Limitations: While image analysis is good at detecting small populations of aneuploid cells, it is less able to discern near-diploid populations[22]. It is a labour-intensive process, as each nucleus of the 200–300 to be analysed must be selected by the microscopist. For an adequate evaluation there must be a distinct image of each nucleus analysed. FNA and brush cytology specimens often contain mucus and other debris, which can inhibit light transmission and clump cells together. Improved methods of specimen preparation and collection will probably overcome these difficulties.

Conclusion

Image cytometry is a promising technique to assist in the diagnosis and management of patients with suspected pancreatic malignancies. In addition to characterizing DNA content, image cytometry can quantify immunohistochemical stains, which has both research and clinical potential.

FLOW CYTOMETRY

Flow cytometry is also capable of quantifying DNA content; specimens must first undergo filtration and protein digestion. Nuclei are then stained with fluorescent intercalating dyes, such as propidium iodide; the amount of staining is proportional to the quantity of DNA present. The solution containing the stained nuclei is passed as a liquid stream into a counting chamber. The cells pass before a laser beam and scatter the laser light, which is detected and described by photosensors. The amount of light scatter and fluorescence intensity is mathematically related to the amount of DNA present; this is used to determine histogram type and ploidy status (Figure 6.6)[22,23]. From the histogram data, the relative constituents of the cell cycle can be calculated. Unlike image cytometry, neither morphometric nor textural parameters can be assessed by flow cytometry.

Applications

The primary clinical use of flow cytometry has been in the evaluation of haematological malignancies. Its application in tissue obtained from solid tumours has been useful in differentiating malignant from non-malignant disease and it may provide insight into the potential biological behaviour of certain malignancies[23]. Of the many potential applications for flow cytometry, only its capacity to assess DNA content and the clinical application of this in the evaluation of pancreatic malignancies will be reviewed here.

Diagnosis and prognosis

Flow cytometric quantification of pancreatic adenocarcinoma nuclear DNA content has been evaluated for its ability to diagnose and predict the outcome of these malignancies. The sensitivity of flow cytometry in detecting pancreatic malignancy from cytology specimens has been shown to be equal to that of standard cytology, but with less specificity. Combining flow cytometry and standard cytology increases the sensitivity but has an unacceptably low specificity[24].

Studies have examined the ability of nuclear DNA content assessed by flow cytometry to provide prognostic information in pancreatic ductal malignancies. Diploid and

Figure 6.6 Flow cytometric DNA histogram patterns. (Left) diploid, (centre) tetraploid, (right) aneuploid. (Adapted from Herrera et al. Ann Surg 1992; 215:120–4).

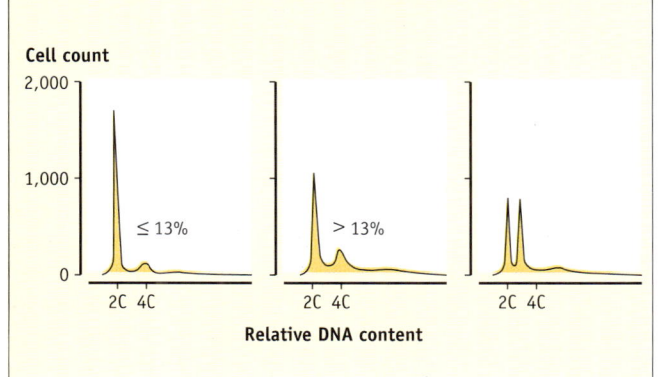

tetraploid tumours appear to have an increased survival over aneuploid tumours, which supports similar image cytometric data. The S-phase fraction also has independent prognostic implications[24–29]. Not all investigators have shown ploidy status or S-phase fraction to be predictors of survival[24,30,31].

Conclusion

Flow cytometry is a process capable of rapidly assessing the DNA content of a large cell population. Currently, flow cytometry does not appear to improve the diagnostic sensitivity of cytology alone in pancreatic adenocarcinoma. Because DNA content may be useful in predicting outcome, flow cytometry, like image cytometry, may be useful in assisting in the clinical management of pancreatic adenocarcinoma.

IMAGE CYTOMETRY *VERSUS* FLOW CYTOMETRY

Flow cytometry is rapid (up to 10,000 nuclei per second evaluated), less labour-intensive and better at detecting near-diploid cell populations than is image cytometry[22,23] (Figure 6.7). Some disadvantages to flow cytometry include its requirement for large numbers of nuclei, lack of sensitivity for small aneuploid populations, and inability to define features other than densitometric parameters[22]. Flow cytometry appears, in early studies, to be less sensitive and specific than image cytometry in differentiating benign from malignant pancreatic disease. This is possibly explained by the fact that image cytometry can assess more nuclear chromatin variables than flow cytometry. In addition, nuclei evaluated by image cytometry are selected by the investigator, eliminating clumped nuclei, other nuclei such as from white blood cells, and other debris. Too few studies have been carried out to make definitive statements about either technology in the evaluation of pancreatic malignancies. Both technologies require strict adherence to standards as many variables exist that can significantly alter the results[32,33].

GENETICS

It is thought that most malignancies develop after a series of genetic alterations have taken place. Numerous gene mutations have been associated with pancreatic adenocarcinoma. Pancreatic malignancies have been shown to have a high rate of K-*ras* gene mutations at codon 12. The K-*ras* oncogene is thought to be involved in cell growth regulation and becomes activated by single point mutations[34]. In addition p53, c-*myc*, c-*erb*B-2 oncogene, DCC (deleted in colon cancer) suppressor gene, and the APC (adenomatous polyposis coli) gene have been suggested to play a role in the development of some pancreatic exocrine malignancies (Figure 6.8)[35–42]. Gene mutations can be assessed in pancreatic cytology specimens with the aim of determining diagnosis and, potentially, prognosis. Early gene mutations could provide a means of screening for resectable pancreatic duct malignancies.

Applications

K-ras Because of the high association of K-*ras* mutations at codon 12 with pancreatic cancer, a number of studies have looked at K-*ras* mutations, using PCR techniques, in pancreatic brushings or fine-needle aspirates [34,43–52] (Figure 6.9). While the presence of K-*ras* mutations in pancreatic brush collections has excellent specificity, nearly 100% for pancreatic cancer, the sensitivity varies between 55% and 100%. The wide range of reported sensitivities may reflect the type of specimens studied or the techniques utilized in detecting K-*ras* abnormalities. In addition it is probable that K-*ras*, while strongly associated with pancreatic adenocarcinoma is not necessary for the development of malignancy[53]. However, cytology specimens have had K-*ras* mutations noted up to 40 months before a diagnosis of pancreatic cancer was made despite negative radiological and surgical evaluations[43]. This suggests that K-*ras* gene mutations at codon 12 are an early marker for pancreatic adenocarcinoma.

Non-K-*ras*

Type 1 growth factor receptor gene abnormalities have also been associated with pancreatic adenocarcinoma. Overexpression of the *erb*B-2 proto-oncogene and *erb*B-3, also felt to be a member of the type 1 growth factor receptor family, has been associated with pancreatic cancer.

Figure 6.7 Comparison of image and flow cytometry.

	Image cytometry	Flow cytometry
Nuclei required	Hundreds	Thousands
Factors assessed	Morphometric, densitometric, textural	Densitometric
Evaluation	Moderately labour-intensive	Rapid
Ploidy assessment	Small aneuploid populations detected	Better for near-diploid populations
Usefulness in:		
Diagnosis	+	–
Staging	±	unknown
Survival	+	+

Figure 6.8 Genetic alterations commonly associated with pancreatic adenocarcinoma.

	K-*ras*	*p53*	*erb*B-2	DCC
Prevalence (%)	80	70	30	50
Early or late marker	Early	Late	?Late	?

APPEARANCE OF THE CONFLUENCE OF THE CBD AND PD

The muscular sphincter structures in the papilla of Vater can be divided into three different parts: the most distal part at the orifice of the common channel; the sphincter of Oddi; and circular and oblique muscle strands that extend more proximally around the distal part of the CBD and main PD. These muscle fibres constitute the sphincter of the CBD and the sphincter of the PD, respectively.

The sphincter of Oddi (common papillary sphincter) consists of a few circular smooth muscle fibres and ramified glands and surrounds the common channel of the CBD and the main PD at the ampulla of Vater. In man, the common papillary sphincter does not seem to be a real anatomical sphincter (the duodenal muscular layer plays this role)[5] and its functional reality is also controversial. However, its pathophysiological role is very important. In fact, the anatomical structures are reported to act as a true sphincter that inhibits the flow of bile from the CBD into the duodenum, to be a propulsive pump that can expel bile by means of an active mechanism, to control gall bladder filling by regulating the flow of bile through the papilla, and to be an anti-reflux mechanism that prevents the duodenal contents from entering the bile duct or PD[6]. Nevertheless, this theory seems to be incompatible with the volume of the cavities of the common papillary sphincter in humans and needs further confirmation. During endoscopic examination, neither spasmodic spurts of bile into the duodenum nor rhythmic contractions of the papillary orifice are seen. With age, the muscle fibres lose their flexibility and extensibility, resulting in increased diameters of both the CBD and the main PD[7].

The ducts join shortly before reaching the duodenal wall, the common channel in the ampulla therefore being very short in most cases. The common channel is observed in 70–80% of subjects and varies from 2 to 15mm in length. Separate openings of the CBD and PD into the papilla of Vater are apparent in 8–18% of subjects, while some investigators report separate papillae in about 2% of cases[8] (Figure 7.5). Hand's analysis[9] of 3000 postmortem specimens showed a common channel in 85% of cases and sep-

Figure 7.6 Anatomical variants of the confluence of the CBD and main PD in the papilla of Vater. (a) Presence of a common channel that prolongs the PD axis (the CBD joining the PD at a right angle. (b) Presence of a common channel that prolongs mainly the CBD. (c) Common channel with ampullary dilatation. (d) Short common channel. (e) Separate openings of CBD and PD in the papilla of Vater. (f) Absence of a common channel, with side-by-side openings of the CBD and PD into the papilla of Vater.

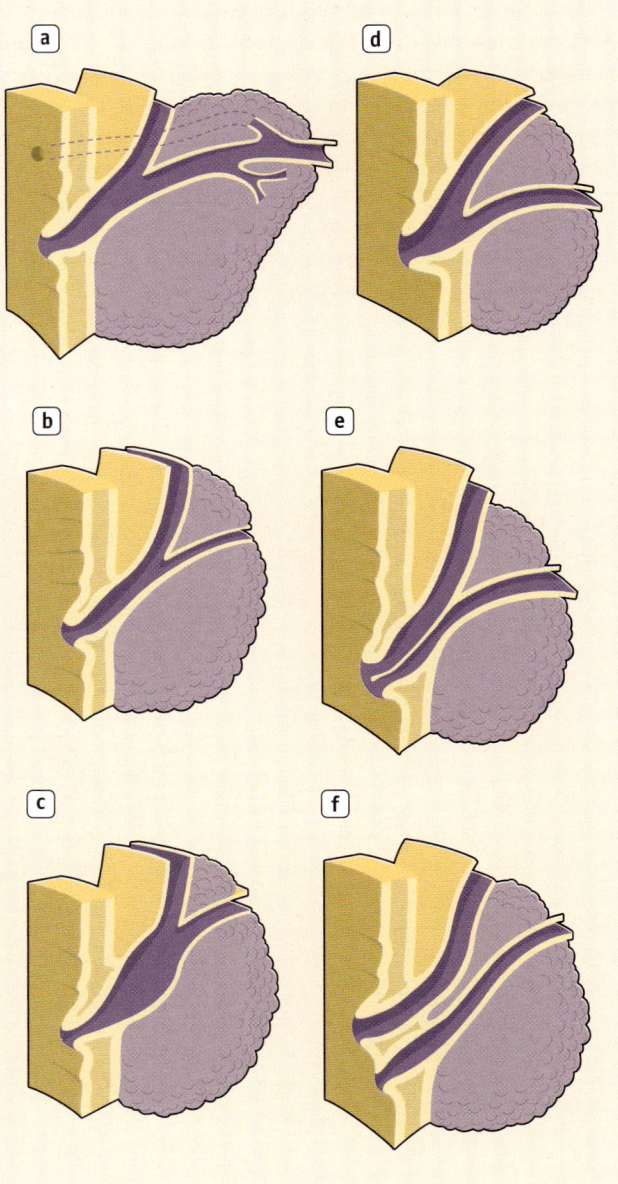

Figure 7.5 Separate openings of the CBD and the PD into the papilla of Vater.

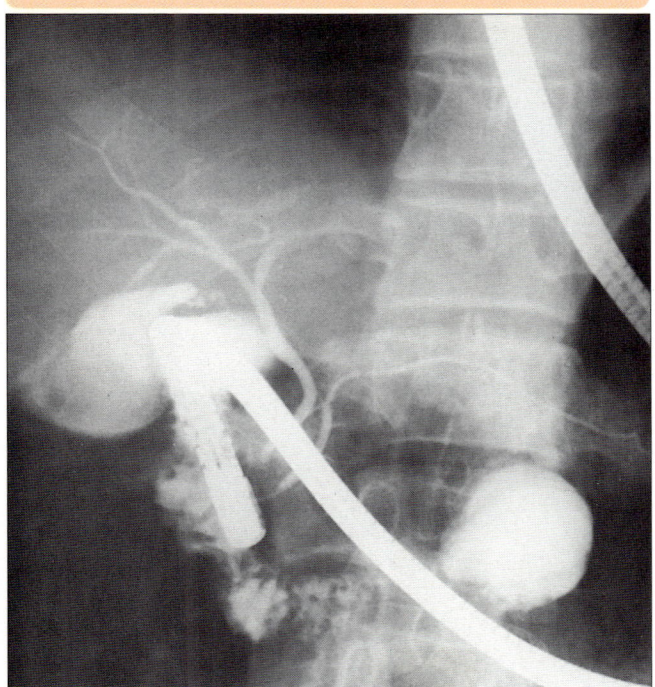

Figure 7.7 Dynamic sphincter function in a normal subject during contraction and relaxation phases, shown by ERCP. There is opacification of both the CBD and the PD. (a) Relaxation phase. (b) Contraction phase.

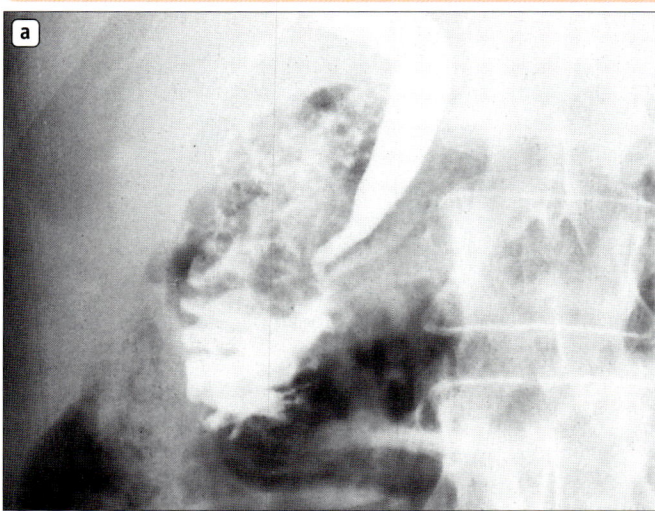

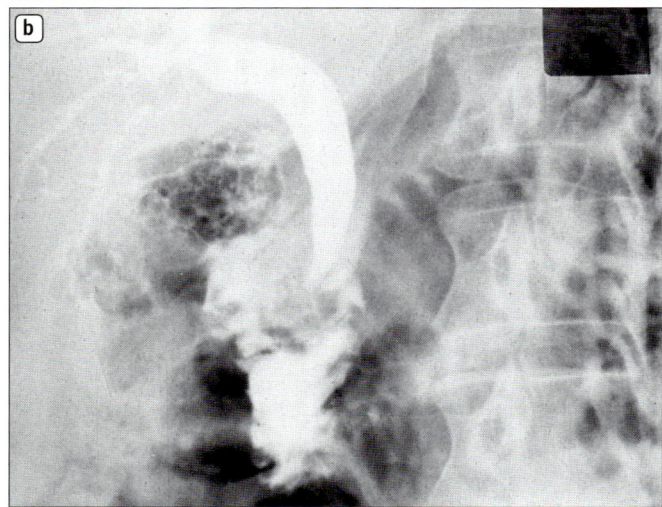

arate terminations in 13%; the duct of Wirsung was absent in 2%, pancreatic drainage taking place via Santorini's duct. Variants of the confluence of the CBD and main PD in the papilla of Vater are listed in Figure 7.6.

The muscle fibres of the sphincter of Oddi extend proximally around the CBD to its oblique entry into the wall of the duodenum to form the biliary sphincter. A short segment of circular smooth muscle also surrounds the PD in the distal part to form the pancreatic sphincter.

Figure 7.8 Contraction of the high-pressure segment of the distal part of the main PD, the so-called pancreatic sphincter, with slight dilatation of the duct.

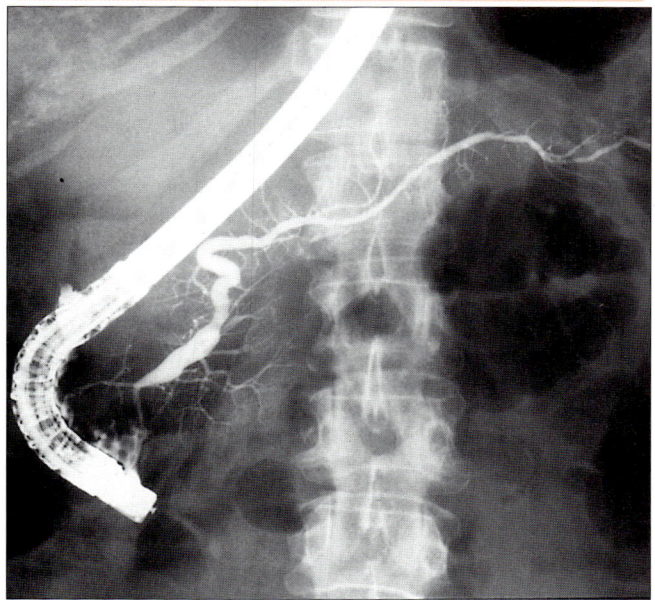

The biliary sphincter is characterized, from a functional point of view, by prominent pressure peaks representing phasic contractions that are superimposed on a low and stable basal pressure (tone), as documented by radiological studies in the past[7,10] and, recently and more accurately, by manometric investigation[11,12]. Dynamic sphincter function in normal subjects during contraction and relaxation phases on ERCP is shown in Figure 7.7.

Several recent studies of the function of the sphincter of Oddi in the interdigestive period have shown a relationship between the sphincter's motility and the phases of the migrating motor complex (MMC): the frequency of contractions gradually increases during phase II and culminates in a short burst of high-frequency contractions just before duodenal phase III activity. The burst of maximal activity lasts throughout phase III of the duodenal MMC (i.e. the activity front in the fasting state) and the sphincter of Oddi returns to its normal contractile activity after the end of phase III[13]. The role of the high-pressure segment of the distal part of the main PD, the so-called pancreatic sphincter, has been discussed and is at present still uncertain. However, the contraction of this segment is clearly defined during ERCP (Figure 7.8) and may play some role in preventing biliopancreatic reflux.

In normal subjects, ERCP may show transient hypertone of the biliary or pancreatic sphincter, with delayed emptying of contrast medium into the duodenum. When there is no dilatation of the CBD or PD system, the finding should not be considered pathological. In the same way, evidence from ERCP of a persistent contraction of the sphincter of Oddi or of the biliary sphincter, even when associated with a moderate dilatation of the CBD which can be seen shortly after an episode of biliary pain, should still be considered within normal limits, as a consequence of a recent passage of stones or biliary sludge (Figure 7.9). In these circumstances, the endoscopist should avoid performing a sphincterotomy unless a previous history of recurrent acute pancreatitis has been reported by the patient.

Figure 7.9 Radiological evidence in ERCP of a persistent contraction of the biliary sphincter associated with a moderate dilatation of the CBD. This is a common finding shortly after an episode of biliary pain and should still be considered within normal limits, and a consequence of a recent passage of stones or biliary sludge. In such a case, in the absence of persistent cholestasis, endoscopic sphincterotomy should be avoided.

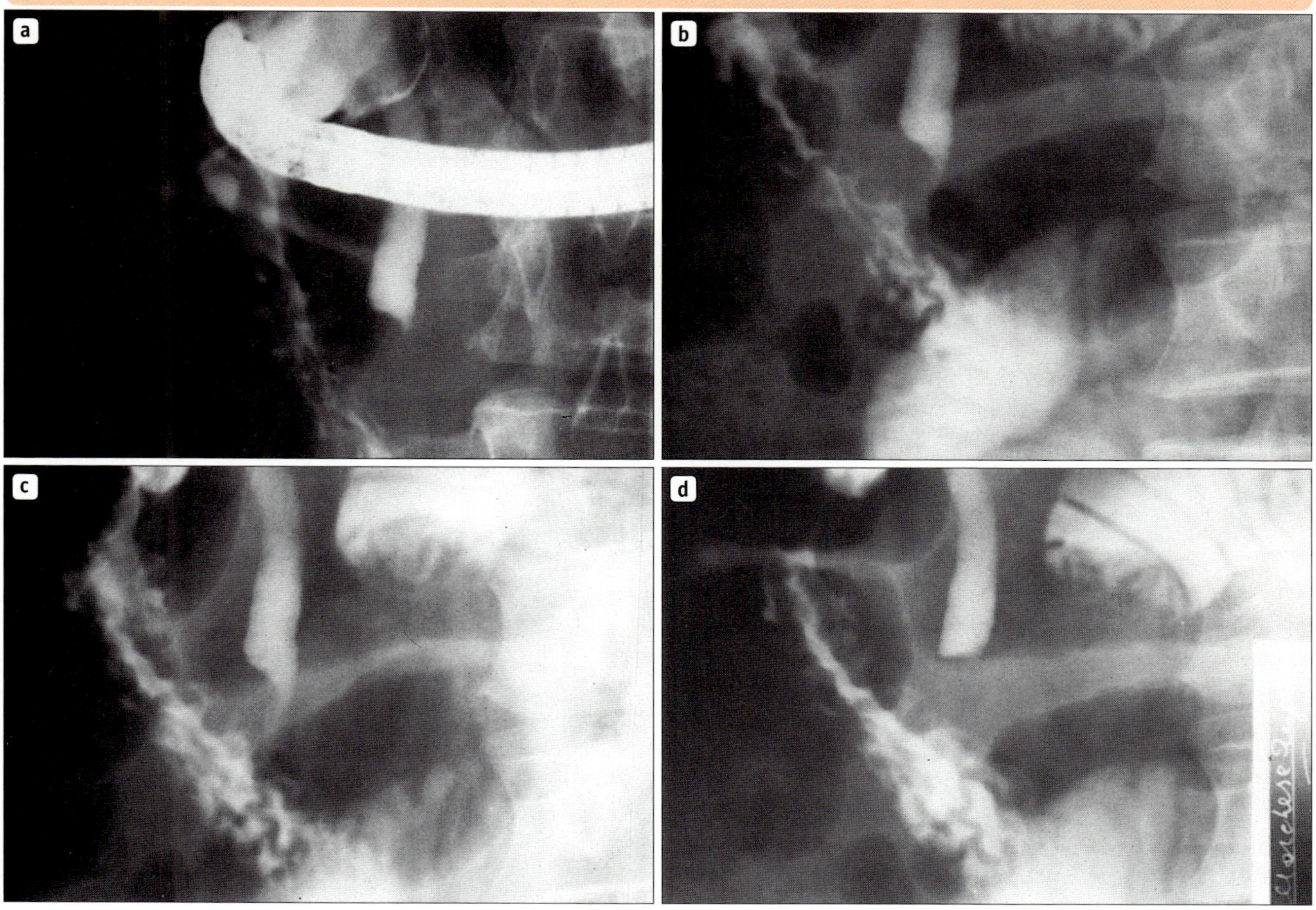

MAIN PD AND ACCESSORY DUCT

Main PD filling

The main PD originates in the vast majority of people between the T-12 and L-1 vertebral bodies, from a radiological point of view. It courses upward, sweeping anteriorly over the spine and aorta, and heads toward the hilum of the spleen. In the passage between the head and body of the gland, it takes a 45 to 90-degree turn, before continuing horizontally in the body and tail (Figure 7.10). The course of the main duct varies, even in subjects with normal pancreatograms. These variations of the head of the pancreas reflect the embryological development of the gland and there is usually no relationship between the course of the duct and pancreatic symptoms or diseases. Four possible overall courses that the main duct may take are: ascending (Figure 7.11); horizontal (Figure 7.12); sigmoid (Figure 7.13) and descending. These are seen in 49.6%, 35.8%, 10.3% and 4.3% of cases, respectively[14]. In 1983 Yatto and Siegel[15] proposed another classification of the normal variations of the main PD (Figure 7.14). This classification identifies, in addition to the normal configuration, the loop and ring variations (Figures 7.15 and 7.16), the N or M configuration (Figure 7.17), bifurcations of the body or tail (Figure 7.18) and angulations (Figure 7.19). In some cases the different configurations of the ductal system produce images of pseudomasses on CT scans, even when the findings of pancreatography correspond to benign variants[16].

The total length of the main PD varies widely, ranging between 95 and 270mm, and it is usually of little clinical diag-

Figure 7.10 Normal pancreatogram. Filling of the main PD is complete to the tail and secondary branches are partially opacified. The contour and configuration of the ducts are normal.

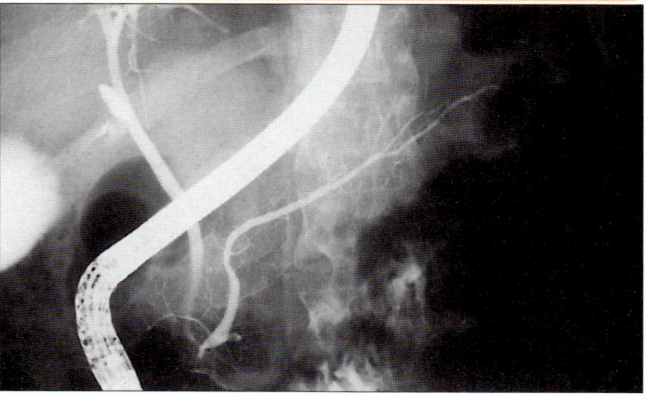

Figure 7.11 Ascending course of a normal main PD, with complete filling of side branches and the duct of Santorini.

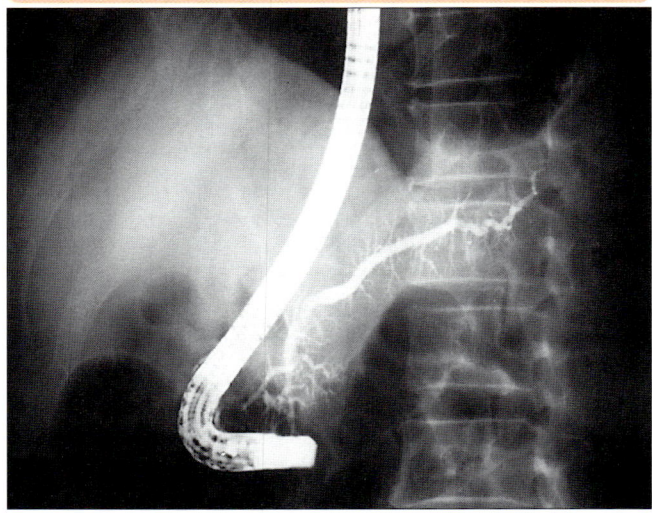

Figure 7.12 Horizontal course of a normal PD, with angulation of the tail and filling of the side branches throughout the length of the duct.

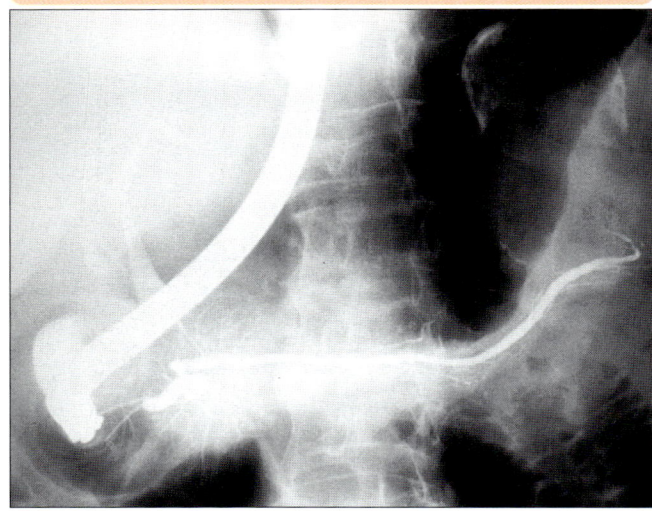

Figure 7.13 Sigmoid course of the normal PD with filling of the main side branches. There is slight dilatation of the cephalic segment in this elderly subject.

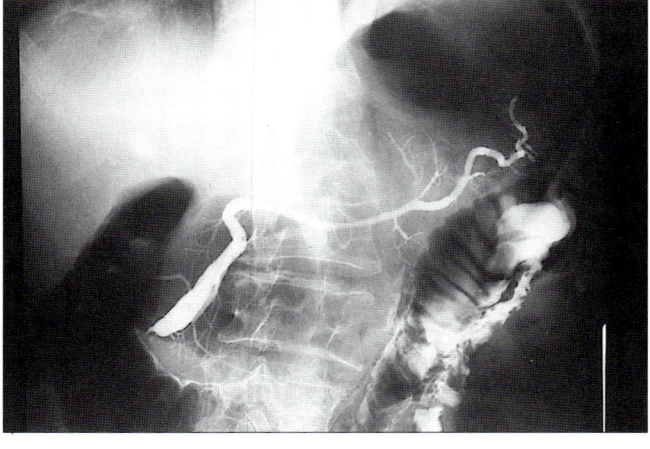

Figure 7.14 Schematic representation of the normal main PD and its variations. (Modified from Siegel[16] with permission.)

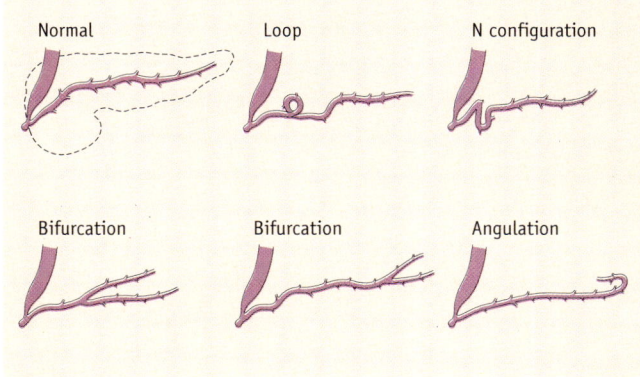

Figure 7.15 A pancreatogram showing a large loop of the main PD at the head of the gland.

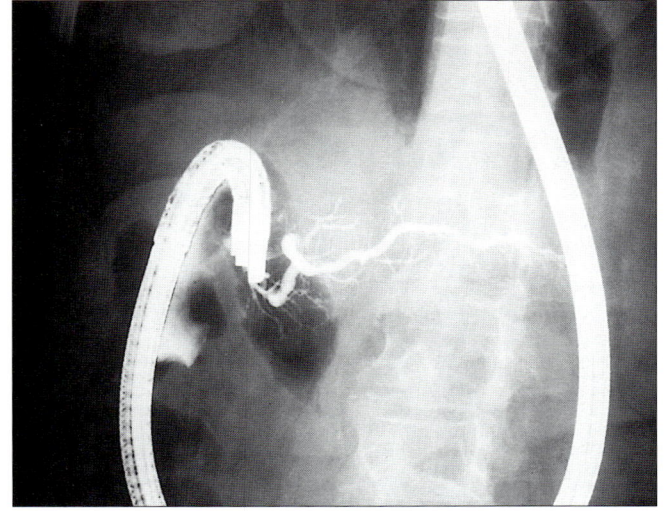

Figure 7.16 Ring variant of the main PD at the head of the pancreas.

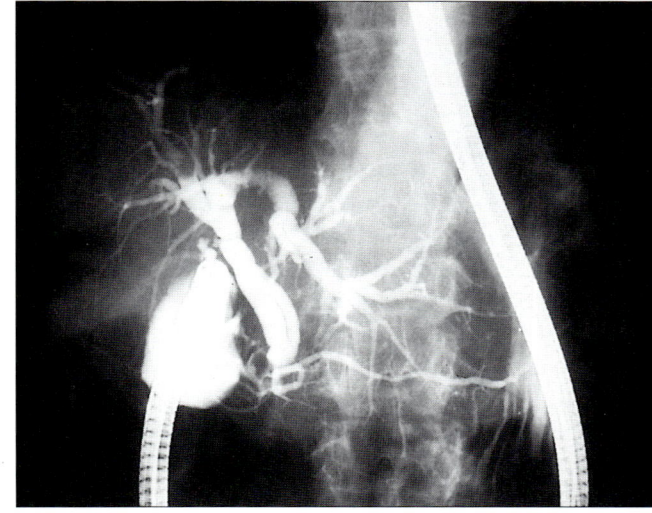

Figure 7.17 M configuration of the course of the main PD, which is also of the descending type.

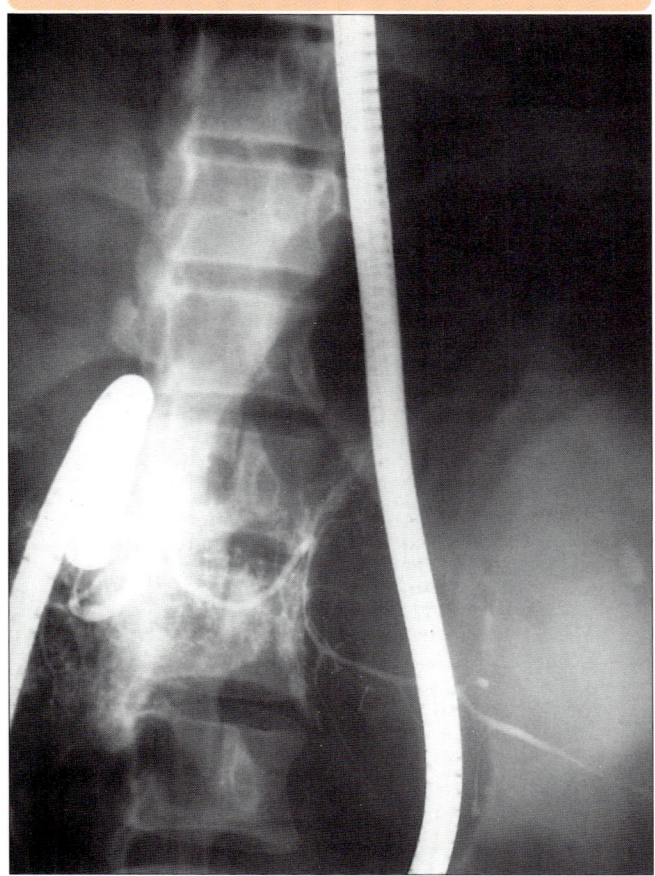

Figure 7.18 Pancreatogram showing bifurcation of the PD at the tail.

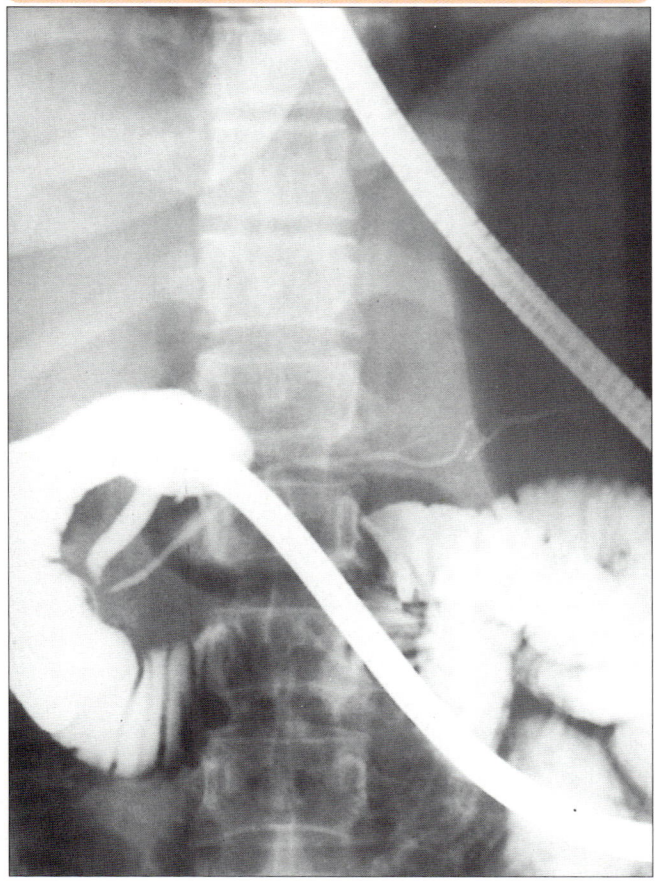

Figure 7.19 Normal pancreatogram showing a large angulation of the PD at the head of the gland.

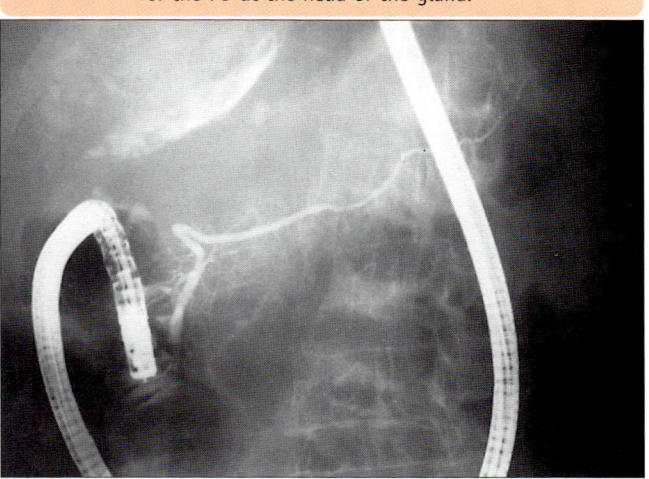

nostic importance. For his series[14] Kizu reported a length of 16.2 ± 1.9cm (mean ± SD) in adult males and of 16.1 ± 1.6 cm in females. There were no statistically significant dfferences between the sexes or with ageing. When there is an apparent short duct, consideration should be given to the possibility that the injection of contrast material was done with inadequate pressure and volume, or that only the biliary duct has been cannulated, with backflow of contrast medium into the PD through the common channel. Other possible reasons for a short main duct are pancreatic malfusion (Figure 7.20) or the presence of a neoplastic lesion in the body or tail of the gland, with complete ductal obstruction (Figure 7.21).

The PD is widest at the head and tapers toward the tail: the accepted normal diameter is approximately 3–5mm at the head, decreasing to 2–4mm in the body and to 1–2mm at the tail. While the increased opacification may result in some dilatation of calibre, the above measures hold for maximum normal values. Figure 7.22 reports the variations in measure-

Figure 7.20 An unusual pancreatogram showing a long ventral duct in pancreas divisum, reaching the body of the gland. The diagnosis of pancreas divisum is based on the presence of a normal distribution of side branches, which can rule out a possible neoplasm. To confirm the diagnosis, opacification of the dorsal duct is mandatory.

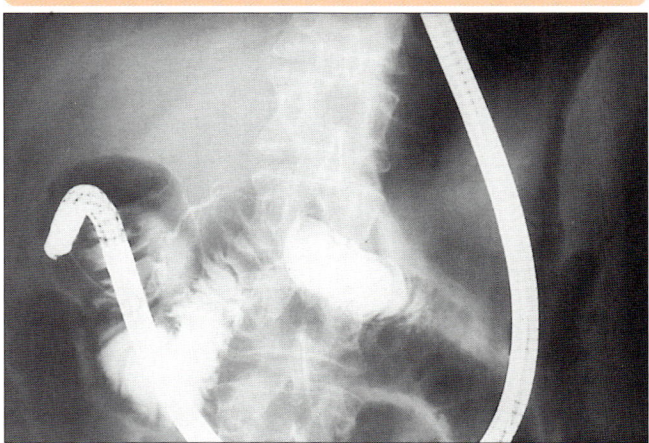

Figure 7.21 A pancreatogram showing a neoplastic interruption of the main PD between the body and tail of the gland. The abrupt obstruction leads to a moderate and regular dilatation of the proximal PD, with side branches filling, due to the elevated pressure of injection of contrast medium.

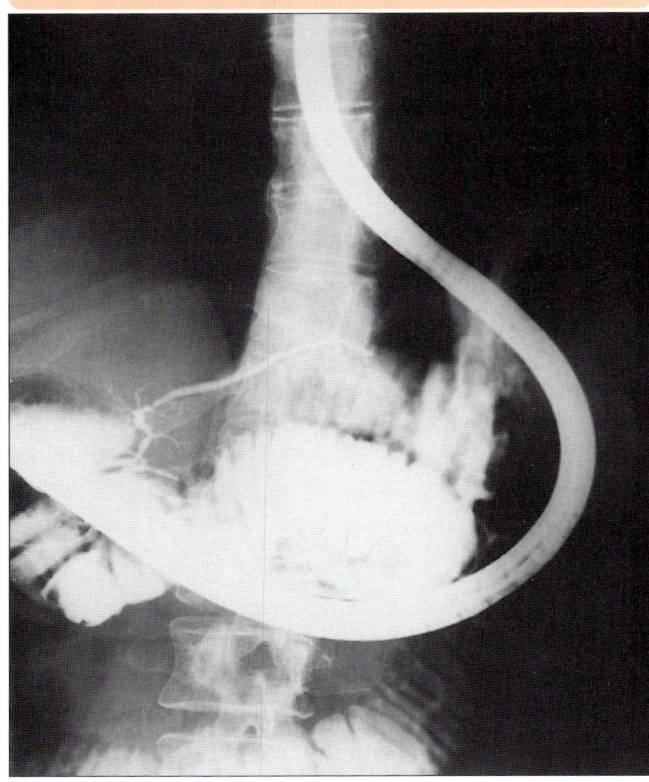

Figure 7.22 Normal variation in mean maximum diameter of the main PD.

Author (ref)	Year	Head	Body	Tail
		(mm)	(mm)	(mm)
Oi (17)	1970	3.6	2.5	1.7
Ogoshi (18)	1970	3.4	2.9	2.0
Kizu *et al.* (19)	1972	3.5	2.9	2.0
Kasugai *et al.* (20)	1972	3.5	2.7	1.7
Watrin (21)	1973	3.5	2.4	1.4
Cotton (22)	1974	4.0	3.0	2.0
Varley *et al.* (23)	1976	3.1	2.0	0.9
Tittobello and Testoni*	1980	3.3	2.7	–

* Unpublished data.

Evaluation of a pancreatogram in which only the main PD is opacified may be hazardous and it should be interpreted with caution to avoid diagnostic pitfalls. An abnormal course may simply correspond to a normal variation or may indicate the presence of an intra- or peripancreatic space-occupying lesion. If the main PD is short and tapers, a congenital anomaly should be considered and an attempt must be made to demonstrate the dorsal PD through the accessory papilla; otherwise a neoplastic lesion occluding the duct must be ruled out. While the diameter of the main PD at the head of the gland is usually greater than that in the body, the reverse may occasionally apply, even in a normal pancreas; in these situations, a pathologically narrowed segment, distal from the ductal dilatation, must be carefully sought and excluded. Finally, assessment of slight duct dilatation, with normal parietal profile, must be made with caution, to exclude the presence of a neoplastic lesion causing stasis in the ductal system (Figures 7.24 and 7.25); in addition, the age of the patient must be taken into account.

ments of the main PD from the literature. Males tend to have a slightly larger duct calibre than females, but the differences are not statistically significant. Ageing may increase the duct diameter, although there is no statistical significance for each age group up to the age of 60 years[14]. Figure 7.23 shows the variations in diameter of the main PD according to age.

Figure 7.23 Mean diameter of the main PD measured at the head, body and tail of the gland. Correlation with sex and age of patients. (Modified from Kizu[14].)

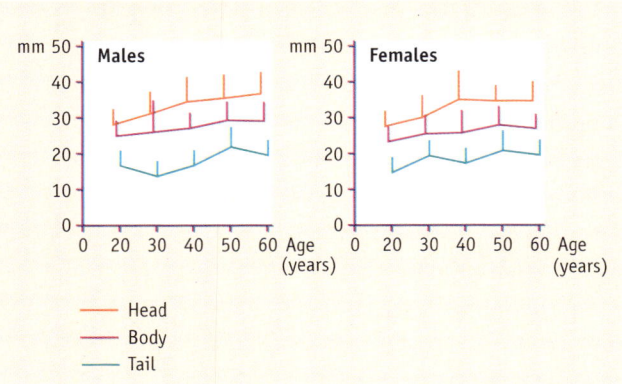

Figure 7.24 Pancreatogram showing slight dilatation of the PD, which maintains a normal contour and configuration throughout the length of the duct. The retrograde dilatation is caused by a small, intraductal protruding neoplasm in the head of the gland.

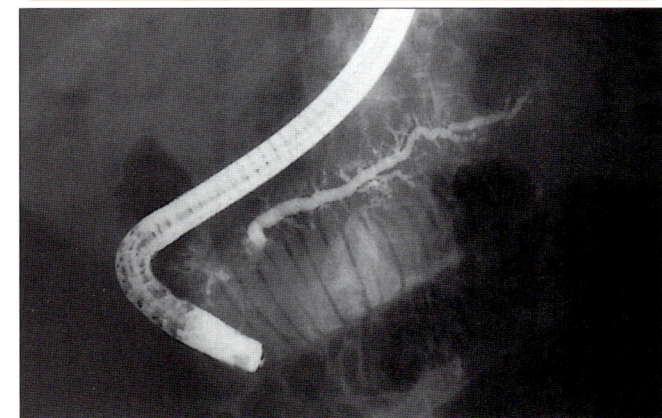

Figure 7.25 Pancreatogram showing a small segmental neoplastic narrowing of the body of the gland, causing a slight dilatation of the distal part of the PD, with normal contour.

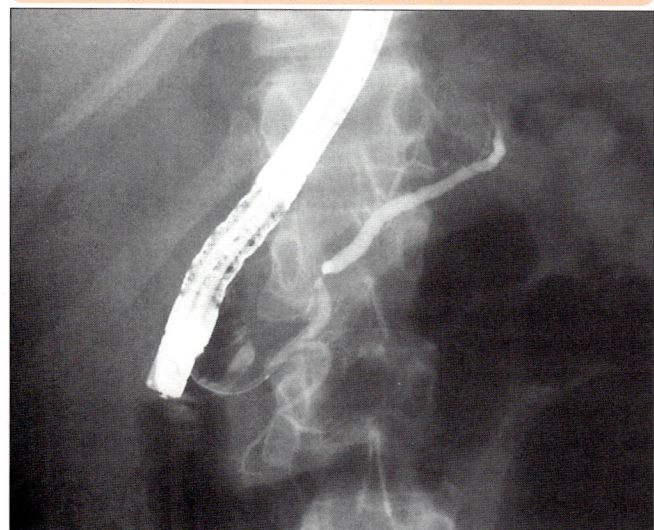

Figure 7.26 Pancreatogram showing the horizontal accessory duct and its branches arising from the minor papilla. There is slight dilatation of the PD with stenosis of the prepapillary portion and tortuous confluence of the accessory duct, which simulates a segmental lesion in the passage of the gland from head and body.

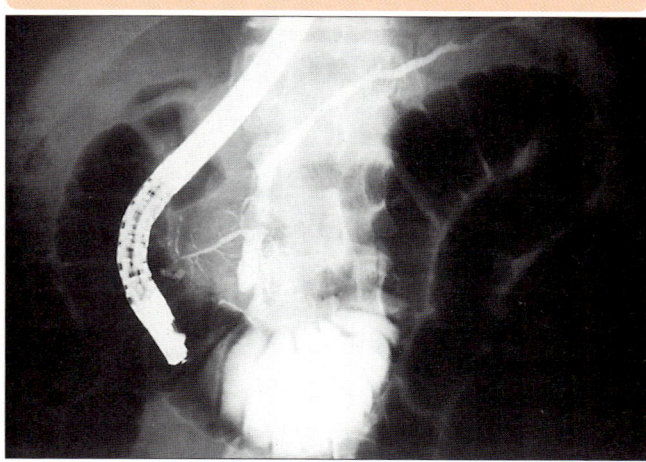

Accessory duct filling

The duct of Santorini is present in 40–80% of all people; it usually communicates with the main duct and passes transversely to the right in the upper part of the head of the pancreas. (Figure 7.26). In about 25% of cases the accessory duct opens into the duodenum through the minor papilla, which is located in the proximal portion of the descending part of the duodenum, proximal to the papilla of Vater (Figure 7.27). In the remaining cases (about 75%) it joins the ductal system from the uncinate process to form a large duct that enters the main PD (Figure 7.28). Berman *et al.*[24] reported the absence of the accessory duct in 48% of cases, in a series of 143 postmortem preparations, the presence of a blind accessory duct in 8% of cases and patency in 33% of cases. The length of the accessory duct is about 2.5cm and the maximum diameter is about 1.5–2.0mm. While the calibre of the duct is usually

smaller than that of the main duct at the head, occasionally this may be reversed in both normal conditions and disease. Variants of the course of the accessory duct in the head of the pancreas are reported in Figure 7.29 and illustrated in Figure 7.30. There is no correlation between the course of the accessory duct and its diameter or length.

Figure 7.28 Opacification of the accessory duct that joins the PD from the uncinate process. The uncinate branches are also visible.

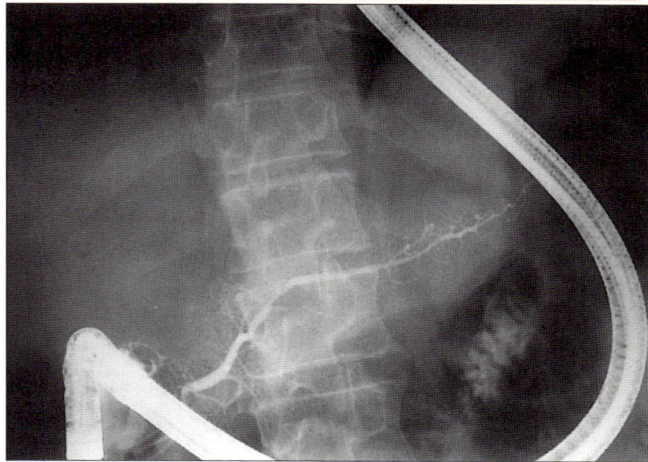

Figure 7.27 A long, vertical and tortuous accessory duct arising from the minor papilla and joining the main PD in the midbody of the gland.

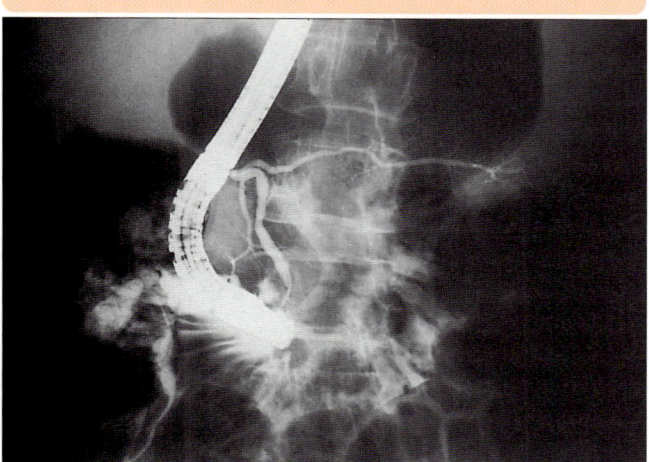

Figure 7.29 Normal variants in the course of the accessory duct.

Course type	Percentage
Parallel	60%
Descending	25%
Arched	10%
Ascending	5%

Unpublished personal data.

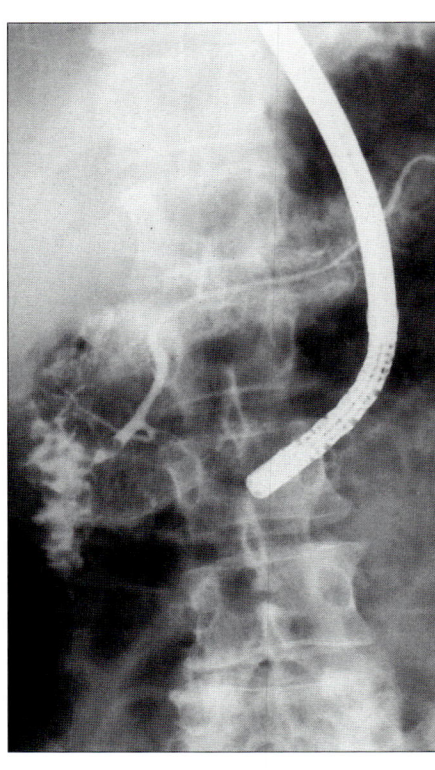

Figure 7.30
Arched course of the accessory duct, arising from the minor papilla. There is an air bubble in the PD.

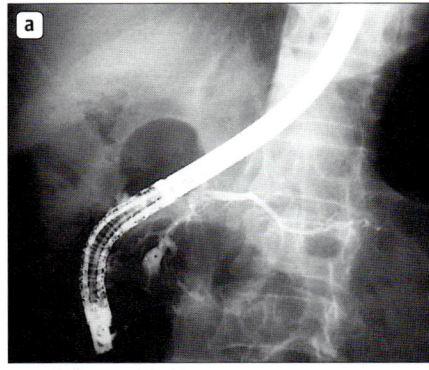

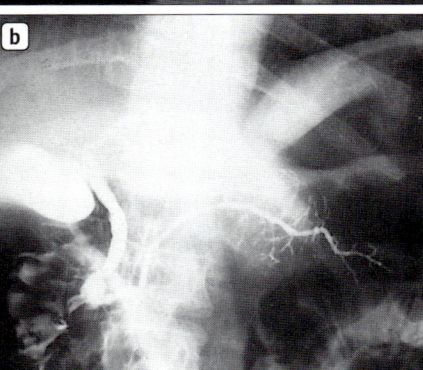

Figure 7.31
Pancreatograms showing opacification of the entire PD and adequate filling of the secondary branches, with normal distribution.

SIDE BRANCHES AND ACINAR TISSUE

Side branch filling

The side branches of the PD should be filled and completely opacified during the injection of contrast medium (Figure 7.31), but avoiding the acinarization that occurs after overfilling of the ductal system. The opacification of major and lesser order branch ducts is the ideal pancreatogram to aim for and for this purpose high-quality, high-resolution fluoroscopic equipment is necessary. In fact, complete opacification of the side branches permits a satisfactory diagnostic evaluation and is the most important finding that distinguishes benign from malignant disease. Loss of side branches or localized filling defects are suggestive of space-occupying lesions, especially in cases with main duct displacement. There is a possibility of identifying even small pancreatic tumours by these changes (Figure 7.32). Cases of 'minimal change' chronic pancreatitis are diagnosed on the basis of morphological abnormalities confined to side branches only, whereas the main PD appears to be radiologically normal (Figures 7.33 and 7.34). However, the normal arrangement of the major branch ducts, the lesser order branch ducts and fine ducts is inconstant in the population, and it is therefore difficult to define the normal pattern.

Figure 7.32 Opacification of the PD with slight segmental narrowing of the contour in the passage between head and body. The complete opacification of the secondary branches shows an irregular distribution in correspondence with the narrowing segment, due to the presence of an early stage neoplasm.

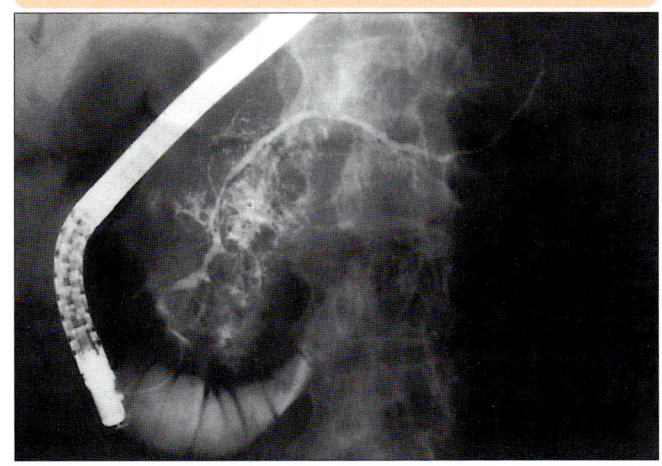

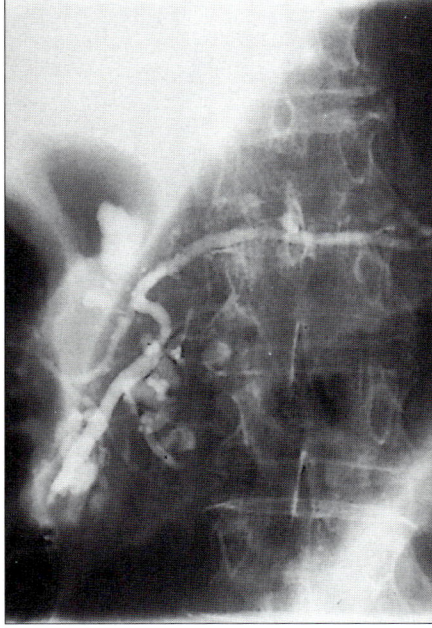

Figure 7.33
Pancreatogram showing normal appearance of the main PD, opacified throughout its total length. Filling of secondary branches shows irregular dilatation in the head of the gland, with stones: 'minimal change' pancreatitis.

Figure 7.34 'Minimal change' pancreatitis: irregular morphology of the secondary branches localized in the head of the gland.

Figure 7.35 Pancreatogram showing overfilling of the tertiary ducts and acinar tissue, which produces a cloudiness (acinarization) that persists for a long period after ERCP.

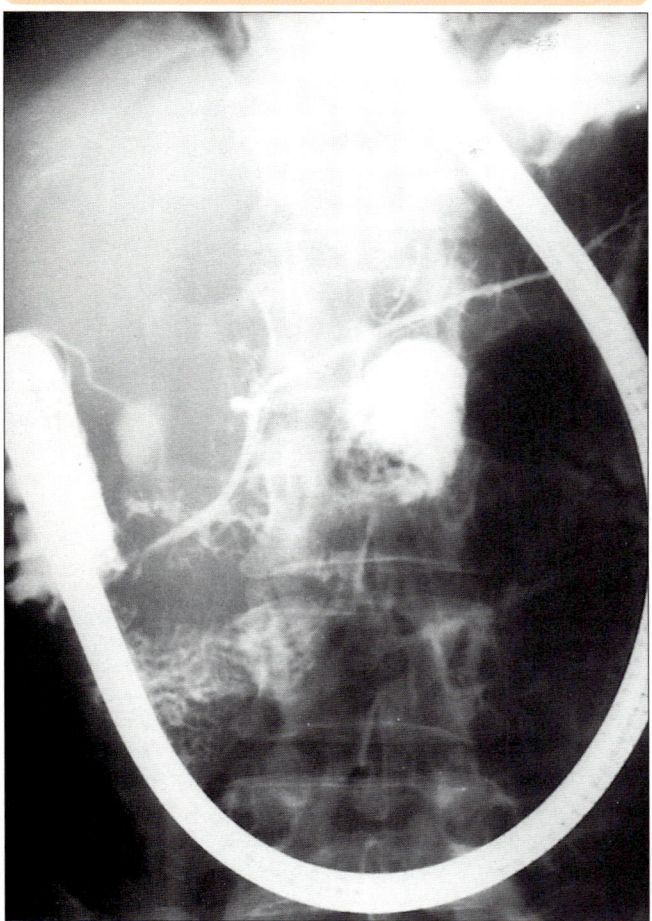

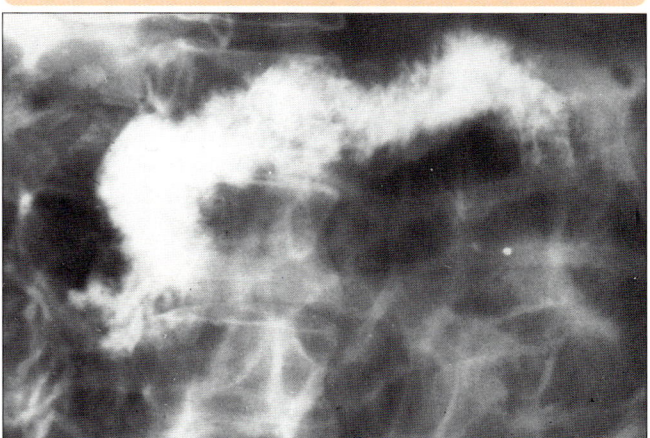

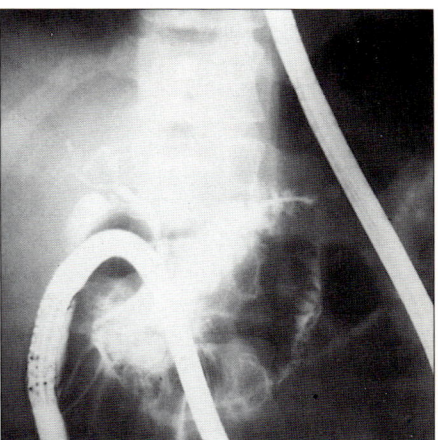

Figure 7.36 Acinarization of the majority of the gland renders it difficult to evaluate the morphology of the PD system.

Acinar filling or parenchymogram

Acinarization is a term applied to the overfilling of the tertiary branches and acinar tissue to produce a parenchymogram that outlines the gland, giving a cloudy appearance (Figure 7.35). Acinarization occurs when excess pressure and contrast material have been used and it is the consequence of the extravasation of the contrast material into the interstitial space. Acinarization during ERCP should be avoided for two reasons: a high percentage of subjects develop a marked rise in serum amylase after the procedure; and the parenchymography renders morphological evaluation of the branch ducts difficult by obscuring them (Figure 7.36). Acute pancreatitis is associated with a high incidence of parenchymography.

A localized parenchymogram may result from complete obstruction of the main PD in the glandular portion that is proximal to the obstructive lesion. When this finding is associated with an irregular appearance of the opacified portion of the main duct and/or side branches, it suggests the presence of a stenotic lesion in chronic pancreatitis; when no abnormalities in proximal ductal system filling are found, the presence of a neoplastic lesion must be considered[25].

Localized parenchymography also occurs as the consequence of main ductal or side branch duct damage during cannulation. It is especially associated with deep cannulation in subjects who have a sharp angulation of the main duct in the head of the pancreas and may result in a localized inflammatory process, followed by a higher incidence of post-ERCP complications[26].

CONGENITAL ABNORMALITIES

In their classification of normal variations of PD morphology seen by pancreatography, Yatto and Siegel[15] identified two categories of variants among the embryological abnormalities: migration variants, which include both the annular pancreas and the aberrant pancreas, and the fusion variants, which include pancreas divisum and incomplete divisum (functional).

Annular pancreas

This is a rare variant that is often associated with duodenal or biliary obstructive symptoms, since both the duodenum and the CBD become entrapped by the annular growth of the gland. Opacification of the PD may show a branch arising from the main PD and curving laterally around the duodenal loop; usually the PD system is normal[27–29].

Figure 7.37 Endoscopic finding of a protruding, umbilicated submucosal lesion located on the greater curvature of the stomach (antral region). The transmucosal biopsy performed during endoscopic ultrasonography reveals the presence of pancreatic tissue (aberrant pancreas).

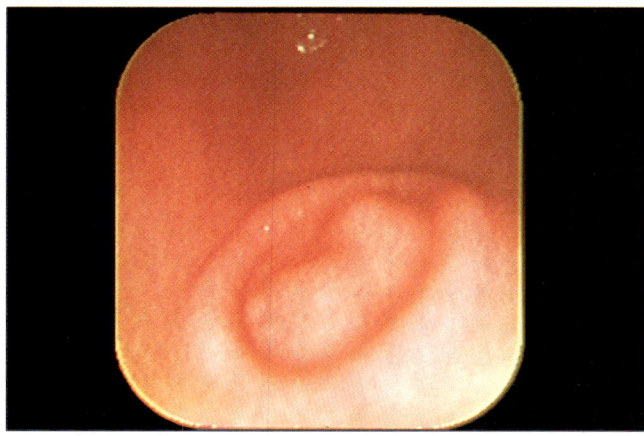

Aberrant pancreas

This congenital variant is without clinical significance and has been described as an umbilicated protruding lesion on the greater curvature of the stomach, which may connect to the pancreatic ductal system (Figure 7.37).

Pancreas divisum

This is the most common congenital variant, occurring in about 5–10% of the population[30,31]. Usually, the ventral PD fuses with the dorsal PD during the seventh to eighth weeks of gestation, giving rise to the normal configuration of the excretory ductal system. The ventral duct forms the main PD (duct of Wirsung), while the dorsal duct forms the accessory duct (duct of Santorini) and the remainder of the main duct in the body and tail of the gland.

When the pancreatic buds fail to fuse, the ventral and dorsal PDs are separate in the head of the gland and the majority of secretions drain through the accessory duct and

Figure 7.38 Pancreatogram showing filling of the ventral duct in pancreas divisum. The side branches of the rudimentary duct are also opacified, with arborization.

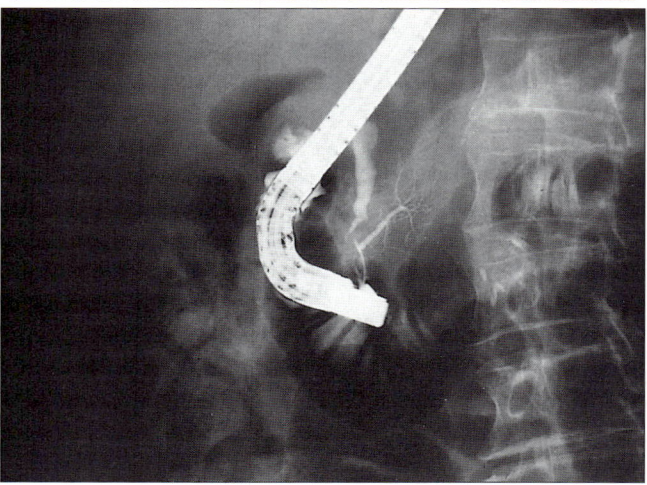

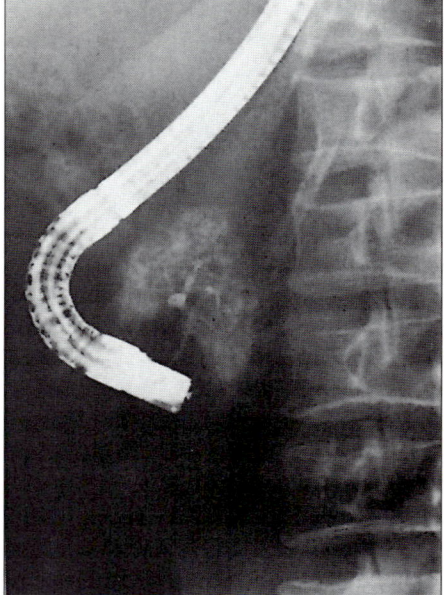

Figure 7.39 Complete acinarization of the ventral ductal system in pancreas divisum as a consequence of the high intraductal pressure induced by the injection of contrast material.

Figure 7.40 Pancreatogram showing complete disruption of the PD and the accessory duct from the uncinate process; the abrupt interruption and absence of secondary duct filling are suggestive of a tumour.

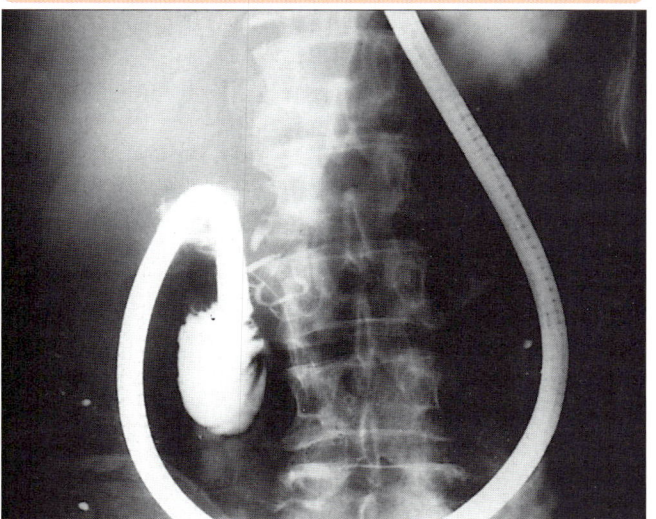

Figure 7.41 Pancreas divisum: a pancreatogram showing opacification of the ventral duct with its side branches and of the dorsal system, throughout the length of the duct. The filling of the dorsal duct make the diagnosis of the fusion variant certain.

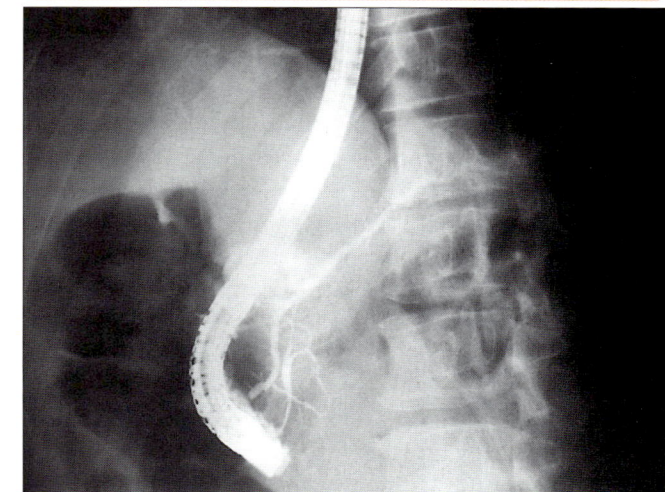

Figure 7.42 Functional divisum variant. Opacification of the dorsal duct is accomplished through the major papilla via a communicating branch.

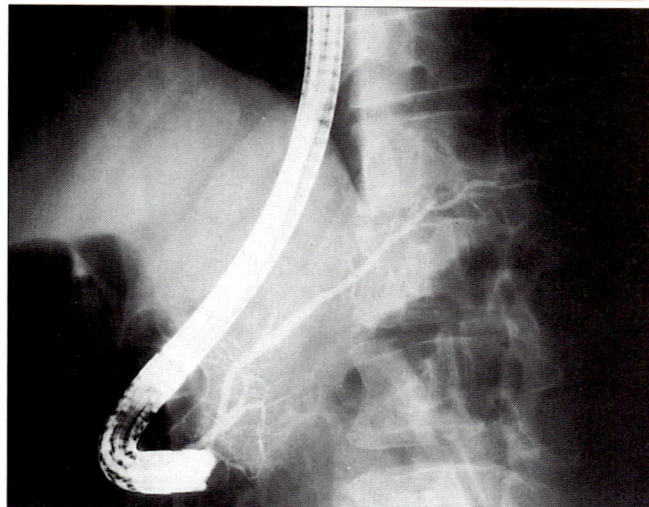

Figure 7.43 Pancreatogram showing an abnormal configuration of the PD, which seems to be completely interrupted between the head and body of the gland, in a subject without symptoms of pancreatic disease. The contour and diameter of the PD are within the normal limits.

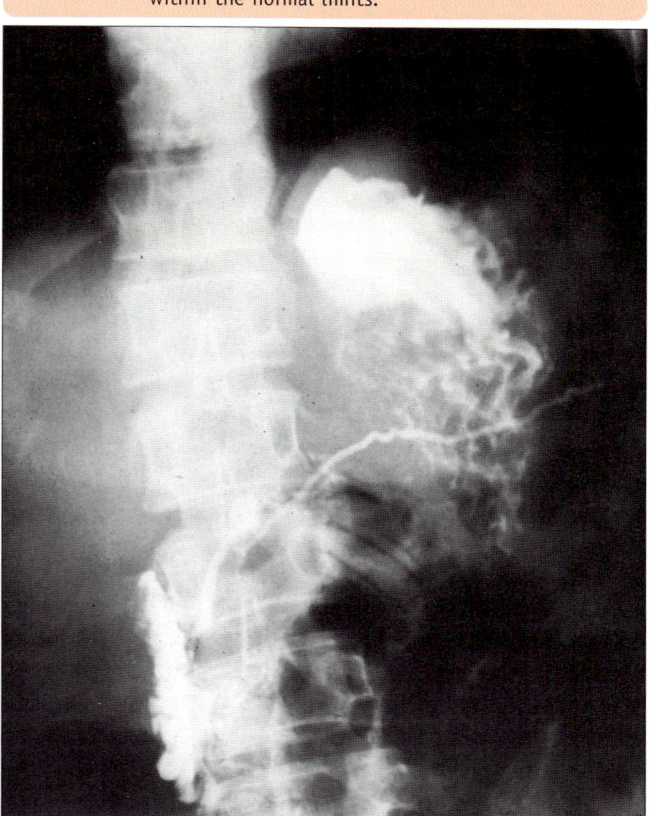

the minor papilla. In such cases, only the ventral duct drains through the major papilla. The ventral duct, as seen by pancreatography, usually terminates within 5–8cm of the major papilla and appears as a rudiment of the duct (Figure 7.38); branching of this duct is a common finding that is a distinguishing characteristic of pancreas divisum (Figure 7.39) and helps to differentiate between the congenital variant and an obstructed PD. In fact, cancer involving the duct usually destroys side branches, whereas in pancreas divisum the side branches are present (Figure 7.40). However, differential diagnosis is often difficult on the basis of radiographical findings until the accessory duct is opacified through the minor papilla. In addition, in several cases the CT scan demonstrates enlargement of the head of the pancreas, which results in confusion of pancreas divisum with neoplasia of the head of the pancreas. The diagnosis of pancreas divisum is definitively confirmed only after cannulating the dorsal duct, with filling of the entire main PD and side branches, both of which taper normally[31,32] (Figure 7.41). The availability of needle-tip catheters makes it possible for the operator to cannulate the minor papilla relatively easily[33].

The congenital variant is associated in some people with recurrent pain shortly after a meal or with a rise in serum amylase. These are attributed to the incapacity of the minor papilla to accommodate the flow of pancreatic juice, when the gland is stimulated[34,35]. The frequency of pancreatitis is also increased in subjects with pancreas divisum[36,37].

Functional pancreas divisum

The functional divisum variant has been described by Siegel[38] as a fusion variant in which opacification of the dorsal duct can be accomplished through the major papilla via a communicating branch of the ventral duct (Figure 7.42). The ventral duct tapers before entering the dorsal duct. However, there is

a narrow communication between the ducts that may be inadequate for draining the increased volume of pancreatic juice and, at times, causes obstructive pain.

OTHER OBSERVATIONS IN THE NORMAL PANCREATOGRAM

Air bubbles in the duct system

This situation arises when air bubbles present in the syringe containing the contrast material are injected into the ductal system (see Figure 7.30). Differential diagnosis from pancreatic stones or mucous plugs is easy in most cases, since the latter two conditions are usually associated with ductal abnormalities.

Cases of difficult differential diagnosis

In some subjects, pancreatography shows irregular distribution of contrast material in the PD system, without evidence of ductal or acinar abnormalities (Figure 7.43). In these circumstances, it is essential to distinguish between a variant of a normal pattern and a neoplastic lesion.

References

1. Classen M, Hellwig H, Roesch W. Anatomy of the pancreatic duct; a duodenoscopic radiological study. *Endoscopy* 1973; 5:14–17.

2. Oi I, Takemoto T, Kondo T. Fiberduodenoscope: direct observation of the papilla of Vater. *Endoscopy* 1969; 1:101–3.

3. Phillip J, Koch H, Classen M. Variations and anomalies of the papilla of Vater, the pancreas and the biliary system. *Endoscopy* 1974; 6:70–7.

4. Kozu T, Oi I, Suzuki S, Takemoto T. Fiberduodenoscopic observation on the dynamics of the duodenal papilla. *Endoscopy* 1970; 2:99–102.

5. Floquet J, Laurent J, Plenat F, Watrin B. Is the sphincter of Oddi a reality in man? In *The Sphincter of Oddi*. Edited by J Delmont. Karger, Basel; 1977: 21–4.

6. Allescher HD. Papilla of Vater: structure and function. *Endoscopy* 1989; 21:324–9.

7. Caroli J, Porcher G, Pequignot G, Delatre M. Contribution of cine–radiography to the study of the function of the human biliary tract. *Am J Dig Dis* 1960; 5:677–96.

8. Geenen JE, Venu RP. Endoscopic retrograde cholangio-pancreatography. In *Bockus Gastroenterology*. Edited by JE Berk. Saunders, Philadelphia; 1985: 601–11.

9. Hand B. Anatomy and function of the extrahepatic biliary system. *Clin Gastroenterol* 1973; 2:3–29.

10. Toouli J, Dodds WJ, Honda R. Motor function of the opossum sphincter of Oddi. *J Clin Invest* 1983; 71:208–20.

11. Torsoli A. Physiology of the human sphincter of Oddi. *Endoscopy* 1988; 20:166–70.

12. Toouli J, Geenen JE, Hogan WJ, Dodds WJ, Arndorfer RC. Sphincter of Oddi motor activity: a comparison between patients with common bile duct stones and controls. *Gastroenterology* 1982; 82:111–17.

13. Worthley CS, Baker RA, Iannos J, Saccone GTP, Toouli J. Human fasting and post-prandial sphincter of Oddi motility. *Br J Surg* 1989; 76:709–14.

14. Kizu M. Normal endoscopic pancreatogram. In *Endoscopic Retrograde Cholangiopancreatography*. Edited by T Takemoto. Igaku-Shoin, Tokyo; 1979: 141–53.

15. Yatto RP, Siegel JH. Variant pancreatography. *Am J Gastroenterol* 1983; 78:115–18.

16. Siegel JH, Yatto RP. Anomalous PDs causing pseudomass of the pancreas. *J Clin Gastroenterol* 1983; 5:33–6.

17. Oi I. Endoscopic pancreato-cholangiography. *Saishin Igaku* 1970; 25:2292–2299. (In Japanese.)

18. Ogoshi K. Endoscopic observation of the duodenum and endoscopic pancreato-cholangiography. *Gastrointest Endosc* 1970; 12:83–94.

19. Kizu M, Kasugai T, Kuno N, Aoki I. A study of pancreatography in the pancreatic neoplasm. *Rinsho Hoshyasen* 1973; 18:1061–70. (In Japanese.)

20. Kasugai T, Kuno N, Kobayashi S, Hattori K. Endoscopic pancreato-cholangiography. I. The normal endoscopic pancreatocholangiogram. *Gastroenterology* 1972; 63:217–26.

21. Watrin B. L'opacification perduodénoscopique des voies pancréatiques normales et pathologiques. *Acta Endoscopica et Radiocinematographica* 1973; 6:143–234.

22. Cotton PB. The normal endoscopic pancreatogram. *Endoscopy* 1974; 6:65–70.

23. Varley PF, Rohrmann CA Jr, Silvis SE, Vennes JA. The normal endoscopic pancreatogram. *Radiology* 1976; 118:295–300.

24. Berman LG, Prior JT, Abramow SM. A study of the pancreatic duct system in man by use of vinyl acetate casts of post-mortem preparations. *Surg Gynecol Obstet* 1969; 110:391.

25. Testoni PA, Masci E, Guslandi M, Tittobello A. The role of pancreatography in differential diagnosis between chronic pancreatitis and pancreatic cancer. *Acta Endosc* 1981; 11:435–41.

26. Bilbao MK, Dotter CT, Lee TG, Katon RM. Complications of endoscopic retrograde cholangiopancreatography (ERCP). A study of 10,000 cases. *Gastroenterology* 1976; 70:314–20.

27. Clifford KM. Annular pancreas diagnosed by endoscopic retrograde cholangiopancreatography (ERCP). *Br J Radiol* 1980; 53:593–5.

28. Yogi Y, Shibue T, Hashimoto S. Annular pancreas detected in adults, diagnosed by endoscopic retrograde cholangio-pancreatography: report of four cases. *Gastroenterol Jpn* 1987; 22:92–9.

29. Dowsett JF, Rode J, Russell RC. Annular pancreas: a clinical, endoscopic, and immunohistochemical study. *Gut* 1989; 30:130–5.

30. Mitchell CJ, Lintott DJ, Ruddell SJ. Clinical relevance of an unfused pancreatic duct system. *Gut* 1979; 20:1066–71.

31. Delhaye M, Engelholm L, Cremer M. Pancreas divisum: congenital anatomic variant or anomaly? Contribution of endoscopic retrograde dorsal pancreatography. *Gastroenterology* 1985; 89:951–8.

32. Siegel JH. Pancreatic disorders: inflammatory, congenital, and malignant. In *Endoscopic Retrograde Cholangiopancreatography: Technique, Diagnosis and Therapy*. Edited by JH Siegel. Raven Press, New York. 1992; 123–74.

33. O'Conner KW, Lehman GA. An improved technique for accessory papilla cannulation in pancreas divisum. *Gastrointest Endosc* 1985; 31: 3–17.

34. Cotton PB. Congenital anomaly of pancreas divisum as a cause of obstructive pain and pancreatitis. *Gut* 1980; 21: 05–14.

35. Staritz M, Meyer zum Buschenfeld KH. Elevated pressure in the dorsal part of pancreas divisum: the cause of chronic pancreatitis? *Pancreas* 1988; 3:108–10.

36. Hayakawa T, Kondo T, Shibata T. Pancreas divisum. A predisposing factor to pancreatitis? *Int J Pancreatol* 1989; 5:317–26.

37. Bernard JP, Sahel J, Giovannini M, Sarles H. Pancreas divisum is a probable cause of acute pancreatitis: a report of 137 cases. *Pancreas* 1990; 5:248–54.

38. Siegel JH. Radiologic interpretation: normal biliary system and variations; normal pancreatic duct and variations. In *Endoscopic Retrograde Cholangiopancreatography: Technique, Diagnosis and Therapy*. Edited by JH Siegel. Raven Press, New York. 1992; 25–59.

8

Chronic pancreatitis

José Sahel & Marc Barthet

INTRODUCTION

Since its introduction into routine gastroenterological practice, endoscopic retrograde cholangiopancreatography (ERCP) has become the most useful tool for the diagnosis of chronic pancreatitis. The first classification of changes seen on the pancreatogram related to chronic pancreatitis was established by Kasugai *et al.* in 1972[1]. Although non-invasive techniques such as endoscopic ultrasonography (EUS) at first appeared promising, ERCP is now the leading technique used in the diagnosis of chronic pancreatitis. However, although ERCP provides precise information concerning the severity and the extent of the disease and its related complications, some difficulties still persist in the diagnosis of early chronic pancreatitis and, in some cases, differential diagnosis when neoplastic disease is involved. The development of endoscopic collection of pancreatic juice for biochemical or cytological analysis may represent one way to improve the diagnosis in such difficult cases.

In the 1988 Marseille–Rome symposium[2], chronic pancreatitis was defined as 'the presence of chronic inflammatory lesions characterized by the destruction of exocrine parenchyma and fibrosis and, at least in the late stages, the destruction of endocrine parenchyma'. Chronic calcifying pancreatitis (CCP), better termed pancreatic lithiasis, is the most frequent form. The calcifications are in reality calcifications of pancreatic plugs, and these intraductal calculi appear as calcifications on plain films of the abdomen in late stages of the disease[3,4]. The irregular patchy localization of the lobular or ductal lesions, the presence of intraductal plugs or stones, and peri- or intralobular fibrosis are the main features of CCP[5]. Obstructive pancreatitis is easily distinguished from CCP by the absence of intraductal plugs or calcified stones and by the presence of an upstream regular dilatation of the main pancreatic dilatation related to a partial or complete ductal obstruction[2].

ERCP FINDINGS IN CHRONIC PANCREATITIS

Several classifications for ductal changes assessed by ERCP have been developed since 1974 in order to evaluate the severity and the extent of the disease, although the relationship between ductal changes at ERCP and the degree of pancreatic functional impairment is still under discussion.

Changes seen on the pancreatogram

Essential features seen on the pancreatogram are dilatation and irregularity of the calibre of the side branches and of the main pancreatic duct. At the onset of disease only some of the side branches are abnormal, with mild or marked irregular dilatation, whereas others are normal (Figures 8.1 and 8.2). Pancreatographic changes seen at this stage are usually termed minimal changes (Figure 8.3)[1,6,7]. The topography of the ductal alterations is variable with patchy, diffuse or, in some cases, segmental distribution. In more advanced stages, the main pancreatic duct is involved and the most characteristic features are: the dilatation and irregular calibre of the main pancreatic duct and of its branches; the tortuous appearance of the main pancreatic duct, mainly in the body or the tail of the pancreas; and the presence of radiolucent stones appearing as small rounded filling defects in the main pancreatic duct or its side branches, or of calcified stones visible on plain films of the abdomen[8] (Figures 8.2 and 8.4–8.6). Pancreatic cysts may be encountered in about 20% of the pancreatograms, even at early stages of chronic pancreatitis (Figure 8.7). In our personal series, 15% of the pancreatograms were considered as normal although chronic pancreatitis could be demonstrated by means of pancreatic function test or by follow-up of the patients.

Chronic obstructive pancreatitis (COP) must be differentiated from CCP. COP refers to lesions resulting from obstruction of the main pancreatic duct antedating the pancreatitis. These lesions are uniformly distributed in the obstructed region of the gland but the exocrine parenchyma downstream from the stricture is normal and no calculi can be

Figure 8.1 Early-stage (Cambridge II) of chronic pancreatitis on the dorsal part of a pancreas divisum.

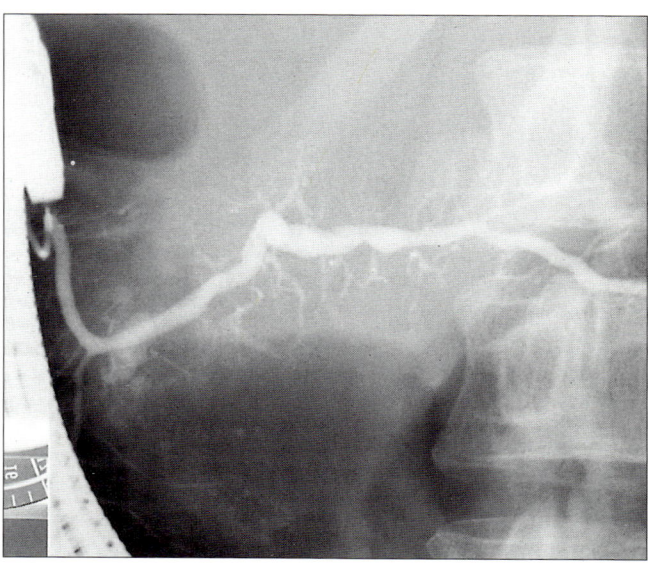

Figure 8.2   Progression of ductal lesions in chronic pancreatitis. (a) Initial ERP showing moderate lesions of side branches of the pancreatic duct and normal bile duct. (b) Four years later: marked changes of the pancreatic ducts, intraductal stones and (stented) stenosis of the bile duct.

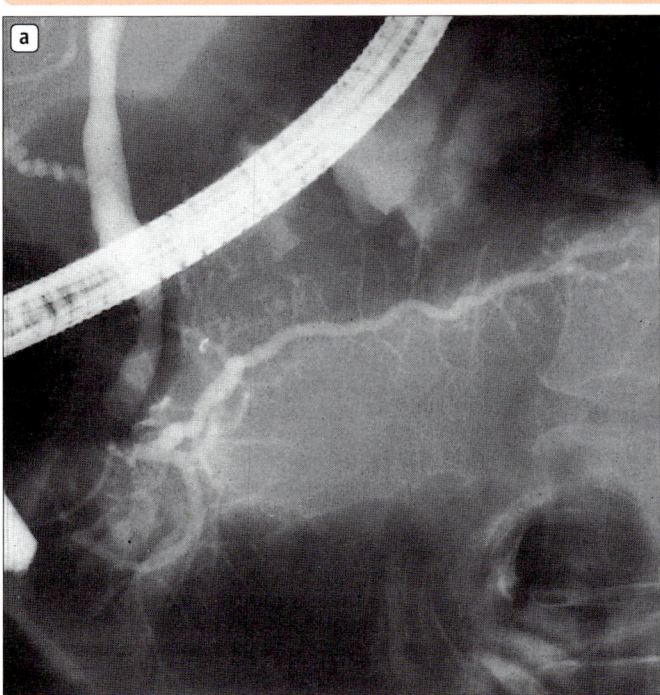

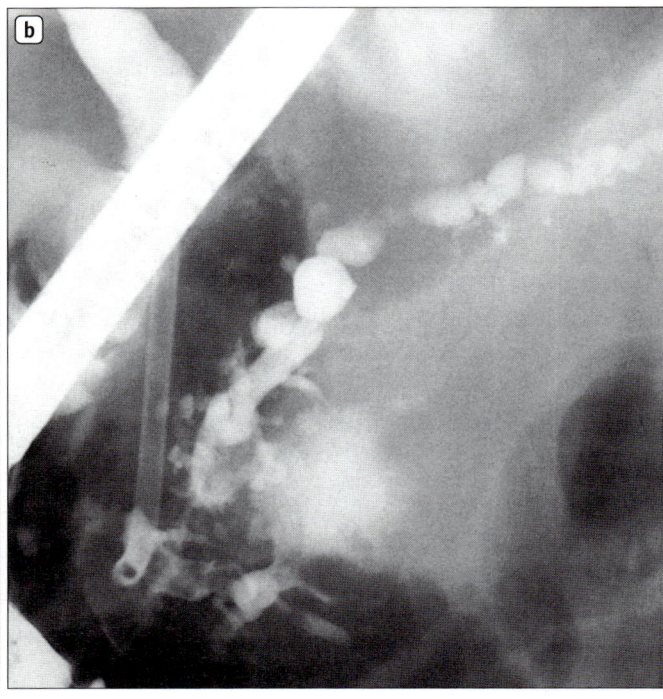

Figure 8.3   Minimal changes at the level of the tail of the pancreas.

Figure 8.4   Marked ductal lesions in a 20-year-old patient with idiopathic pancreatitis.

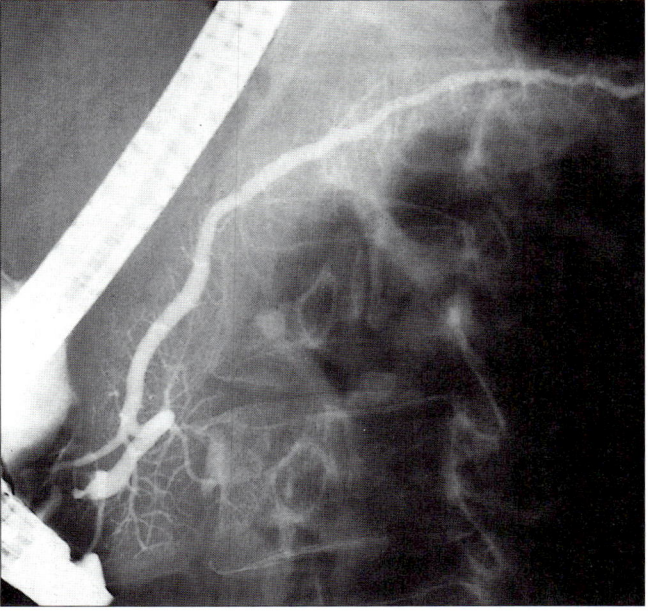

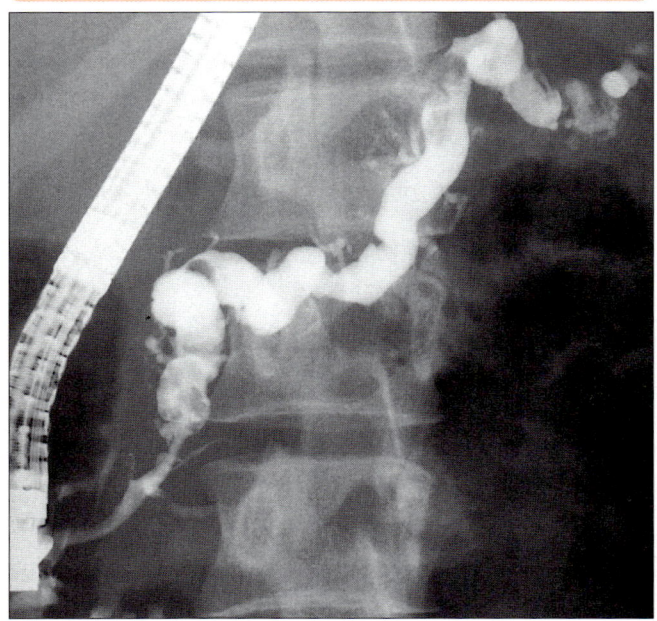

found. On endoscopic retrograde pancreatography (ERP) the ductal dilatation is found predominantly in the main pancreatic duct; it has a regular shape and antedates the dilatation of side branches. The pancreatic ductal system between the papilla and the duct obstruction is normal (Figures 8.8 and 8.9). COP is mainly due to neoplastic causes (ampullary carcinoma, slowly growing pancreatic cancer) but may be secondary to fibrotic stenosis of the pancreatic duct (Figure 8.10) (for instance, following the resorption of a pancreatic pseudocyst complicating acute pancreatitis).

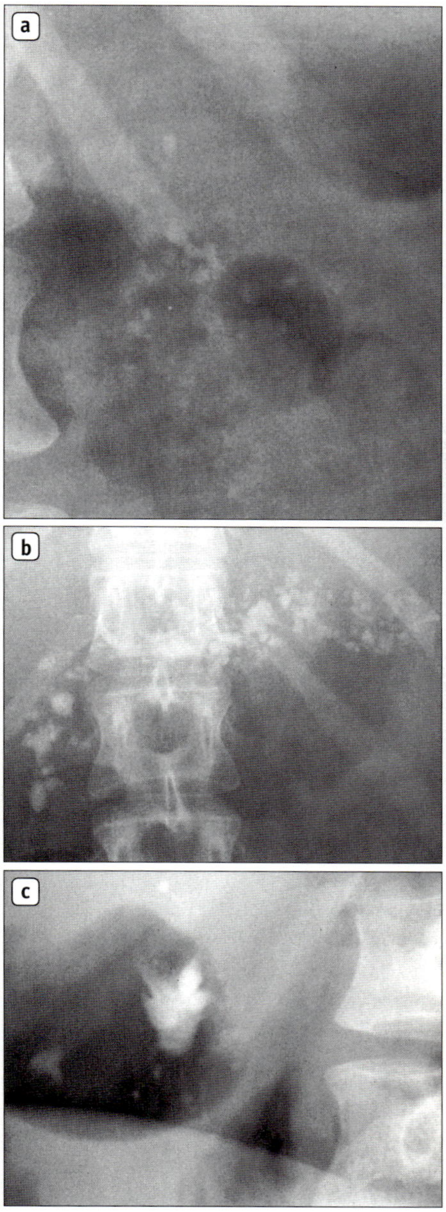

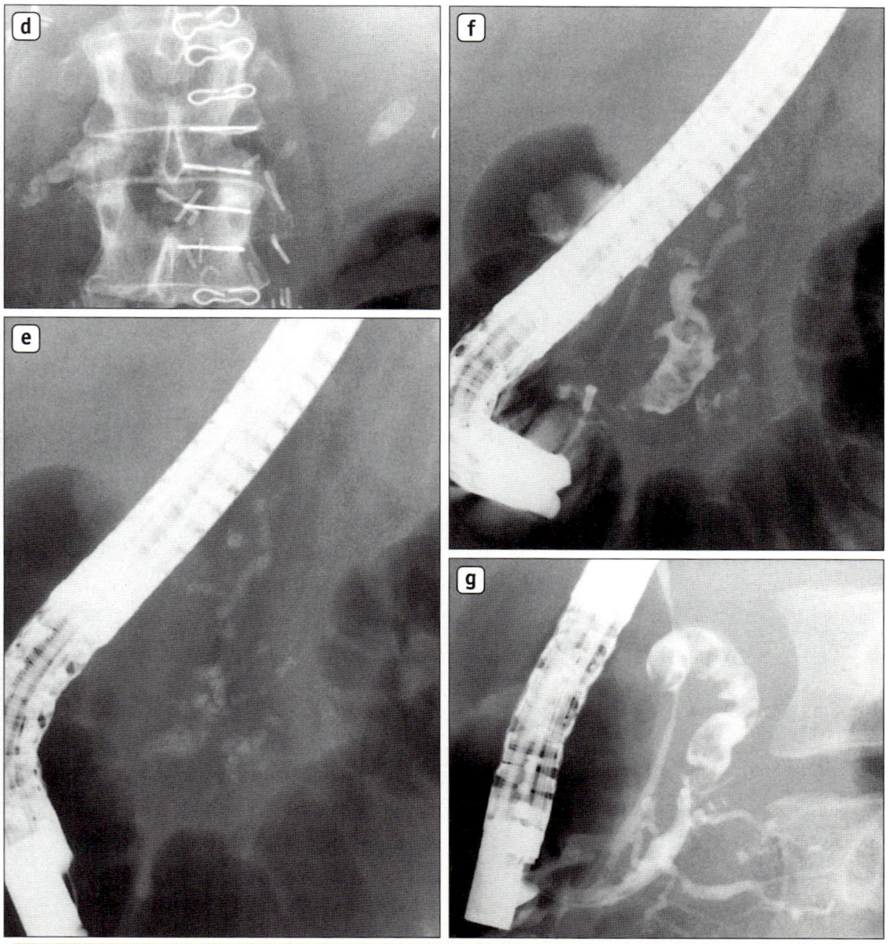

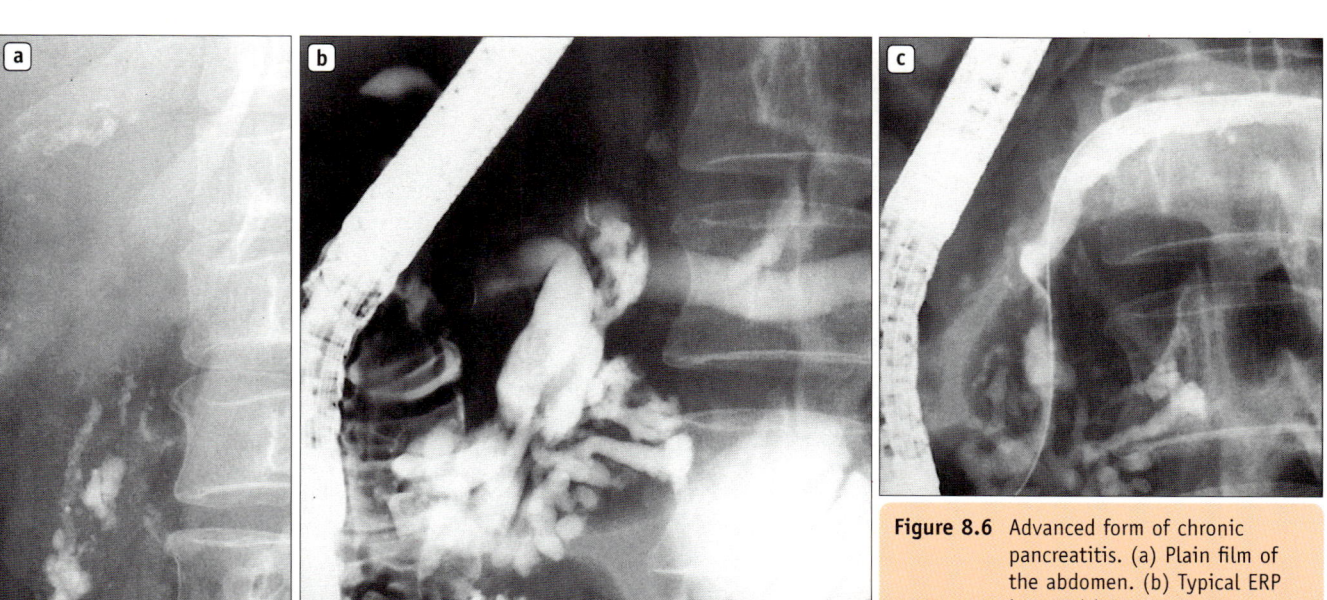

Figure 8.5 Different appearances of pancreatic stones. (a) Small calcified stones in the head of the pancreas. (b) Diffuse stones in the main duct and side branches. (c) Large 'coralliform' stone in the main pancreatic duct. (d) Pancreatic stones in a case of hyperparathyroidism, some appearing as target calculi. (e,f) Stones delineating the main pancreatic duct and side branches. (g) Large radiolucent stones in a case of idiopathic chronic pancreatitis.

Figure 8.6 Advanced form of chronic pancreatitis. (a) Plain film of the abdomen. (b) Typical ERP image. (c) Improvement following extracorporeal shock-wave lithotripsy.

Figure 8.7 Moderate lesions; note the presence of a small cyst in the head of the pancreas which contains stones.

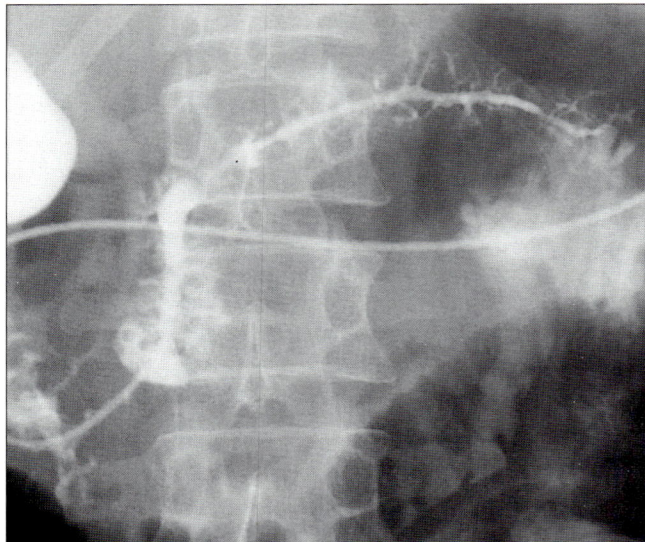

Figure 8.8 Cancer of the head of the pancreas: the 'double duct' sign.

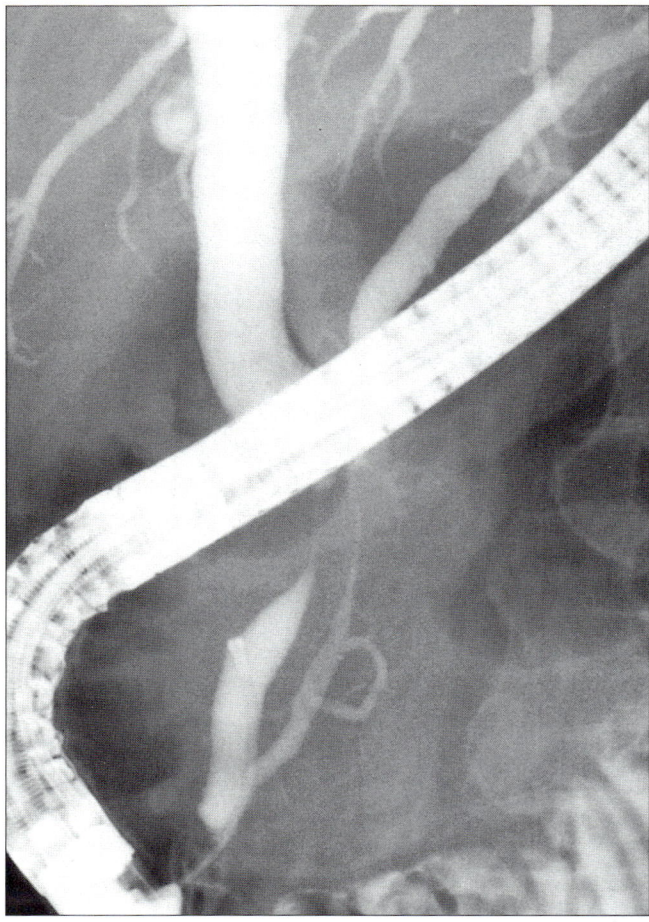

Biliary stenosis

Biliary stenosis may occur in chronic pancreatitis with a prevalence ranging from 10 to 60% depending on the diagnostic imaging procedure used and the duration of follow-up. Symptoms are rare and the most frequent feature is anicteric cholestasis[9,10]; however, severe complications such as jaundice or secondary biliary cirrhosis have been reported. Extended pancreatic fibrosis represents the main mechanism for biliary stenosis but pancreatic cysts located in the head of the pancreas can also be responsible. Several appearances of the common bile duct (CBD) have been described in chronic pancreatitis. The type I described by Caroli and Nora more than 40 years ago consists of a smooth stenosis of the intrapancreatic course of the choledochus, associated or not with an upstream dilatation of the bile ducts[11]. This pattern is encountered in about 40% of cases (Figures 8.11–8.13). Type

III, described by Sarles *et al.* is an hourglass stenosis of the CBD located at the upper part of the pancreas and is observed in about 15% of cases[12] (Figure 8.14). Type IV, also reported by Sarles *et al.*, is an arched compression of the choledochus; caused by a pancreatic cyst located in the head

Figure 8.9 Chronic pancreatitis: difficult differential diagnosis from pancreatic cancer. There is a stenosis at the neck of the pancreas, with proximal dilatation.

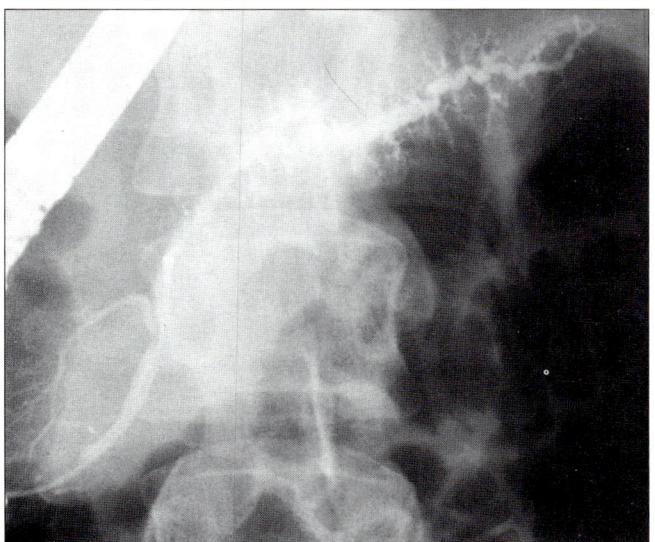

Figure 8.10 Benign stenosis at the level of the body of the pancreas, of unknown origin.

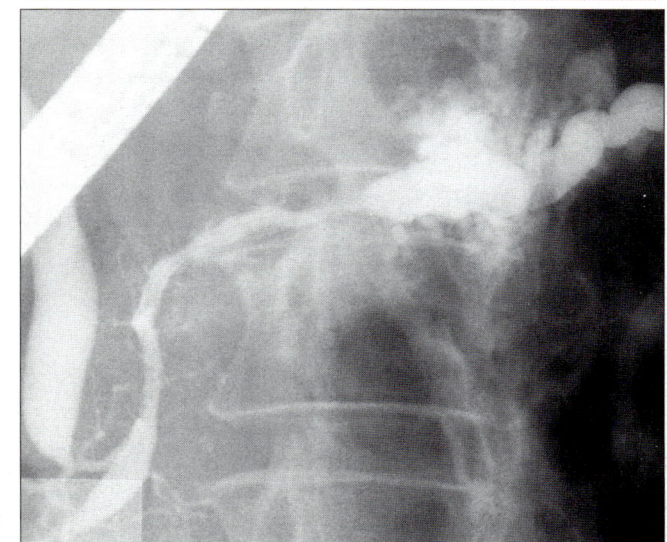

Figure 8.11 Typical stenosis of the choledochus (Caroli type I).

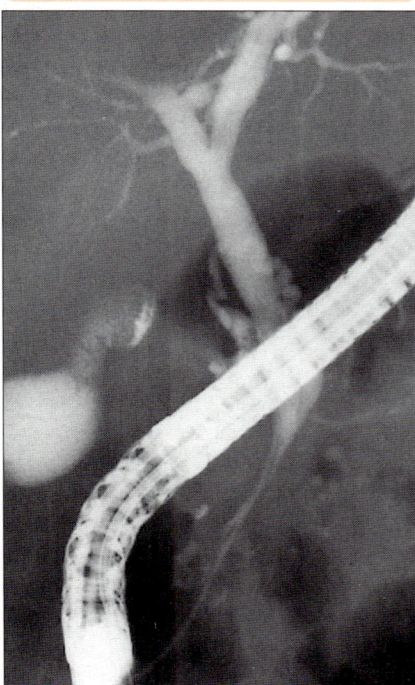

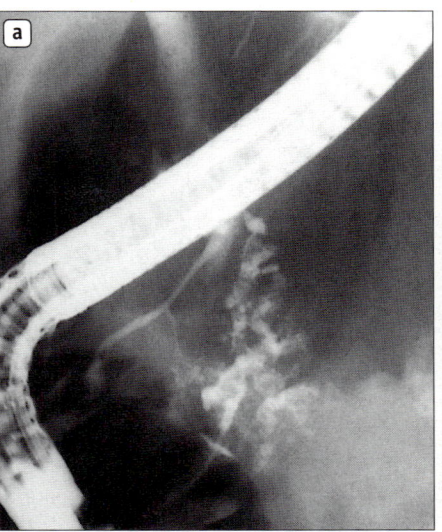

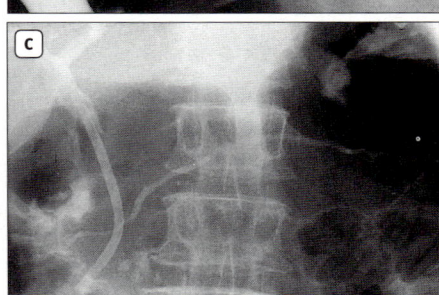

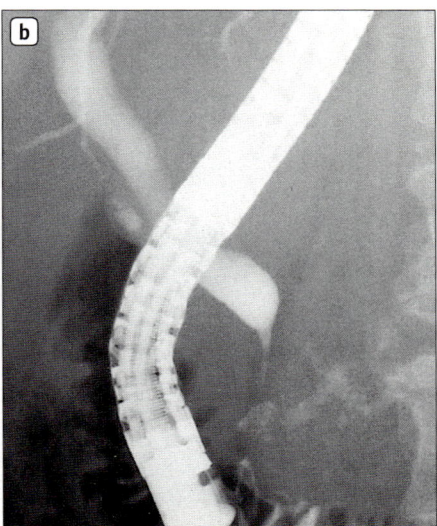

Figure 8.12 (a) Chronic pancreatitis in pancreas divisum: ductal lesions are located only on the ventral part. (b) Typical type I stenosis of the bile duct. (c) Normal dorsal ducts; note the stent in the bile duct.

of the pancreas (Figure 8.15). This pattern is common in pancreatic cancer. The presence of biliary stenosis is not always correlated with the severity of the disease and type I stenosis, for instance, may be observed at early stages of chronic pancreatitis. The evidence of biliary stenosis may facilitate the diagnosis of chronic pancreatitis, especially in the case of minimal pancreatic duct changes. In addition, biliary lithiasis (gallstones) occurs frequently in cases of chronic pancreatitis (about 15%)[13].

Disease severity and pancreatographic classifications

Several classifications of ERCP features in chronic pancreatitis have been proposed in order to judge the severity of the disease and more recently to plan management. Kasugai *et al.* established the first classification on the basis of the pancreatograms of 55 patients presenting with chronic pancreatitis[1]. The abnormalities varied from mild irregular distribution of the side branches to marked strictures or dilatation with obstruction of various parts of the

Figure 8.13 (a) Chronic pancreatitis with tight stenosis of the pancreatic duct on the head of the pancreas and intraductal stones. Note the stenosis of the choledochus (Caroli type I). (b) Balloon dilatation of the pancreatic stenosis. (c) Stenting of the main pancreatic duct and bile duct.

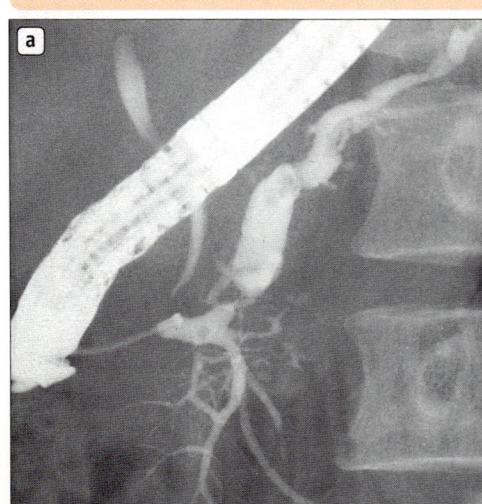

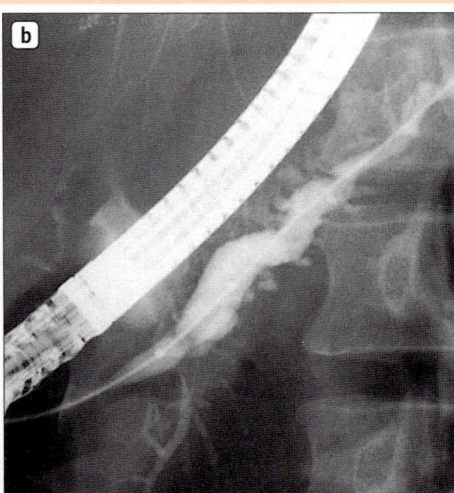

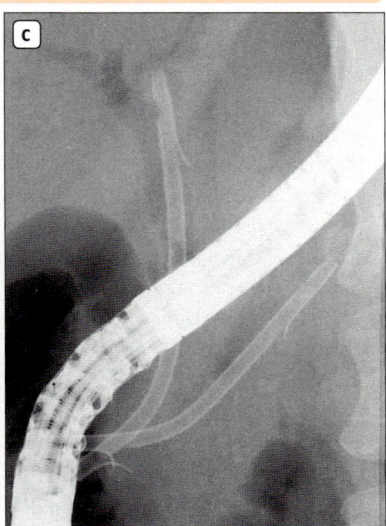

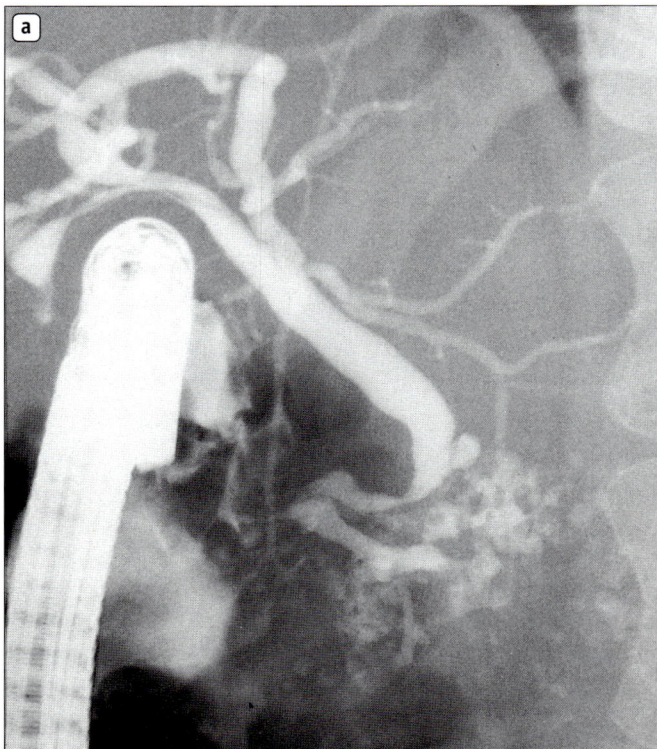

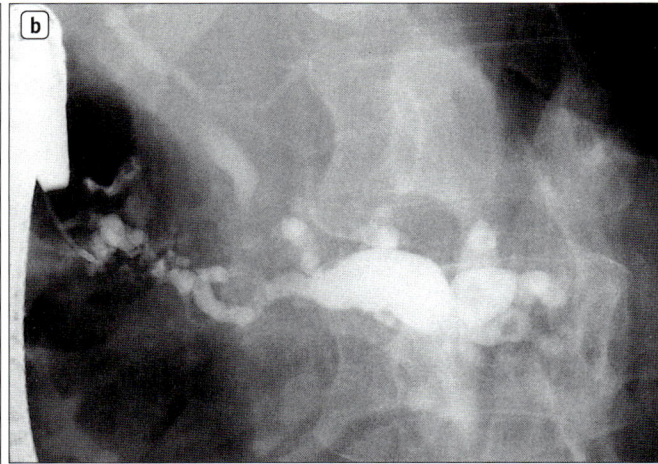

Figure 8.14 Chronic pancreatitis in a case of pancreas divisum.
(a) Cannulation of the major papilla: typical changes on the ventral pancreas. There is an hourglass stenosis of the choledochus (Caroli type III).
(b) Lesions on the dorsal pancreatic duct system.

pancreatic ducts and, on occasion, acinar opacification, cysts and calculi. These abnormalities were classified into three groups: minimal, moderate and advanced pancreatitis. Minimal pancreatitis was represented by changes at the level of side branches (irregular distribution, dilatation, stenosis and obstruction). Moderate pancreatitis was represented by marked changes at the level of side branches and by tortuous appearance, dilatation and stenosis of the main pancreatic duct. Advanced pancreatitis corresponded to marked changes at the level of both the side branches and the main pancreatic duct, associated with cysts and calculi.

In each category lesions can be diffuse, segmental or sub-segmental (occupying less than one third of the pancreas).

Cremer et al.[6] proposed an analytical classification of chronic pancreatitis into six types: minimal changes with only alterations of ductules; type I (minor pancreatitis), with irregularly outlined main pancreatic duct and alterations of ductules; type II (focal pancreatitis), with macrocystic dilatations of one or several ductules, localized in one segment of the gland; type III (diffuse pancreatitis), with one or several stenoses of the main pancreatic duct without any dilatation upstream; type IV (segmentary pancreatitis of the

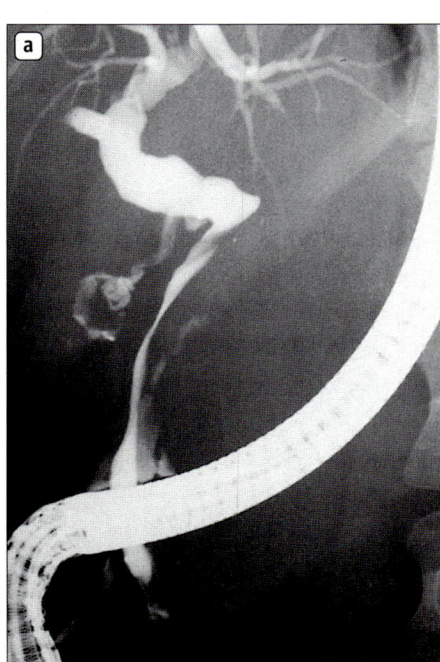

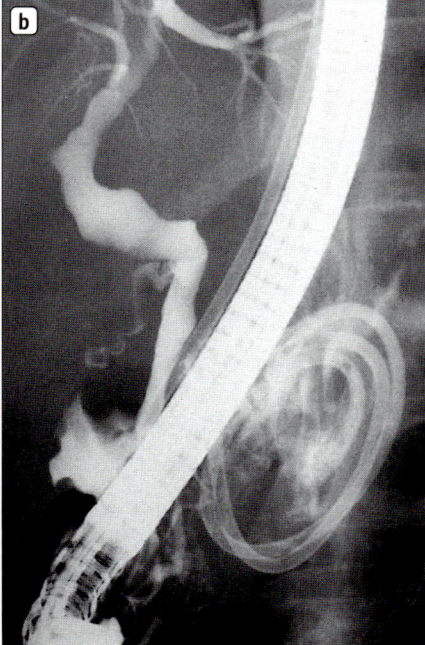

Figure 8.15 Bile duct lesions.
(a) Compression of the choledochus by a large cyst of the head of the pancreas (Caroli type IV).
(b) After endoscopic cyst-duodenostomy and drainage via a nasocystic catheter.

head), with stenosis of the main pancreatic duct with remarkable proximal dilatation; and type V (pancreatitis with a stop in the head of the pancreas). Frequencies of alcoholism, diabetes mellitus and pain increased from type I to type V[6].

An international conference has proposed a simplified classification, the so-called Cambridge classification[7]. The grading severity is as follows: Equivocal pancreatic changes (Cambridge I), fewer than three abnormal branches. Mild to moderate pancreatic changes (Cambridge II), more than three abnormal branches; abnormal main duct and branches. Marked pancreatic changes (Cambridge III), abnormal main duct and branches; ductal obstruction with stricture; intraductal calculi; gross irregularity of main duct; large cavities[7].

In our personal experience, calcified forms of chronic pancreatitis may belong to the moderate pancreatitis group as classified by Kasugai whereas precalcified forms of chronic pancreatitis may be found in the advanced pancreatitis group. In addition, pancreatic pseudocyst or ductal leakage may be observed at the onset of chronic pancreatitis, although such features are classified as end stages of the Cambridge classification. This underlines the fact that there is no strict parallel between the course of the disease and the intensity of the lesions as assessed by ERCP. In addition, serum levels of amylase, trypsin and trypsin inhibitor do not appear to correlate well with pancreatographic changes demonstrated by ERCP, since the sensitivity for these three proteins was 40% and the specificity 80%[14]. However, many previous series established a strong correlation between pancreatic ductal changes and the degree of functional exocrine impairment. The Lundh test and ERP were significantly correlated and minimal changes or gross radiographic changes correlated with varying degrees of mean trypsin activity[15]. By means of discriminant analysis, the maximal bicarbonate concentration obtained by duodenal suction allowed a correct classification of 46% of patients according to a four-stage classification of pancreatograms (initial classification of Cremer[6]), whereas the maximum bicarbonate concentration and the maximum bicarbonate output in pure pancreatic juice after secretin stimulation provided a correct classification of 70% of patients[16]. Comparison of functional impairment assessed by duodenal intubation with the Cambridge classification showed a good correlation: no patients with normal pancreatograms had exocrine functional impairment; all the patients with marked pancreatic duct changes had global pancreatic insufficiency; 30% of patients with equivocal changes and 50% of patients with mild to moderate changes had global functional impairment[17]. In a series of 75 patients evaluated by the means of pancreolauryl test and ERP (Cambridge classification), the odds ratio calculated by stepwise multivariate logistic regression analysis demonstrated a strong association (OR = 5.8)[18]. Therefore it can be concluded that the degree of exocrine functional impairment correlates relatively well with the severity of pancreatic ductal changes assessed by ERP, although the clinical course does not.

Special forms

Pancreas divisum and chronic pancreatitis: The frequency of pancreas divisum ranges from 1.3% to 7.5% on ERCP[19–22]. The clinical relevance of pancreas divisum is still controversial. On the basis of the hypothesis of a functional or organic obstruction at the level of the minor papilla, some authors postulate that pancreas divisum is a cause of acute recurrent pancreatitis; however, the dorsal pancreatogram is usually normal in cases of acute pancreatitis. On rare occasions, pancreas divisum may induce obstructive pancreatitis[23] with pancreatographic changes rather evocative of obstructive pancreatitis seen on the dorsal pancreatogram. The relationship with CCP (pancreatic lithiasis) has been evaluated recently[24]. Pancreas divisum was diagnosed in 5% of a series of 411 patients with CCP, which is nearly the same incidence oberved in a control population[24,25]. Clinical course and morphological features did not differ in patients with pancreas divisum and chronic pancreatitis compared to patients with chronic pancreatitis but with a normally fused pancreas[24]. However, segmental lesions could be demonstrated on either the ventral pancreas alone or on the dorsal part alone in about half of the cases (Figures 8.16 and 8.17).

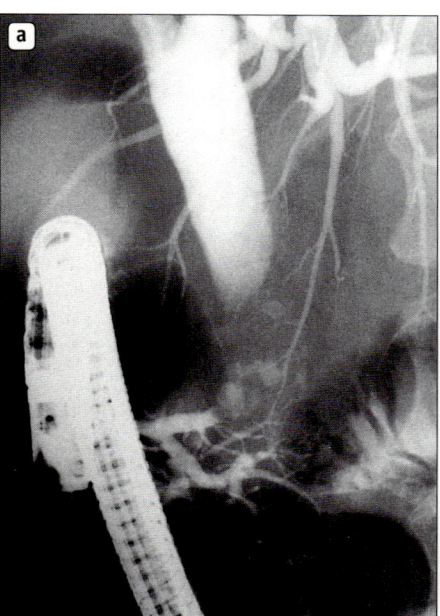

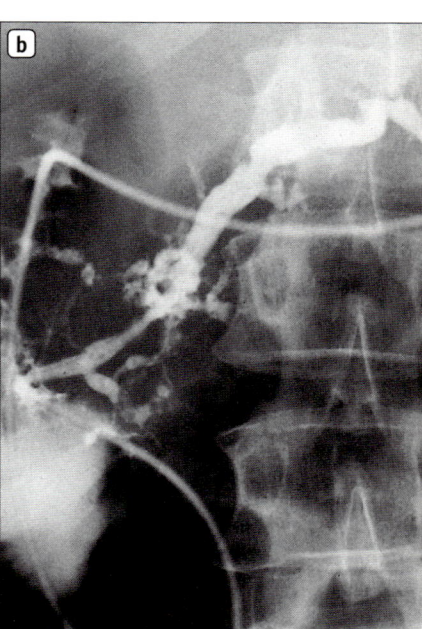

Figure 8.16 Chronic pancreatitis and pancreas divisum.
(a) Obstruction of the ventral duct by stones. (b) Typical changes; on the dorsal duct system.

Figure 8.17 Chronic pancreatitis and pancreas divisum. (a) Plain film of the abdomen, showing a densely calcified stone. (b) Cannulation of the main papilla; the ventral pancreas is annular. (c) Dorsal pancreatography: tight stenosis, with acinar filling up to the stone.

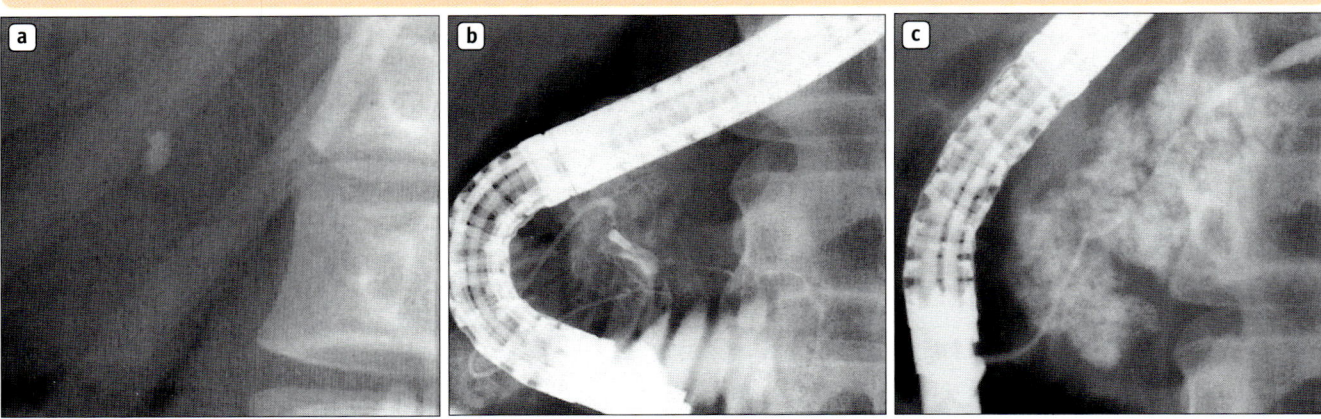

Radiolucent stones:

Radiolucent stones: Whether radiolucent stones are a precursor stage for calcified pancreatic lithiasis or a new entity is still a matter of controversial debate (Figures 8.5g and 8.18). A working hypothesis suggests that radiolucent stones may correspond to the precipitation of a protein whose major component might be lithostatin[26]. Radiolucent pancreatic lithiasis accounted for about 15% of pancreatic lithiasis in one series of 278 consecutive patients[27]. In some cases, pure radiolucent stones may evolve toward more calcified stages such as target calculi (radiolucent core with calcified shell)[26,27]. The lack of calcium carbonate in the composition of most radiolucent stones and epidemiological differences, such as three different age categories (juvenile form (<20 years), older form (>60 years) and intermediate form (20–40 years)), lower consumption of alcohol, and more frequent familial history of pancreatitis or diabetes, suggest that radiolucent pancreatic lithiasis is a different disease from calcified pancreatic lithiasis[26,27]. However, the complication rate is similar to that of CCP and the pancreatograms do not differ except in terms of the calcifications present.

Figure 8.18 A large radiolucent stone in the ventral duct of a pancreas divisum. The bile ducts are normal.

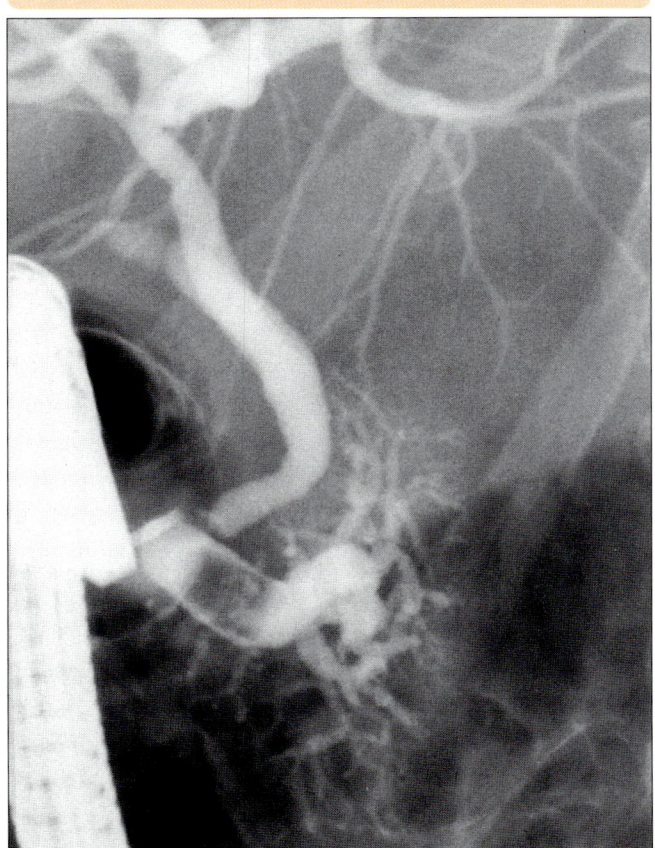

Cystic dystrophy of the duodenal wall: In some cases chronic pancreatitis, especially in non-alcoholic patients, may be associated with cystic dystrophy of the duodenal wall[28]. Conversely, cystic dystrophy of the duodenal or gastric wall can be demonstrated without chronic pancreatitis. Thickening of the duodenal wall with nodular and inflammatory patterns is highly suggestive of cystic dystrophy and is shown by ERCP. If CCP is associated with cystic dystrophy, pancreatograms show the changes usually observed during chronic pancreatitis. The best imaging procedure for cystic dystrophy of the duodenal wall, associated or not with chronic pancreatitis, seems to be endoscopic ultrasonography[28].

Complicated forms

Cysts and pseudocysts: Pancreatic cysts and pseudocysts are collections of pancreatic juice, either pure or containing necrotizing fragments of the pancreas or blood, and restricted or otherwise to the area of the pancreas from which they arise[29]. They may complicate chronic pancreatitis in 20–38% of cases[30–32]. Different pathogenetic mechanisms may be recognized and pancreatic pseudocysts may or may not communicate with the pancreatic ductal system. Retention cysts result from ductal obstruction caused by plugs, calculi or ductal .stenosis (Figures 8.19–8.21). Pseudocysts may result from solitary or repeated attacks of acute pancreatitis, which may complicate the course of chronic pancreatitis (Figure 8.22). ERCP provides detailed information on pancreatic and biliary duct characteristics

Figure 8.19 Retention cyst in chronic pancreatitis. (a) ERP image showing a cyst communicating with the pancreatic ductal system. (b) Disappearance of the cyst following endoscopic transpapillary drainage.

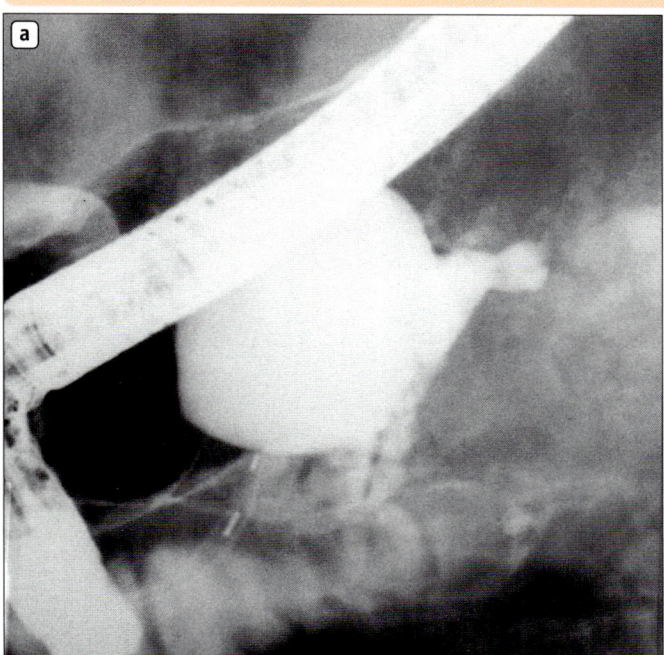
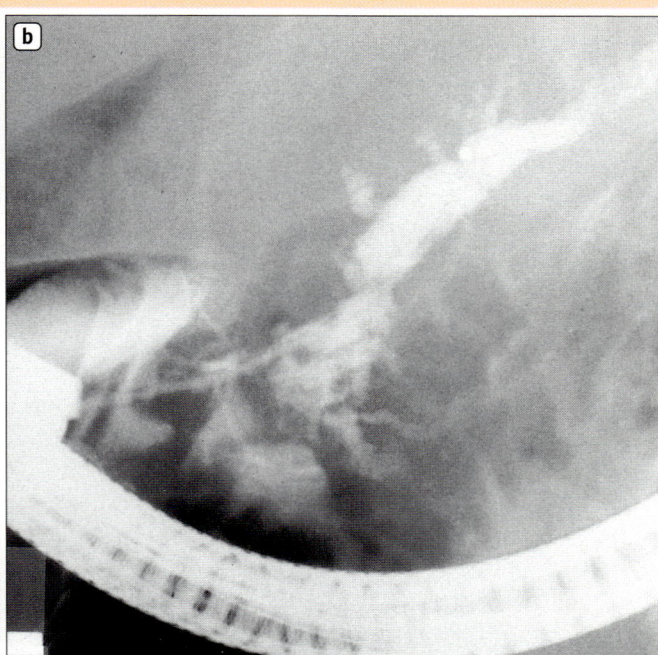

that influence the choice of therapy. On endoscopy, a compression of the duodenal or gastric wall is observed in about 50% of patients that allow endoscopic cystenterostomies. On pancreatography, cystic communication between cysts and the ductal system is demonstrated in about 50% of patients presenting with chronic pancreatitis, which makes possible eventual endoscopic transpapillary

Figure 8.20 Chronic pancreatitis with a small cyst in the head of the pancreas and ductal lesions dominant in the ventral part in a case of rudimentary fusion of the pancreas. The dorsal duct is slightly stenosed in the head of the pancreas.

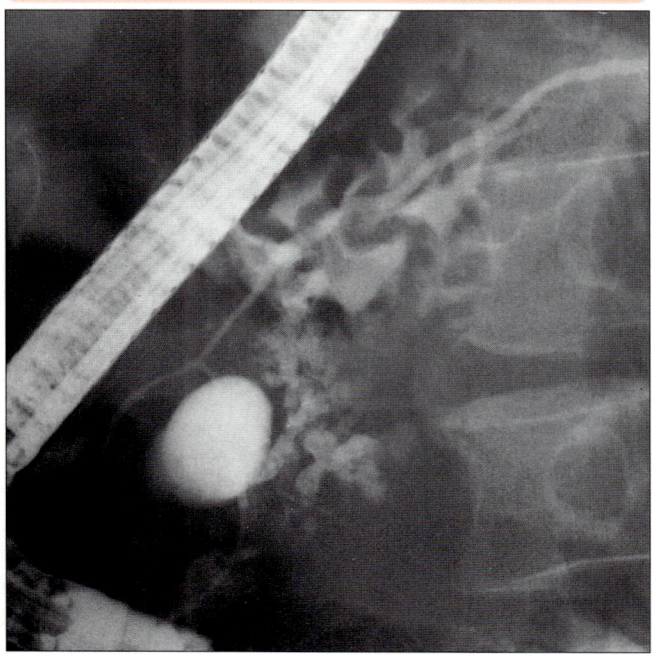

drainage (Figures 8.19 and 8.23). Retention cysts mostly appear with homogeneous content and regular shape whereas pseudocysts have irregular shape and heterogeneous content due to the presence of necrotizing fragments. Pancreatic cysts and pseudocysts are mainly located in the head of the pancreas (two thirds of cases) and may be multiple in 15% of cases[33]. Non-communicating cysts or pseudocysts may result in a lack of opacification, dislocation of side branches close to the cyst or compression of the main pancreatic duct. Rarely, complete obstruction of the main pancreatic duct due to compression by a pancreatic cyst may occur. In addition, compression of the choledochus (type IV of Caroli–Sarles classification) may be observed related to a pancreatic cyst located in the head of the pancreas (see Figure 8.15). Superinfection of pancreatic pseudocysts or cysts may occur in about 15% of cases, particularly where cysts communicate with the ductal system[34].

Serosal effusions: Pleural or peritoneal effusion may be demonstrated at ERP if communication exists between the pancreatic ductal system and the pleural or peritoneal cavity. The pathogenetic mechanisms for this communication may be a direct disruption of the main pancreatic duct or its side branches, or the rupture of a communicating pseudocyst. This may lead to an endoscopic drainage procedure being carried out[35].

Wirsungorrhagia: During chronic pancreatitis, digestive haemorrhage may be caused by either oesophageal or gastric varices secondary to splenoportal venous obstruction, duodenal ulcer or Wirsungorrhagia[36,37]. Blood can enter the pancreatic ductal system via a pseudocyst that previously eroded a pancreatic or peripancreatic vessel, through the

Figure 8.21 Cyst in the body of the pancreas, following blunt trauma of the pancreas. (a) Complete stenosis of the pancreatic duct in the body of the pancreas. (b) Opacification of the cyst after endoscopic cyst-gastrostomy.

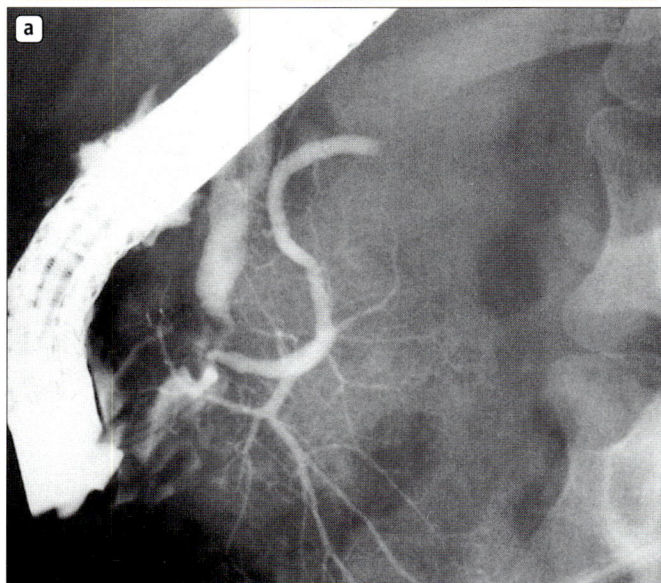

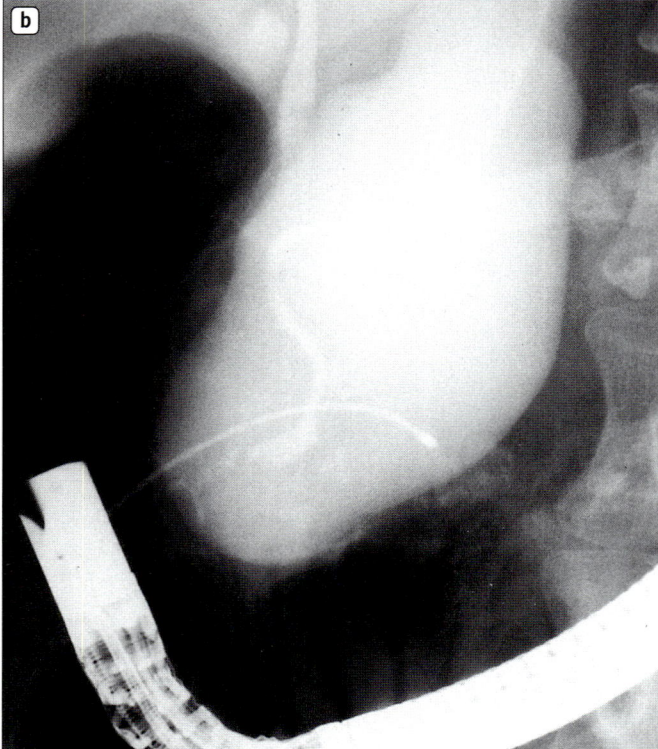

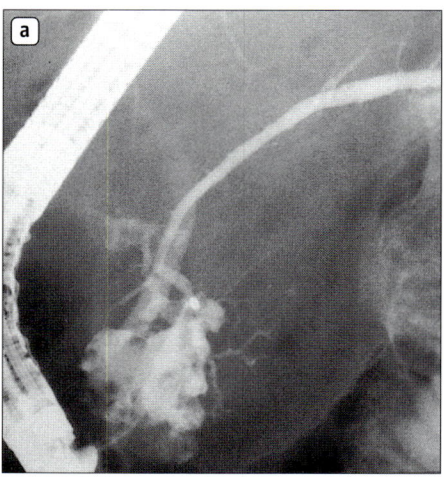

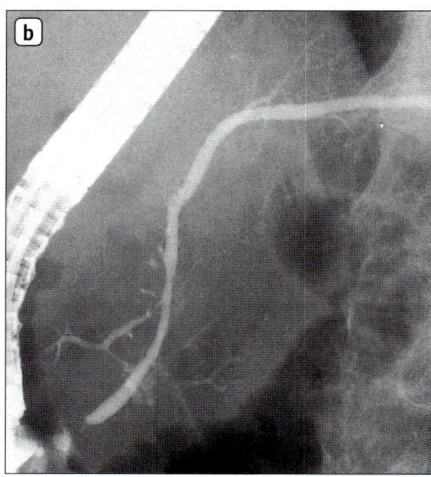

Figure 8.22 Post-acute pancreatitis pseudocyst. (a) Initial ERP image. (b) Following endoscopic transpapillary drainage of the pseudocyst: slight stenosis of the main pancreatic duct in the head of the pancreas.

Figure 8.23 Pseudocyst in the tail of the pancreas following left pancreatectomy. Note the pseudocystocutaneous fistulous tract.

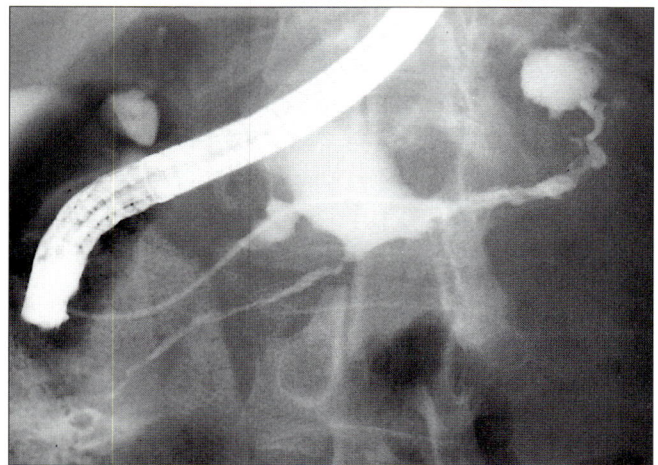

ductal disruption, resulting in a flow of blood into the duodenum. Emergency duodenoscopy may show blood flowing through the papilla in some cases. On ERP, contrast filling defects may be demonstrated in the lumen of the main pancreatic duct, corresponding to blood clots. It may be difficult to differentiate this pancreatographic pattern from intraductal calculi if no blood flow can be seen at the level of the papilla.

Pancreatic cancer: Pancreatic cancer is a rare complication arising during chronic pancreatitis, and may occur with estimated prevalence rates of 1.8% at 10 years and 4% at 20 years after the diagnosis of chronic pancreatitis[38]. The diagnosis of pancreatic cancer complicating chronic pancreatitis remains very difficult since many symptoms (jaundice, weight loss) and morphological features (stenosis or obstruction of the main pancreatic duct or stricture of the choledochus) are commonly seen in advanced chronic pancreatitis and pancreatic cancer complicating chronic pancreatitis. In our experience, it may be impossible to distinguish between the conditions and in many cases only pathology after surgical resection allows the right conclusion to be made. It is possible that the measurement of Ki-*ras* protein levels in pure pancreatic juice will facilitate the diagnosis of pancreatic cancer complicating chronic pancreatitis[39].

LIMITATIONS OF ERCP INTERPRETATION

As the sensitivity of ERCP for the diagnosis of chronic pancreatitis reaches more than 85%, some points are still a matter of debate. The distinction between COP and CCP is not always easy to make. The presence of calcified stones has a positive predictive value of 100% but they are observed in only 62% of cases at 5 years after onset of the disease and in 80% 10 years after onset[3]. Moreover, pancreatograms of some patients presenting with CCP present an obstructive component since a tight stenosis in the proximal part of the main pancreatic duct may be present.

In order to aid the diagnosis of chronic pancreatitis, some medical teams proposed to analyse pure pancreatic juice. Lactoferrin assessment is no longer used as a specific marker for chronic pancreatitis. Lithostatin levels measured by high-pressure liquid chromatography were decreased in the pure pancreatic juice of patients with alcoholic and non-alcoholic chronic pancreatitis but also in alcoholic patients without evidence of chronic pancreatitis[40]. Complementary studies are required to evaluate the accuracy of determination of lithostatin levels in pure pancreatic juice for the diagnosis of chronic pancreatitis. In addition, other teams have proposed to measure Ki-*ras* protein levels in pure pancreatic juice to confirm or to establish the diagnosis of pancreatic cancer in cases of difficult diagnosis. This procedure seems to be fairly accurate for the diagnosis of pancreatic cancer and may be a promising method for differentiating early chronic pancreatitis from pancreatic cancer[39,41].

Pancreatic duct damage may be observed after acute pancreatitis. Severe pancreatic duct damage may lead to the development of pancreatic duct stricture and subsequently to an obstructive pancreatitis[42]. ERCP changes have been described in several autoimmune disorders such as primary biliary cirrhosis, sclerosing cholangitis and Gougerot–Sjögren syndrome[43–44].

The main difficulty in interpreting changes seen on pancreatography is probably the effect of patient age on the pancreatographic results. Many studies performed at necropsy, with or without postmortem pancreatography, have shown that the incidence of abnormalities of the pancreatic duct and its side branches increases with age[45–47]. Dilatation of the pancreatic duct and ductular ectasia (mainly located in the head of the pancreas), pancreatic lithiasis with calculi <3mm in side branches, lipomatosis and fibrosis, were the main pathological features observed to increase with age[45–47]. At ERCP, the existence of a linear correlation between age and the diameter of the main pancreatic duct has been demonstrated[48–49]. In addition, an undulating main pancreatic duct, ectatic side branches, filling defects in the main pancreatic duct, and cavity formations, have been described from pancreatograms of patients aged 75 years or above[50]. The proportion of abnormal pancreatograms in a series of 218 patients was 15% in subjects aged between 20 and 40, 25% between 40 and 60, 53% between 60 and 80 and 78% above 80 years[51]. These abnormalities were enlargement of the main pancreatic duct, irregularities of the main pancreatic duct, dilatation of side branches, irregularities of side branches and the presence of cysts (ranging from 2 to 11mm)[52]. The abnormalities increased linearly with the age of the patients. Thus interpretation of abnormal pancreatograms in the elderly must be done with care.

References

1. Kasugai T, Kuno N, Kizu M, Koboyashi S, Hattori K. The pathological endoscopic pancreatocholangiogram. *Gastroenterology* 1972; 63:227–34.
2. Sarles H, Adler G, Dani R. The classification of pancreatitis and definiiion of pancreatic diseases. *Digestion* 1989; 43:234–6.
3. Bernades P, Belghiti J, Athouel M, Mallardo N, Breil P, Fekete F. Histoire naturelle de la pancréatite chronique: étude de 120 cas. *Gastroenterol Clin Biol* 1983; 7:8–13.
4. Sarles H. Etiopathogenesis and definition of chronic pancreatitis. *Dig Dis Sci* 1986; 31:91S–107S.
5. Sahel J, Cros C, Durbec JP *et al.* Multicenter pathological study of chronic pancreatitis. Morphological regional variations and differences between chronic calcifying pancreatitis and obstructive pancreatitis. *Pancreas* 1986; 1:471–7.
6. Cremer M, Toussaint J, Hermanus A, Deltenre M, De Toeuf J, Engelholm L. Les pancréatites chroniques primitives. Classification sur base de la pancréatographie endoscopique. *Acta Gastroenterol Belg* 1976; 34:522–46.
7. Axon ATR, Classen M, Cotton PB, Cremer M, Freeny PC, Lees WR. Pancreatography in chronic pancreatitis: international definitions. *Gut* 1984; 25:1107–12.
8. Sahel J Endoscopic retrograde pancreatography findings and their grading in chronic pancreatitis. In *Diagnostic Procedures in Pancreatic Disease*. Edited by P Malfertheiner, H Ditschuneit. Springer-Verlag, Heidelberg. 1986;169–72.
9. Petrozza JA, Dutta SK, Latham PS. Prevalence and natural history of distal common bile duct stenosis in alcoholic pancreatitis. *Dig Dis Sci* 1984; 29:890–5.
10. Wisloff F, Jakobsen J, Osnes M. Stenosis of the common bile duct in chronic pancreatitis. *Br J Surg* 1982; 69:52–4.
11. Caroli J, Nora J. L'hépatocholédoque dans les pancréatites. *Semin Hôp Paris* 1953; 29:575–80.
12. Sarles H, Sarles JC, Guien C. Etudes des voies biliaires et pancréatiques au cours de la pancréatite chronique. *Arch Fr Mal App Dig Nutr* 1958; 47:664–83.
13. Lamarque D, Dutreuil L C, Moulin C, Soule JC, Delchier JC. Pathogénie de la lithiase biliaire au cours de la pancréatite chronique. *Gastroentérol Clin Biol* 1992; 16:869–74.

14. Borgstrom A, Wehlin L. Correlations between serum concentrations of three specific exocrine pancreatic proteins and pancreatic duct morphology at ERCP examinations. *Scand J Gastroenterol* 1984; 19:220–7.

15. Ashton MG, Axon ATR, Lintott DJ. Lundh test and ERCP in pancreatic disease. *Gut* 1978; 19:910–15.

16. Deviere J, Gulbis B, Delhaye M, Quenon M, Cremer M. Relation entre la morphologie canalaire et la fonction exocrine du pancréas: une méthode originale d'estimation linéaire de la fonction pancréatique. *Acta Endosc* 1985; 15:1–12.

17. Bozkurt T, Braun U, Lefrink S, Gilly G, Lux G. Comparison of pancreatic morphology and exocrine functional impairment in patients with chronic pancreatitis. *Gut* 1994; 35:1132–6.

18. Dominguez-Munoz JE, Manes G, Pieramico O, Buchler RM, Malfertheiner P. Effect of pancreatic ductal changes on exocrine function in chronic pancreatitis. *Pancreas* 1995; 10:31–5.

19. Sugawa C, Walt AJ, Nunez DC, Masuyama H. Pancreas divisum: is it a normal anatomic variant? *Am J Surg* 1987; 153:62–7.

20. Burtin P, Person B, Carneau J, Boyer J. Pancreas divisum and pancreatitis: a coincidental association? *Endoscopy* 1991; 23: 55–8.

21. Delhaye M, Engelholm L, Cremer M. Pancreas divisum: congenital anatomic variant or anomaly? Contribution of endoscopic retrograde dorsal pancreatography. *Gastroenterology* 1985; 89:951–8.

22. Cotton PB. Congenital anomaly of pancreas divisum as cause of obstructive pain and pancreatitis. *Gut* 1950; 21:105–14.

23. Lehman GA, Sherman S, Nisi R, Hawes RH. Pancreas divisum: results of minor papilla sphincterotomy. *Gastrointest Endosc* 1993; 39:1–8.

24. Barthet M, Valantin V, Spinosa S, Bernard JP, Sahel J. Clinical course and morphological features of chronic calcifying pancreatitis associated with pancreas divisum. *Eur J Gastroenterol Hepatol* 1995; 7:993–8.

25. Bernard JP, Sahel J, Giovanini M, Sarles H. Pancreas divisum is a probable cause of acute pancreatitis: a report of 137 cases. *Pancreas* 1990; 5:248–54.

26. Sarles H, Camarena J, Gomez–Santana C. Radiolucent and calcified pancreatic lithiasis: two different diseases. Role of alcohol and heredity. *Scand J Gastroenterol* 1992; 27:71–6.

27. Barthet M, Daniel R, Bernard JP, Laugier R, Sahel J. Radiolucent pancreatic lithiasis: a precursor stage for calcified pancreatic lithiasis or a new entity? *Pancreas* 1995; 11:420.

28. Flejou JF, Potet F, Molas G, Bernades P, Amouyal P, Fekete F. Cystic dystrophy of the gastric and duodenal wall developing in heterotopic pancreas: an unrecognised entity. *Gut* 1993; 34:343–7.

29. Sarles H, Martin M, Camatte R, Sarles JC. Le démembrement des pancréatites aiguës et des pancréatites chroniques. *Presse Med* 1963; 5:237–40.

30. Elliott DW. Pancreatic pseudocysts. *Surg Clin North Am* 1975; 55:339–62.

31. Frey CF. Pancreatic pseudocysts. Operative strategy. *Ann Surg* 1978; 188:652–62.

32. Staub JL, Le Genissel H, Sarles H. Etude de la séméiologie et des résultats du traitement chirurgical de 103 cas de pancréatites chroniques compliquées de kystes ou de pseudokystes. *Gastroenterol Clin Biol* 1981; 5:433–9.

33. Barthet M, Bugallo M, Moreira LS, Bastid C, Sastre B, Sahel J. Management of cysts and pseudocysts complicating chronic pancreatitis. *Gastroenterol Clin Biol* 1993; 17:270–6.

34. Laxson LC, Fromkes JJ, Cooperman M. Endoscopic retrograde cholangio-pancreatography in the management of pancreatic pseudocysts. *Scand J Gastroenterol* 1986; 21(S123):123–9.

35. Kozarek R, Ball T, Patterson D, Freeny P. Endoscopic transpapillary therapy for disrupted pancreatic duct and peripancreatic fluid collections. *Gastroenterology* 1991; 100:1362–70.

36. Bernades P, Baetz A, Levy P, Belghiti J, Menu Y, Fekete F. Splenic and portal venous obstruction in chronic pancreatitis. A prospective longitudinal study of a medical–surgical series of 266 patients. *Dig Dis Sci* 1992; 37:340–6.

37. Camishion RC, Pello MJ, Spence RK. Hemoductal pancreatitis. *Surgery* 1992; 111:86–9.

38. Lowenfels AB, Maisonneuve P, Cavallini G *et al*. Pancreatitis and the risk of pancreatic cancer. *New Engl J Med* 1993; 328:1433–7.

39. Kondo H, Sugano K, Fukayama N *et al*. Detection of point mutation K-ras oncogene at codon 12 in pure pancreatic juice for diagnosis of pancreatic carcinoma. *Cancer* 1994; 73:1589–94.

40. Bernard JP, Barthet M, Gharib B, *et al*. Quantification of human lithostatin by high performance liquid chromatography. *Gut* 1995; 36:630–6.

41. Berthelemy P, Bouisson M, Escourrou J, Vaysse N, Rumeau JL, Pradayrol L. Identification of K-ras mutations in pancreatic juice in the early diagnosis of pancreatic cancer. *Ann Intern Med* 1995; 123:188–91.

42. Singer MV, Gyr K, Sarles H. Revised classification of pancreatitis: a report of the second international symposium on the classification of pancreatitis in Marseille, France, March 28–30,1984. *Gastroenterology* 1985; 89:683–90.

43. Epstein O, Chapman RW, Lake–Bakaar G, Rosalki SB, Sherlock S. The pancreas in primary biliary cirrhosis and primary sclerosing cholangitis. *Gastroenterology* 1982; 83:1177–82.

44. Palmer KR, Cotton PB, Chapman M. Pancreatogram in cholestasis. *Gut* 1984; 25:424–7.

45. Nagai H, Ohtsubo K. Pancreatic lithiasis in the aged. Its clinicopathology and pathogenesis. *Gastroenterology* 1984; 86:331–8.

46. Stamm BH. Incidence and diagnostic significance of minor pathologic changes in the adult pancreas at autopsy: a systematic study of 112 autopsies in patients without known pancreatic disease. *Hum Pathol* 1984; 15:677–83.

47. Kreel L, Sandin B. Changes in pancreatic morphology associated with aging. *Gut* 1973; 14:962–70.

48. Ananad BS, Phil D, Vij JC, Mac HS, Chowdhury V, Kumar A. Effect of aging on the pancreatic ducts: a study based on endoscopic retrograde pancreatography. *Gastrointest Endosc* 1989; 35:210–13.

49. Neoptolemos JP, Carr–Locke DL, Kelly KA. Factors affecting the diameter of the common bile duct and pancreatic duct using endoscopic retrograde cholangiopancreatography. *Hepatogastroenterology* 1991; 38:243–7.

50. Jones SN, McNeil NI, Lees WR. The interpretation of retrograde pancreatography in the elderly. *Clin Radiol* 1989; 40:393–6.

51. Barthet M, Affriat C, Bernard JP, Berthezene P, Dagorn JC, Sahel J. Is biliary lithiasis associated with pancreatographic changes? *Gut* 1995; 36:761–5.

52. Barthet M, Affriat C, Bernard JP, Spinosa S, Sahel J. Aspects de la pancréatographie rétrograde endoscopique au cours de la sénescence pancréatique. *Gastroenterol Clin Biol* 1994: 18:A74.

9

Minimal change pancreatitis

Marc Barthet & José Sahel

INTRODUCTION

Despite the advent of more sophisticated techniques, endoscopic retrograde cholangiopancreatography (ERCP) remains the reference diagnostic tool that provides detailed information on the severity of chronic pancreatitis. Its capacity for diagnosing early stages of chronic pancreatitis, however, is still under discussion and many studies have tried to correlate the presence of minimal changes seen on pancreatography with changes associated with other diagnostic procedures (such as endoscopic ultrasonography (EUS), pancreatic function tests and sampling of pure pancreatic juice) in order to improve the capacity of endoscopic retrograde pancreatography (ERP) to diagnose early stages of chronic pancreatitis.

DEFINITION AND NATURAL HISTORY OF MINIMAL CHANGES ON ERP

Kasugai first introduced the concept of minimal pancreatographic changes, in which radiological abnormalities were slight and confined to the side branches[1]. This concept is still questionable since the histological interpretation and correlations are not available[2–4], differential diagnosis from changes due to ageing is still difficult, and pancreatogram interpretation is not completely reliable, especially in the early stages of chronic pancreatitis. The lack of histological assessment procedures for the diagnosis of chronic pancreatitis is a major problem for early stages of chronic pancreatitis and is partially responsible for the confusion existing between acute alcoholic chronic pancreatitis and early chronic pancreatitis[5]. When histology has been available in patients with mild pancreatographic changes, only about 50% have shown histological evidence of chronic pancreatitis[6,7]. The definitive diagnosis of chronic pancreatitis may not be possible in the absence of histological proof, since patients may have normal or abnormal pancreatic function tests[4–8]. In such cases, the confirmation of chronic pancreatitis requires long-term follow-up before detecting genuine abnormalities in pancreatic structure or function. In some cases, alterations of pancreatic exocrine function or apparitions of pancreatic stones may still be lacking after 12 years[9,10].

In some circumstances pancreatographic changes due to age (Figure 9.1) may mimic the features of early stages of chronic pancreatitis, with either minimal or mild changes[11–13]. Severe ductal alterations may be demonstrated in old patients and the incidence and severity of abnormal pancreatograms increase with age[12,13]. In the age class ranging from 40 to 60 years, 18% of patients without chronic pancreatitis presented with equivocal or mild changes, and 34% of

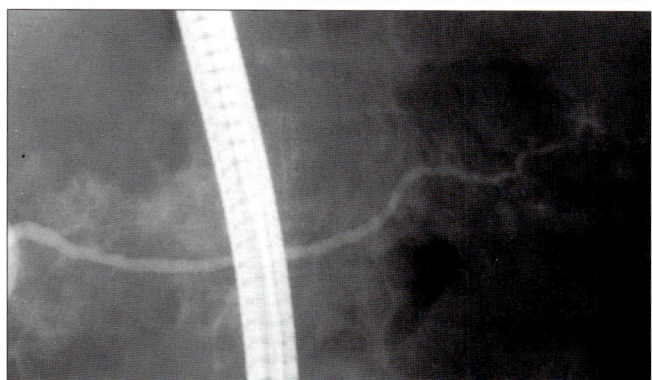

Figure 9.1 Pancreatographic changes due to advancing age.

patients had equivocal, mild, moderate or severe pancreatographic changes. However, since the mean age at onset of chronic pancreatitis is about 40 years[14], in many cases age does not really affect the interpretation of the pancreatogram. In older patients (late pancreatitis), the differential diagnosis between early chronic pancreatitis and senile abnormalities of the pancreatic ductal system may be rather difficult to make.

In addition, observer variation in the interpretation of ERP has to be taken into account. In a study of 40 pancreatograms (20 pancreatic cancer, 20 chronic pancreatitis), unanimous and correct opinions were given by four observers in only 53% of cases[15]. The diagnostic accuracy was significantly increased by providing clinical information. It is probable that interobserver variability is maximal in the case of minimal changes confined to side branches and this may lead to false conclusions at early stages of chronic pancreatitis.

MINIMAL CHANGES AND ERCP CLASSIFICATIONS

Minimal changes have been defined by Kasugai *et al.* as ductal changes confined to side branches with irregular distribution, dilatation, stenosis and obstruction[1] (Figure 9.2). In the first report, only two thirds of the patients presenting with minimal changes had a confirmed chronic pancreatitis. In the first report of Cremer's classification, six categories were established from a series of 2371 ERCPs of which 158 cases presented with chronic pancreatitis (minimal changes and types I to V pancreatitis)[16]. Minimal changes, characterized by alterations to ductules only, were demonstrated in 30% of cases, of which 49% were considered as showing idiopathic pancreatitis; the mean age of this group was greater than

Figure 9.2 Minimal changes: the Wirsung duct is normal in calibre, but its edges are irregular. Irregularities of side branches are also present.

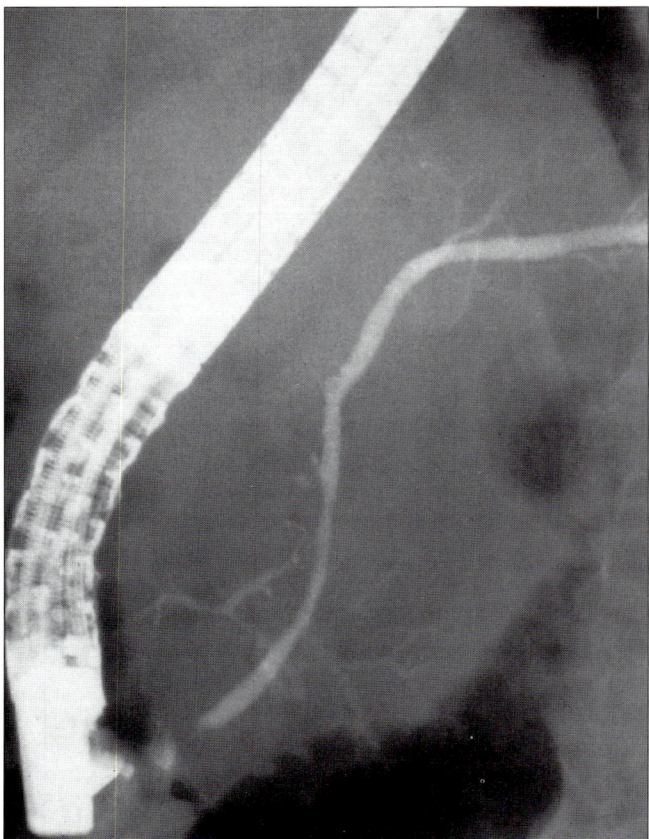

Figure 9.3 Typical features of early chronic pancreatitis: irregularities of side branches and slight enlargement of the PD.

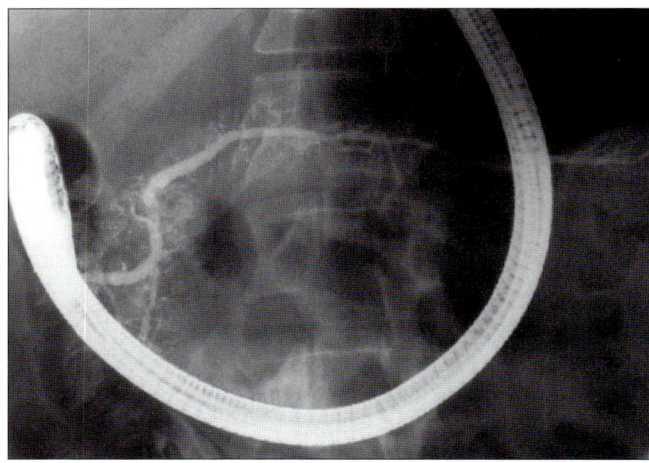

Figure 9.4 Early stage of chronic pancreatitis: the Wirsung duct is moderately dilated, side branches are irregular. A small cyst containing radiolucent stones is visible in the head of the pancreas.

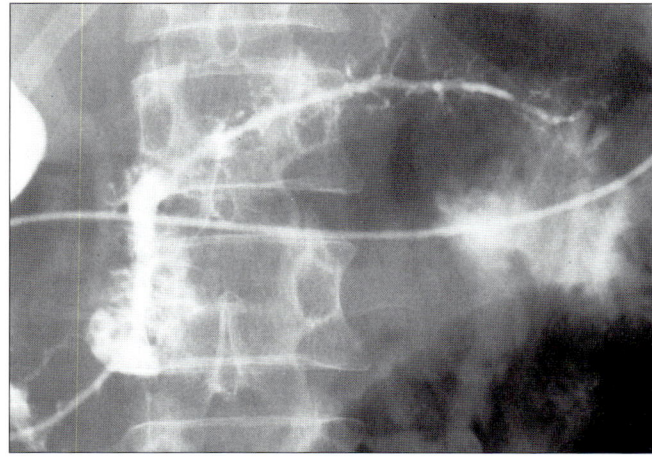

that for types I to V pancreatitis. This may be related to the presence of pancreatographic changes due to the effect of ageing. The Cambridge classification established three different stages: equivocal (Cambridge I, Figure 9.2), mild to moderate (Cambridge II, Figure 9.3), and marked changes (Cambridge III, Figure 9.4)[17]. The Cambridge I stage corresponds to pancreatograms with fewer than three abnormal branches, which is closer to the definition of minimal changes of Kasugai et al. than that of Cremer et al. Therefore minimal changes seen on pancreatography concern radiological features but are not always consistent with the diagnosis of chronic pancreatitis. If they are suggestive of early stages of chronic pancreatitis, in half to two thirds of cases they require additional diagnostic procedures such as pancreatic function tests, long-term follow-up or the development of other imaging procedures to confirm the diagnosis of chronic pancreatitis.

RELATIONSHIP OF MINIMAL CHANGES ON ERP TO OTHER DIAGNOSTIC PROCEDURES

Endoscopic ultrasonography

ERP provides detailed information on the pancreatic ductal system but appears to be of limited value in demonstrating lesions or tumours located in the pancreatic parenchyma. Endoscopic ultrasonography (EUS) appears to show some promise in this regard. The possibility of placing the trans-ducer in close relation to the pancreas, through the duodenal or the gastric wall, allows high-resolution imaging, enhanced by high ultrasound frequencies. This is clearly demonstrated with the high sensitivity of EUS for diagnosing endocrine tumours of the pancreas and small tumours of the exocrine parenchyma[18–20].

Even though chronic calcifying pancreatitis (CCP) appears to be initially a ductal disease characterized by the precipitation of plugs or pancreatic stones[21], the capacity of EUS to diagnose early stages of chronic pancreatitis has been evaluated in three studies[22–24]. EUS was compared with ERCP, with or without pancreatic exocrine function testing. In a prospective study, Wiersema et al. identified 22 patients with chronic pancreatitis based on clinical, pure pancreatic juice data and minimal (11 patients) or no (11 patients) changes on pancreatography[22]. In these patients, the sensitivity of EUS for diagnosing chronic pancreatitis was 86% versus 50% for ERCP. The EUS predictors of chronic pancreatitis were assessed by a stepwise logistic regression. Focal areas of reduced echogenicity, irregular calibre of the main

Figure 9.5 EUS appearance of chronic pancreatitis with two small calculi in side branches (arrow head) (calculi were not detectable on plain films of the abdomen and CT).

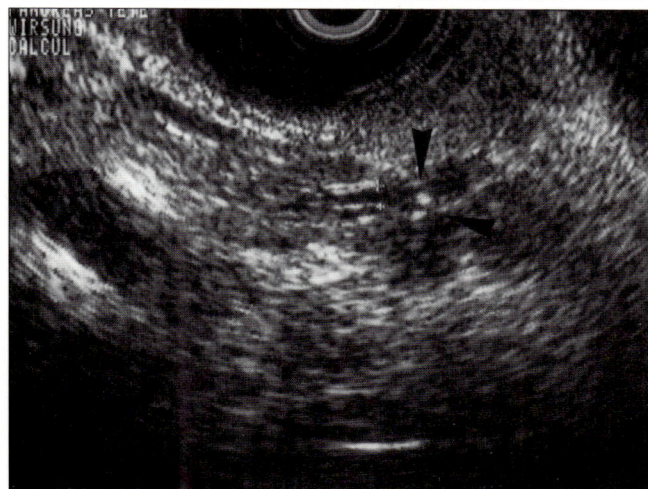

pancreatic duct, dilatation of side branches and echogenic foci were the strongest statistically significant predictive factors. However, the most useful EUS feature relevant to chronic pancreatitis (positive predictive value of 100%) was the demonstration of calculi (Figure 9.5). In a series of 114 patients who had inflammatory pancreatic disease (either chronic pancreatitis or post-acute oedematous pancreatitis), Natterman et al. found abnormal EUS features in 88% of patients with Cambridge stage I and in 63% of patients with Cambridge stage 0[23]. EUS features in patients presenting with Cambridge stage I or 0 consisted mainly in alternating echo-poor and echo-rich areas and in a lobulated parenchymal pattern (Figure 9.6). Isolated side branch alterations, as detected in stage I, escaped EUS (Figure 9.7). Changes of the main pancreatic duct were mainly found in stages II and III. However, EUS was also positive in a considerable number

of patients with a recent attack of acute pancreatitis and normal ERCP but without evidence of chronic pancreatitis. This fact may underline a lack of specificity of EUS in the diagnosis of chronic pancreatitis, even if its sensitivity appears to be higher than that of ERCP.

In a series of 44 patients with chronic pancreatitis, Buscail et al. identified 20 patients with non-calcified forms who were followed up for 14 ± 5 months[24]. EUS features seen were a heterogeneous pattern and/or cystic lesions of the pancreas; two cases showed a hyperechoic parenchyma and three patients appeared normal. Among the 20 patients ERCP was normal in five cases; EUS changes were observed in four of these five. It was concluded that EUS has a higher sensitivity than ERCP for diagnosing early stages of chronic pancreatitis and might resolve diagnostic problems in patients suspected of having chronic pancreatitis.

The major criteria of EUS features at early stages of chronic pancreatitis are subjective, since they are represented by the demonstration of a heterogeneous pattern, irregular delimitation of the pancreas or lobulated pancreatic pattern. Interobserver variation in evaluation of EUS features was tested by Natterman et al. in 18 patients but should be tested in larger series. The specificity of EUS appears to be questionable since patients presenting with alcohol abuse or recent attacks of acute pancreatitis had changes similar to those observed in patients presenting with proven early chronic pancreatitis[24,25]. More studies with long-term follow-up and systematic evaluation of the exocrine secretion are required to assess the specificity and the positive predictive value of EUS at early stages of chronic pancreatitis.

Minimal change pancreatitis and exocrine function tests

Patients with minimal changes on pancreatography require further investigation since this pancreatographic pattern has a lack of specificity. Numerous studies based on either ERCP or autopsy have shown alterations of the pancreatic ductal system increasing with age[26,30]. Many studies have tried to

Figure 9.6 Areolar features suggestive of chronic pancreatitis.

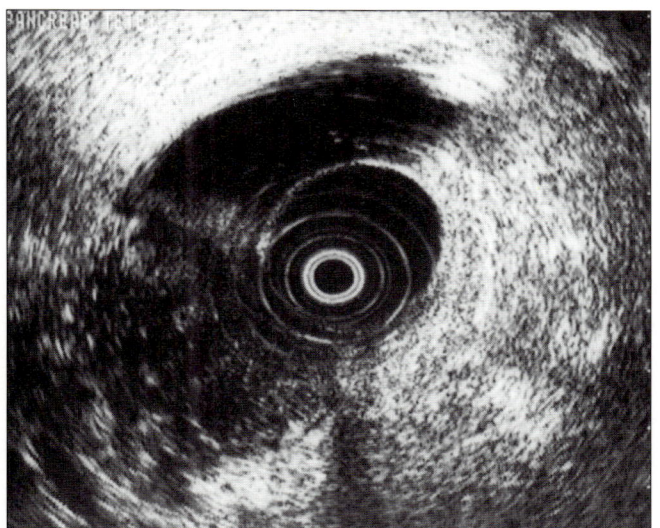

Figure 9.7 Ductal changes: hyperechoic wall of the Wirsung duct and of side branches (arrow heads).

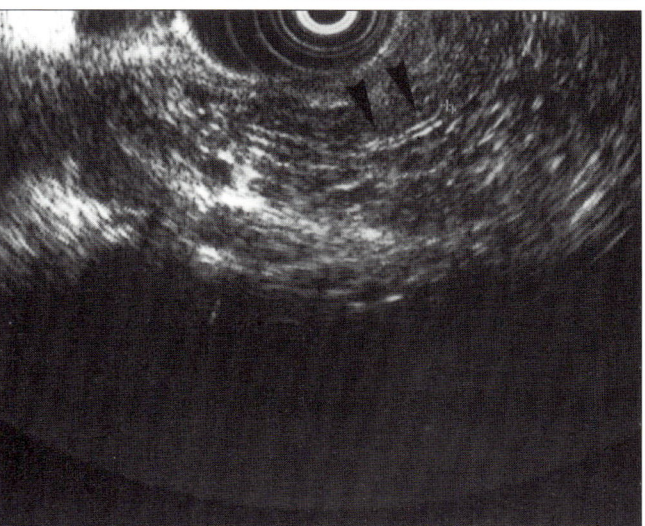

correlate pancreatic exocrine function tests and minimal changes demonstrated on pancreatograms[8,31–38]. Pancreatic function tests were performed by using either Lundh test meal or secretin–CCK test. In these studies there was evidence of impaired pancreatic function in 56% of patients studied with the secretin–caerulein test and 42% of patients studied using the Lundh test meal. More recently, Bozkurt *et al.* found 70% of patients with equivocal pancreatic duct changes (Cambridge classification) had dissociated pancreatic insufficiency and 30% had global pancreatic insufficiency, as assessed by the secretin–caerulein test[39]. The pancreolauryl test appeared to correlate well with alterations of the pancreatograms classified according to the Cambridge classification (odds ratio 5.8, stepwise multiple logistic regression) but no detailed information concerning patients with minimal changes was provided in the study[40]. The faecal elastase test has recently been evaluated[41,42] and its sensitivity appears to be better than that of the faecal chymotrypsin test and its specificity better than that of the pancreolauryl test[42]. However, in patients with equivocal or mild changes the latter three pancreatic function tests were normal in one large series whereas a good correlation was demonstrated between the secretin–caerulein and faecal elastase tests in another series. Therefore, more studies are required to assess the value of the faecal elastase test in early stages of chronic pancreatitis. Whereas studies using pancreatic function tests showed impaired pancreatic function in approximately 50–70% of patients with equivocal or mild changes on pancreatography, studies where histological data were available demonstrated pancreatic alterations in about 50% of patients with similar pancreatographic features[1,6,7]. This result highlights the value of pancreatic function tests in making the diagnosis of chronic pancreatitis, especially in patients with minimal pancreatography changes.

Pure pancreatic juice sampling

Pure pancreatic juice sampling is rarely performed as the technique is invasive with technical difficulties and a rate of complications that is not negligible. Some assays have been performed, however. The measurement of lactoferrin appeared to be promising, since concentrations of lactoferrin were significantly increased compared to controls in three alcoholic groups (asymptomatic alcoholics, alcoholics with acute pancreatitis, alcoholics with established chronic pancreatitis) and the lactoferrin output clearly differentiated asymptomatic from symptomatic alcoholics[43]. Surprisingly, this test has not been intensively studied in recent years.

Based on the demonstration that lithostatin may inhibit the precipitation and development of calcium carbonate crystals, Bernard *et al.* showed that lithostatin levels in pancreatic juice assessed by HPLC were 3 times lower in patients with chronic pancreatitis than in patients without pancreatic disease[44]. Similar levels were found in chronic alcoholics without evidence for chronic pancreatitis and in patients with chronic pancreatitis. Further developments are necessary for a better understanding of the precise role of lithostatin in the pathogenesis of chronic pancreatitis.

References

1. Kasugai T, Kuno N, Kizu M, Kobayashi S, Hattori K. The pathological endoscopic pancreatocholangiogram. *Gastroenterology* 1972; 63:227–34.
2. Sarner M, Cotton PB. Classification of pancreatitis. *Gut* 1984; 25:756–9.
3. Singer MV, Gyr K, Sarles H. Revised classification of pancreatitis: report of the second international symposium on the classification of pancreatitis in Marseille, France; March 28–30 1984. *Gastroenterology* 1985; 89:683–90.
4. Chari ST, Singer MV. The problem of classification and staging of chronic pancreatitis: proposals based on current knowledge of its natural history. *Scand J Gastroenterol* 1994; 29:949–60.
5. Ammann RW, Muellhaupt B, Meyenberger C, Heitz PU. Alcoholic non progressive chronic pancreatitis: prospective long–term study of a large cohort with alcoholic acute pancreatitis (1976–1992). *Pancreas* 1994; 9:365–73.
6. Kizu M, Newmann J, Cotton PB, Kasugai T. Histological correlation with pancreatography in necropsy specimens. *Gut* 1977; 18:399–400.
7. Trapnell JE. Chronic relapsing pancreatitis: a review of 64 cases. *Br J Surg* 1979; 66:471–5.
8. Boyd EJS, Rinderknecht H, Wormsley KG. Laboratory tests in the diagnosis of the chronic pancreatic diseases. Comparison between function tests and morphological investigation in the diagnosis of pancreatic disease. *Int J Pancreatol* 1988; 3:301–8.
9. Marks IN, Bank S, Louw JH. Chronic pancreatitis in the Western Cape. *Digestion* 1973; 9:447–53.
10. Ammann RW, Muellhaupt B. Progression of alcoholic acute to chronic pancreatitis. *Gut* 1994; 35:552–6.
11. Jones SN, McNeil NI, Lees WR. The interpretation of retrograde pancreatography in the elderly. *Clin Radiol* 1989; 40:393–6.
12. Barthet M, Affriat C, Bernard JP, Berthezene P, Dagorn JC, Sahel J. Is biliary lithiasis associated with pancreatographic changes? *Gut* 1995; 36:761–5.
13. Barthet M, Affriat C, Bernard JP, Spinosa S, Sahel J. Aspects de la pancréatographie rétrograde endoscopique au cours de la sénescence pancréatique. *Gastroenterol Clin Biol* 1994; 18:A74.
14. Bernades P, Belghiti J, Athouel M, Mallardo N, Breil P, Fekete F. Histoire naturelle de la pancréatite chronique: étude de 120 cas. *Gastroenterol Clin Biol* 1983; 7:8–13.
15. Reuben A, Johnson AL, Cotton PB. Is pancreatogram interpretation reliable? A study of observer variation and error. *Br J Radiol* 1978; 51:956–62.
16. Cremer M, Toussaint J, Hermanus A, Deltenre M, De Toeuf J, Engelholm L. Les pancréatites chroniques primitives. Classification sur base de la pancréatographie endoscopique. *Acta Gastroenterol Belg* 1976; 34:522–46.
17. Axon ATR, Classen M, Cotton PB, Cremer M, Freeny PC, Lees WR. Pancreatography in chronic pancreatitis: international definitions. *Gut* 1984; 25:1107–12.
18. Glover JR, Shorvon PJ, Lees WR. Endoscopic ultrasound for localisation of islet cell tumors. *Gut* 1992; 33:108–10.

19. Rosch T, Lightdale CJ, Botet JF. Localization of pancreatic endocrine tumors by endoscopic ultrasonography. *New Engl J Med* 1992; 326:1721–6.

20. Palazzo L, Roseau G, Salmeron M. Endoscopic ultrasonography in the preoperative localization of pancreatic endocrine tumors. *Endoscopy* 1992; 24:350–3.

21. Sarles H. Etiopathogenesis and definition of chronic pancreatitis. *Dig Dis Sci* 1986; 31:91S–107S.

22. Wiersema MJ, Hawes RH, Lehman GA, Kochman ML, Sherman S, Kopecky KK. Prospective evaluation of endoscopic ultrasonography and endoscopic retrograde cholangiopancreatography in patients with chronic abdominal pain of suspected pancreatic origin. *Endoscopy* 1993; 25:555–64.

23. Natterman C, Goldschmidt AJW, Dancygier H. Endosonography in chronic pancreatitis. A comparison between endoscopic retrograde pancreatography and endoscopic ultrasonography. *Endoscopy* 1993; 25:565–70.

24. Buscail L, Escourrou J, Moreau J *et al*. Endoscopic ultrasonography in chronic pancreatitis: A comparative study with conventional ultrasonography, computed tomography and ERCP. *Pancreas* 1995; 10:251–7.

25. Wiersema MJ, Schwartz SM, Hawes RH, Rex DK. Abnormalities of pancreas parenchyma and ductular features detected by endosonography in asymptomatic subjects with a history of moderate to heavy alcohol use. *Gastrointest Endosc* 1993; 39:A563.

26. Anand BS, Phil D, Vij JC, Mac HS, Chowdhury V, Kumar A. Effect of aging on the pancreatic ducts: a study based on endoscopic retrograde pancreatography. *Gastrointest Endosc* 1989; 35:210–13.

27. Neoptolemos JP, Carr-Locke DL, Kelly KA. Factors affecting the diameter of the common bile duct and pancreatic duct using endoscopic retrograde cholangiopancreatography. *Hepatogastroenterol* 1991; 38:243–7.

28. Stamm BH. Incidence and diagnostic signifiance of minor pathologic changes in the adult pancreas at autopsy: a systematic study of 112 autopsies in patients without known pancreatic disease. *Hum Pathol* 1984;15:677–83.

29. Nagai H, Ohtsubo K. Pancreatic lithiasis in the aged. Its clinicopathology and pathogenesis. *Gastroenterology* 1984; 86:331–8.

30. Kreel L, Sandin B. Changes in pancreatic morphology associated with aging. *Gut* 1973; 14:962–70.

31. Rolny P, Lakes PJ, Gaurklou R, Jagenburg R, Nilson A. A comparative evaluation of endoscopic retrograde pancreatography and secretin–CCK test in the diagnosis of pancreatic disease. *Scand J Gastroenterol* 1978; 13: 777–81.

32. Braganza JM, Hunt LP, Warwick F. Relationship betwwen pancreatic exocrine function and ductal morphology in chronic pancreatitis. *Gastroenterol* 1982; 82:1341–7.

33. Girwood AH, Hatfield ARW, Bornman PC, Denyer ME, Kottler R, Marks IN. Structure and function in non-calcific pancreatitis. *Am J Dig Dis* 1984; 29:721–6.

34. Salmon PR, Baddley H, Machado G, Low–Beer T, Rhys-Davies E, Trapnell J. Endoscopic pancreatography, scintigraphy and exocrine function in pancreatitis: a comparative study. *Gut* 1975; 16:830.

35. Seligson L, Che JW, Ihre T, Lundh G, Pyk E. Evaluation of the diagnosis of pancreatitis. *Scand J Gastroenterol* 1982; 17:905–11.

36. Ashton MG, Axon ATR, Lintott DJ. Lundh test and ERCP in pancreatic disease. *Gut* 1978;19:910–15.

37. Elsborg L, Bruusgaard A, Strangaard L, Reinicke V. Endoscopic retrograde pancreatography and the exocrine pancreatic function in alcoholism. *Scand J Gastroenterol* 1981; 16:941–4.

38. Deviere J, Gulbis B, Delhaye M, Quenon M, Cremer M. Relation entre la morphologie canalaire et la fonction exocrine du pancréas: une méthode originale d'estimation linéaire de la fonction pancréatique. *Acta Endosc* 1985; 15:1–12.

39. Bozkurt T, Braun U, Lefrinks S, Gilly G, Lux G. Comparison of pancreatic morphology and exocrine functinal impairment in patients with chronic pancreatitis. *Gut* 1994; 35:1132–6.

40. Dominguez-Munoz JE, Manes G, Peramico O, Buchler M, Malfertheiner P. Effect of pancreatic ductal changes on exocrine function in chronic pancreatitis. *Pancreas* 1995; 10:31–5.

41. Dominguez-Munoz JE, Hieronymus C, Sauerbruch T, Malfertheiner P. Accuracy of the fecal elastase test (FET) for the diagnosis of chronic pancreatitis. *Gut* 1995; 37:A130.

42. Loser CHR, Molgaard A, Folsch UR. Fecal elastase 1: An easy, inexpensive and highly sensitive and specific tubeless routine test in pancreatic insuficiency. *Gut* 1995; 37:A140.

43. Brugge WR, Burke CA. Lactoferrin secretion in alcoholic pancreatic disease. *Dig Dis Sci* 1988; 33:178–84.

44. Bernard JP, Barthet M, Gharib BB *et al*. Quantification of human lithostatin by high performance liquid chromatography. *Gut* 1995; 36:630–6.

10

Pancreatic cancer

Antonio Russo, Clara Virgilio & Francesco Russo

INTRODUCTION

The pancreas is one of the intra-abdominal organs that is most difficult to study with non-invasive tests. Imaging by ultrasonography (US) and computed tomography (CT) scan have relatively low sensitivity for the correct diagnosis of pancreatic disease[1-4] and frequently need the use of invasive methods. While in the future magnetic resonance imaging (MRI)[5-11] or positron emission tomography[12] may add significantly to the diagnostic potential of non-invasive imaging modalities, at present endoscopic retrograde cholangiopancreatography (ERCP) is often the best next step in the confirmation of pathological CT scans or in the clarification of uncertain images[13].

For neoplastic diseases of the pancreas the diagnostic potential of ERCP consists in visualizing either the main pancreatic duct (MPD) or the secondary branches. Eighty per cent of pancreatic neoplasms arise from the MPD, and the 20% arising peripherally from the side branches or acini eventually compress or alter the MPD. Therefore, less than 3% of patients with pancreatic cancer have a normal pancreatogram[14,15].

There are three limitations to the sensitivity of ERCP in the diagnosis of pancreatic cancer. ERCP has a high diagnostic accuracy, especially for neoplasms that are already clinically suspected[1]; the sensitivity and specificity are 94% and 97%, respectively; and the positive/negative predictive values are 83% and 99%[16]. Lesions arising in the pancreatic tail, the uncinate process and around the duct of Santorini can grow quite large before compressing the MPD or common bile duct (CBD) and causing symptoms[17]. A definitive diagnosis of malignancy cannot be made strictly from radiographs, but must depend on tissue sampling by cytological or histological means[18,19].

Despite these drawbacks, since the majority of pancreatic cancers begin in the main ducts, ERCP provides, for pancreatic neoplasms < 2cm in diameter, a correct diagnosis in 94.1% of patients with jaundice and in 100% of patients without jaundice[20,21].

ENDOSCOPIC DIAGNOSIS OF PANCREATIC CANCER

Gastroduodenoscopy

Before visualizing the ducts with pancreatography, careful endoscopic examination of the stomach, duodenal C-loop, papilla, and periampullary areas must be carried out to look for secondary changes of pancreatic neoplasia[22-24]. In the stomach, pancreatic neoplasia must be considered in the presence of fundic varices (secondary to thrombosis of the splenic vein), or compression or rigidity of the posterior wall

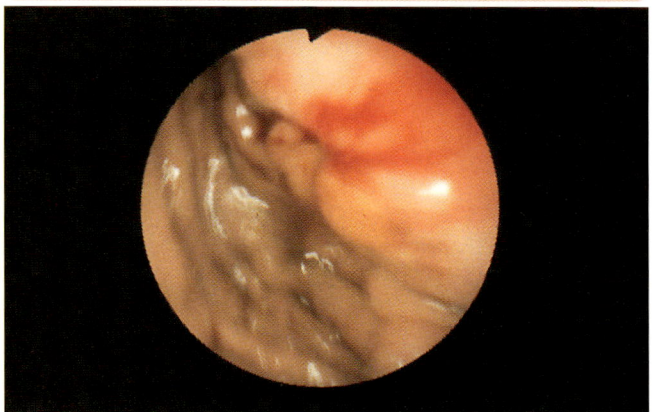

Figure 10.1 Pancreatic carcinoma. Endoscopic view, showing compression and submucosal invasion of the posterior wall of the gastric body.

of the antrum and body, especially associated with central ulceration (Figure 10.1). In the duodenum, tumour infiltration at the apex of the bulb or descending duodenum is seen when the neoplasm arises in the head of the pancreas[25]. In these situations biopsy or aspiration on biopsy[26] of abnormal mucosa is recommended. Compression or infiltration is seen in the transverse duodenum and the ligament of Treitz[25] when the tumour arises from the uncinate process or the body of the pancreas.

ERCP

The radiological diagnosis of pancreatic cancer is manifest by alterations in the morphology of the pancreatic duct, main duct and side branches. These pancreatoductal lesions may be seen alone or in association with parenchymal and/or common bile duct alterations.

Morphology of pancreatic ducts

The alterations of the MPD and the second- and third-order side branches from pancreatic cancer vary with the site or origin of the neoplasm and the size of the mass[16,23]. In the past these variations led to the development of several classification schemes[13,25,27-30]. One of these[30] divides the pancreatographic images into five major types (Figure 10.2). Figure 10.3 shows the prevalence of the various morphological contours of the pancreatic duct seen in 129 cases of pancreatic neoplasia.

Stenosis: Stenosis of the MPD is one of the most common abnormalities seen with pancreatic cancer[24,25]. The stenosed ductal segment varies in length.

Figure 10.2 Pancreatographic images in pancreatic carcinoma.

Stenosis
Complete obstruction
   abrupt
   tapering type ('rat tail')
Side branch deviation
Cyst formation

Figure 10.3 Prevalence of abnormal ERP findings in pancreatic carcinoma.

ERP finding	n	%
Stenosis	65	50.2
Complete obstruction	54	
abrupt	34	26.4
tapering	20	15.3
Side branch deviation	8	6.2
Cyst formation	2	1.9
Total	**183**	**100.0**

Strictures longer than 10mm are generally of malignant aetiology (Figure 10.4), whereas strictures shorter than 10mm are likely to be benign[31]. Data from neoplasia diagnosed in an advanced stage show a correlation between the length of the stricture and the size of the neoplastic mass[32]. In advanced diseases the contour of the lumen in the narrowed zone is generally irregular, nodular and eccentric (Figure 10.5). Typically, the MPD downstream (toward the papilla) from the neoplasm is normal (Figure 10.6) whereas the upstream duct is uniformly dilated. Secondary branches around the neoplastic area are decreased in number, absent, distorted, or displaced. Early or small neoplasms cause only minimal ductal narrowing and are therefore difficult to diagnose correctly (Figure 10.7). Rarely in early lesions the MPD appears normal, but subtle compression from adjacent neoplasm may cause delayed drainage of contrast medium from the upstream duct, as seen on delayed films.

It must be taken into account that a pancreatic tumour set in the region of the accessory pancreatic duct, which is in close proximity to the intrapancreatic portion of the CBD, may cause biliary obstruction but no abnormalities in the MPD[33]. Care must be taken during ductography to visualize completely the accessory ductal system to avoid missing lesions[34–36]. Occasionally this requires supplemental ductography via the minor papilla.

Figure 10.4 Pancreatic carcinoma. Pancreatography shows a long stenosis of the MPD, acinarization downstream from the neoplasia and absence of secondary branches around the neoplastic area.

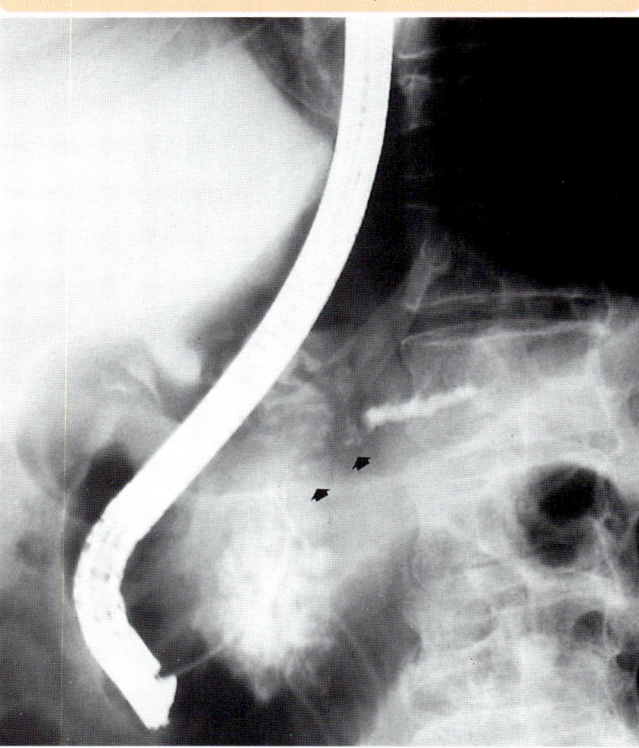

Figure 10.5 Pancreatic carcinoma: stenosis of the MPD. The lumen downstream from the neoplasia is regular; absence of secondary branches around the narrowed segment; dilatation of the duct upstream of the stenosis.

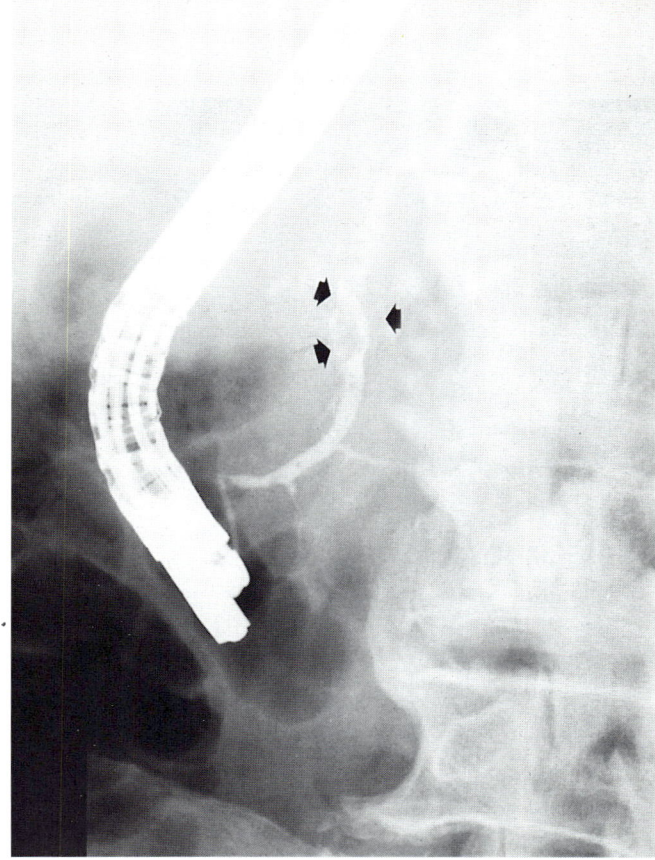

Figure 10.6 Pancreatic carcinoma: stenosis of the MPD. The lumen in the narrowed zone is irregular and eccentric and there is a small focal dye collection around the stricture.

Figure 10.7 Pancreatic carcinoma: stenosis of the MPD with uniformly dilated duct upstream of the neoplasia. The secondary branches around the neoplastic area are decreased in number. (Courtesy of G.Lehman.)

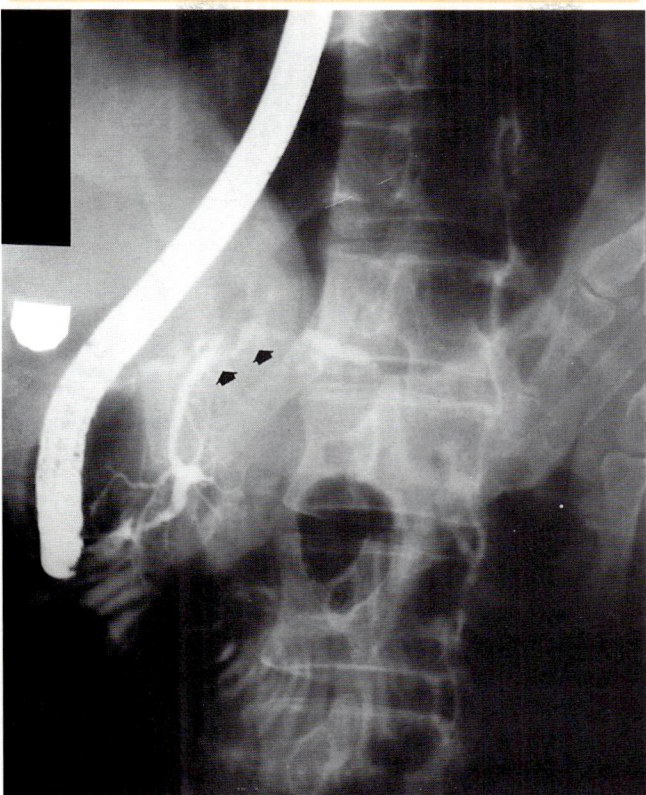

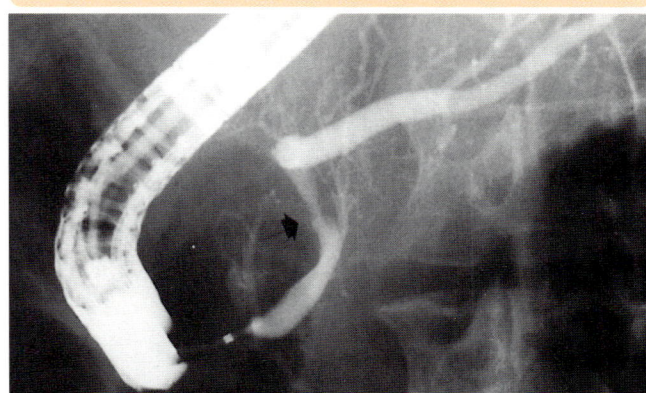

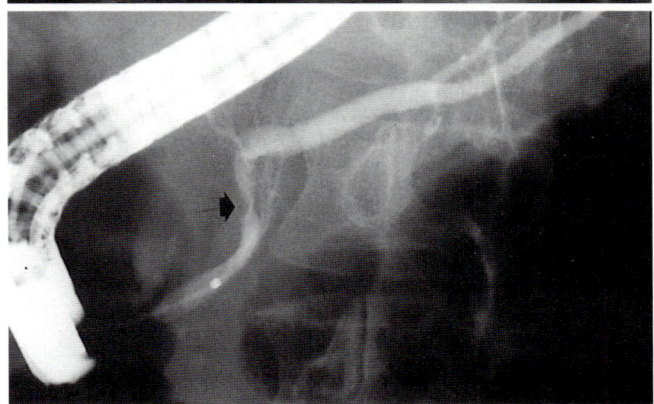

Figure 10.8 Pancreatic carcinoma. The MPD is abruptly and totally obstructed (cut-off). The occlusion is irregular and 'mouse-bitten'. Downstream from the obstruction the duct is normal and the side branches are filled with a generous amount of contrast medium.

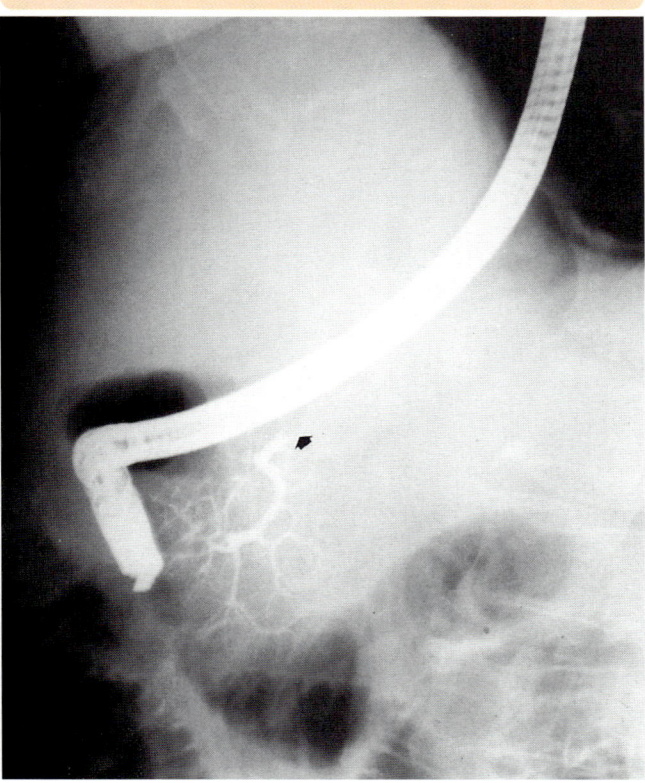

Obstruction: Obstruction is a result of the natural progression of a stricture and is one of the more common and typical lesions seen in a neoplastic pancreatic duct[14,37,38]. An obstructed duct is more frequently observed in neoplasms at the head of the pancreas. It may appear either as an abrupt cut-off or as a termination seated at the end of a constantly narrowed segment (tapered type or rat-tail stenosis). In the abrupt occlusion the main duct between the papilla and the narrowing is generally normal. The narrowed segment is typically irregular or sawtooth (Figure 10.8). In this situation, before making a diagnosis of neoplasm, care must be taken to assure an adequate injection volume of contrast medium and the absence of unintentional air bubbles[39]. To reduce the number of interpretive errors it is mandatory that the ERCP be performed using optimal technique, with attention focused on the morphology of the stricture and the secondary branches near the narrowing, as well as downstream[34,40]. Downstream side branches generally fill with a generous amount of contrast medium, even to the point of acinarization as the contrast medium follows the route of least resistance into these branches.

The secondary ducts near the stricture are absent, compressed or displaced and occasionally show small cystic dilatation. When the neoplastic occlusion occurs very near the major papilla the visualized ductal system may mimic a ventral pancreas or pancreas divisum. This situation can be clarified by cannulating the accessory papilla. If a full dorsal ductogram is obtainable, the patient probably has pancreas divisum; if the dorsal ductogram is cut off in the region corresponding to the head of the gland, a neoplasm is strong-

Figure 10.9 Pancreatic carcinoma. There is a tapering-type complete obstruction present. Secondary branches are present downstream from the occlusion. There is parenchymal staining with small dye collections around the tapered segment.

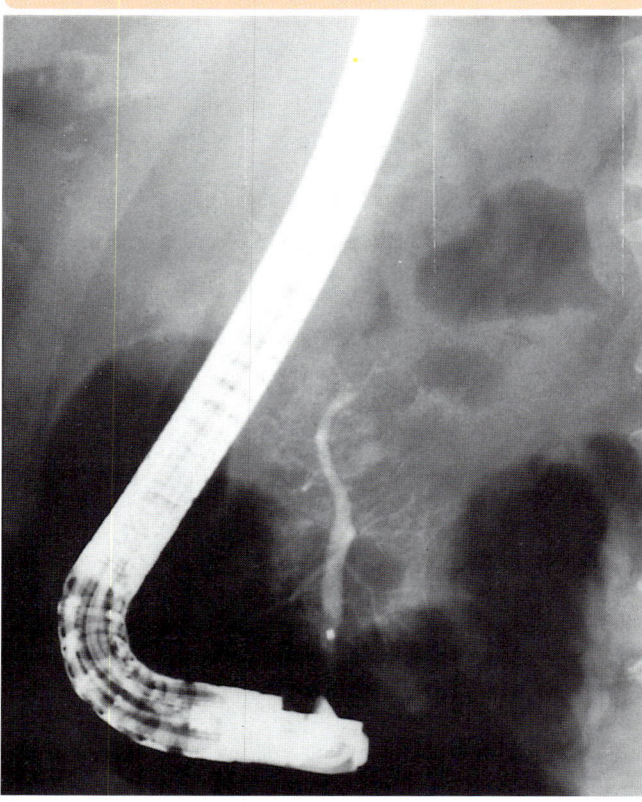

Figure 10.10 Pancreatic carcinoma: pancreatographic appearance of cyst formation.

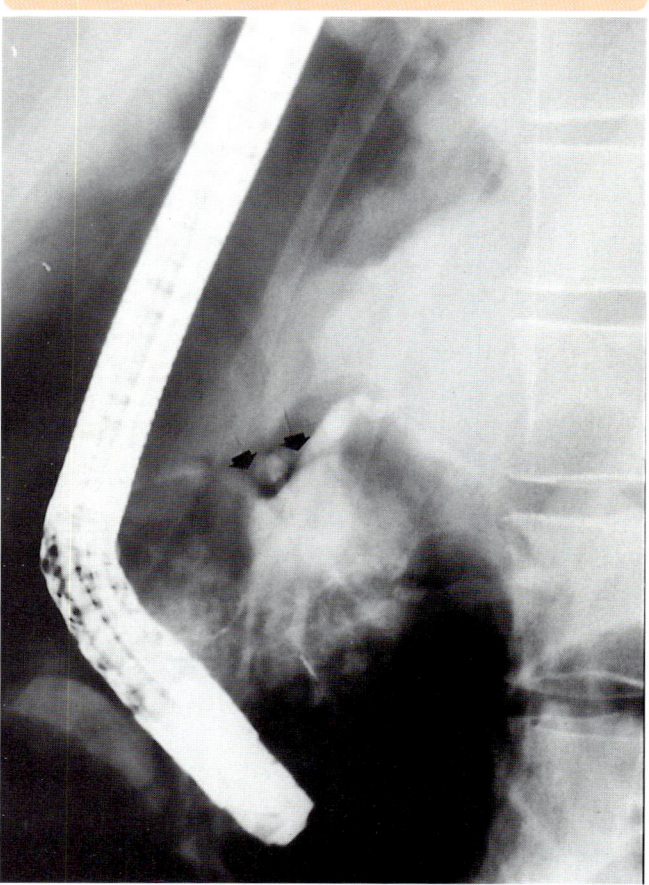

ly suggested. In the rat-tail form (Figure 10.9), the MPD tapers terminally, progressively to the point of complete occlusion. The abnormal segment of the duct appears scirrhous and thin. Secondary branches are preserved in the downstream duct, but diminish in number and finally disappear at the point of cut-off. Parenchymal staining with small focal dye collections is occasionally seen in the tapered segment. The tapering-type pancreatic duct may be related to the peripheral growth of neoplasms that lead to progressive invasion of the MPD.

Side branch changes: Pancreatic neoplasia growing from the ducts of the second and third order, and rare acinar cell neoplasia[41], undergo morphological changes initially evident only if visualized by detailed side branch ductography or even parenchymatography. The absence of side branches over a short segment combined with distortion of these branches in adjacent areas is strongly suggestive of a neoplastic lesion[30]. Only later, after further neoplastic invasion, may the MPD appear displaced, twisted or angulated. When parenchymatography is obtained (intentionally or unintentionally), the neoplasia appears as a large filling defect within the more normal parenchymal filling. Neoplastic lesions on the peripheral pancreatic ducts can be identified if complete filling of side branches occurs; attention must be paid to avoiding technical errors that lead to side branch incomplete filling[34].

Cyst formation: Approximately 2–5% of pancreatic neoplasms have a pancreatographic appearance of cyst formation[13,14]. The cyst generally represents an area of necrotic neoplasm that communicates with an excretory duct[14]. The collection of contrast medium assumes an amorphous contour (Figure 10.10) as it fills the interstices of the irregular necrotic cavity[28]. The margins of the cystic cavity are generally irregular and indistinct.

The differential diagnosis of such cystic lesions includes pancreatic abscess, pseudocyst and cystic tumours. If the outer contour of the cystic structure is smooth and regular and precisely defined, this suggests a pseudocyst, though in pancreatic abscess the margins are very similar. The clinical presentation will help differential diagnosis.

Cystic tumours (serous microcystic and mucinous macrocystic neoplasms) account for approximately 1% of pancreatic malignancies[42,43] and often are confused with benign pancreatic cysts[44]. The majority of tumours do not communicate with the pancreatic ducts[45,46] and therefore the pancreatographic appearance depends on the relationship between the tumour and the pancreatic ducts[36]. If the tumour is peripheral and small the ductogram will be normal. If the tumour is large, displacement or compression of the MPD and side branches will be seen.

At the point of the cystic lesion seen by non-invasive imaging (CT scan), the MPD may appear narrowed or displaced. Aggressive cystic neoplasms that invade the MPD

Figure 10.11 Mucinous ductal ectasia. Duodenoscopic view, showing mucus exuding through the enlarged papillary orifice.

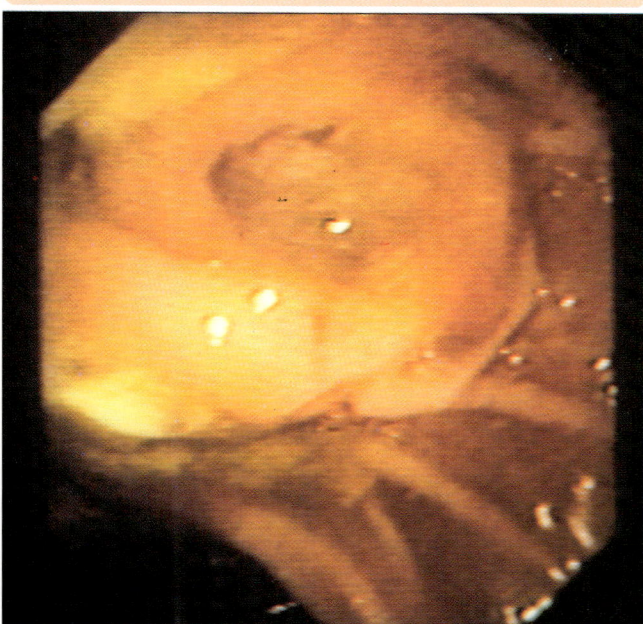

may cause frank obstruction, or strictures, or other distortions described above for adenocarcinoma.

Mucinous ductal ectasia[47], termed in reports with an emphasis on pathology as intraductal papillary mucinous neoplasm[48,49], represents a distinct subset of the mucinous type of cystic pancreatic tumour. The diagnosis is commonly made by duodenoscopy, as the major and minor papilla orifices may be dilated and a clear or milky mucus may ooze (Figure 10.11) from these orifices[49–51].

Pancreatography shows either dilated side branches of the MPD limited to the uncinate process (Figure 10.12) or diffuse dilatation and cystic appearance of the MPD and side branches (Figure 10.13). Filling defects are generally present within the dilated ducts, corresponding either to tumour nodules or to mucinous material[36,45,50–52].

Thick mucus may give the appearance of complete duct cut-off; the passage of a guide wire up through the mucus, and further extraction of mucus with a balloon, permit a detailed ductography which shows the correct diagnosis[50].

Common bile duct

A close anatomical relationship between the CBD and the head of the pancreas helps explain the observation that 90%

Figure 10.12 Mucinous ductal ectasia. There is marked dilatation of the side branches of the MPD in the uncinate process. (Courtesy of G. Lehman.)

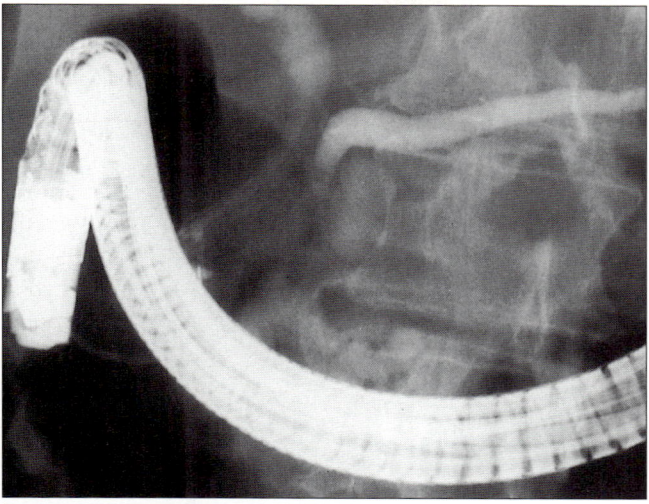

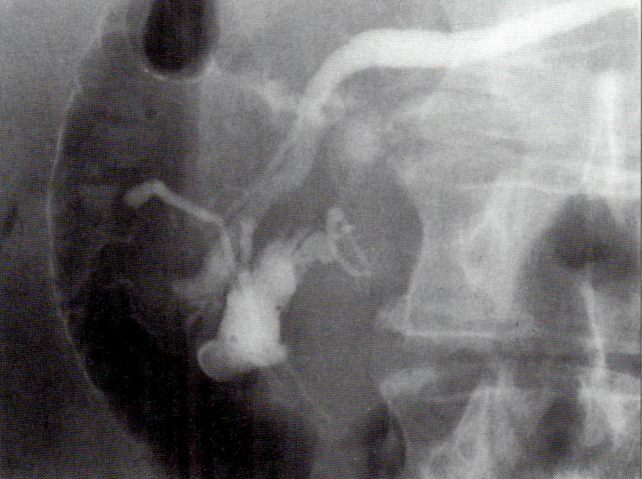

Figure 10.13 Mucinous ductal ectasia. The main duct and side branches are both dilated and cystic in appearance. (Courtesy of G. Lehman.)

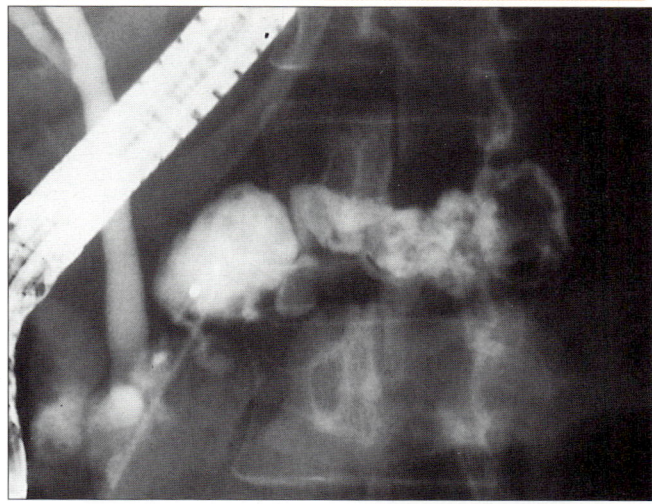

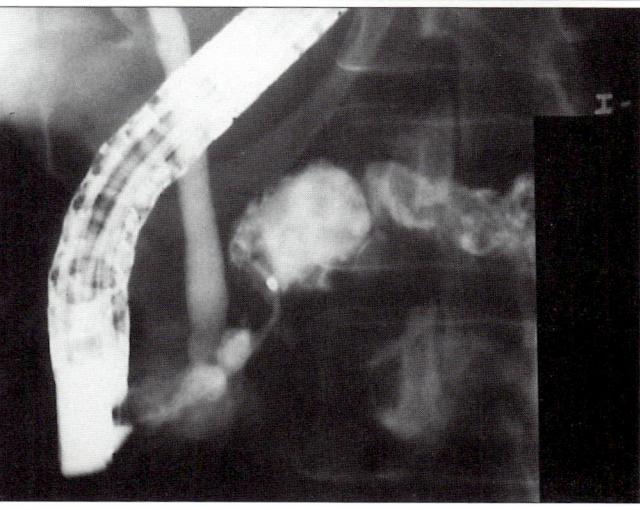

of pancreatic head cancers and a small portion of pancreatic body cancers present with obstructive jaundice. The CBD involvement on ERCP appears as a stricture, a compression, or a complete obstruction at the level of the superior margin of the pancreas[13–15,17]. A stricture (Figure 10.14) is the most frequent abnormality of the CBD seen on ERCP in the presence of pancreatic head cancer.

Stenosis: The stricture is generally intrapancreatic and may appear simply as a narrowing or with additional angulation or deviation from mass effect[23]. The stricture may be of variable length, from a few millimetres to the involvement of the entire intrapancreatic segment of duct. The margin of the stricture is abrupt or tapered and the luminal contour within the stricture is variably smooth or irregular. The abrupt (shelved) contour at the upper margin strongly suggests a malignant process, whereas a more gradually tapered margin favours a benign process[13]. The upstream bile duct is virtually always dilated if the patient has been jaundiced for more than a few days. If the CBD narrowing shows non-specific changes, these must be interpreted in the light of the accompanying pancreatographic changes; the combination may point more strongly toward neoplasia[23].

If ERCP shows an apparent malignant stricture of the intrapancreatic portion of the CBD but pancreatography has failed, the aid of non-invasive images often helps to clarify the origin of the neoplasm; brush cytology of the bile duct is recommended[19]. It must be remembered that occasionally pancreatic neoplasms arising from the region of the accessory duct of Santorini present with neoplastic stenosis of the CBD but with a normal-appearing MPD. Less frequently the pancreatic mass will laterally compress the CBD in similar fashion to that seen with a pseudocyst and further studies are then needed to make the diagnosis.

Obstruction: When the CBD shows complete obstruction to the flow of contrast media this nearly always indicates malignant obstruction[16,29,36]. The neoplastic obstruction is usually abrupt (shelved, square-edged, blunt) and irregular, nodular, encased or eccentric[23].

One of the most specific signs of pancreatic cancer is the 'double duct sign', defined as a stricture (Figure 10.15) or obstruction of the MPD and the contiguous portion of the intrapancreatic CBD[53,54].

The two ducts are normal in their downstream portions for a variable length, varying with the site of the tumour origin. The double duct sign *per se* is not disease-specific and may be seen in benign or malignant diseases[53]. However, if frank

Figure 10.14 Pancreatic carcinoma: cholangiographic pattern. There is irregular stricture of the main bile duct, which is dilated upstream of the stenosis.

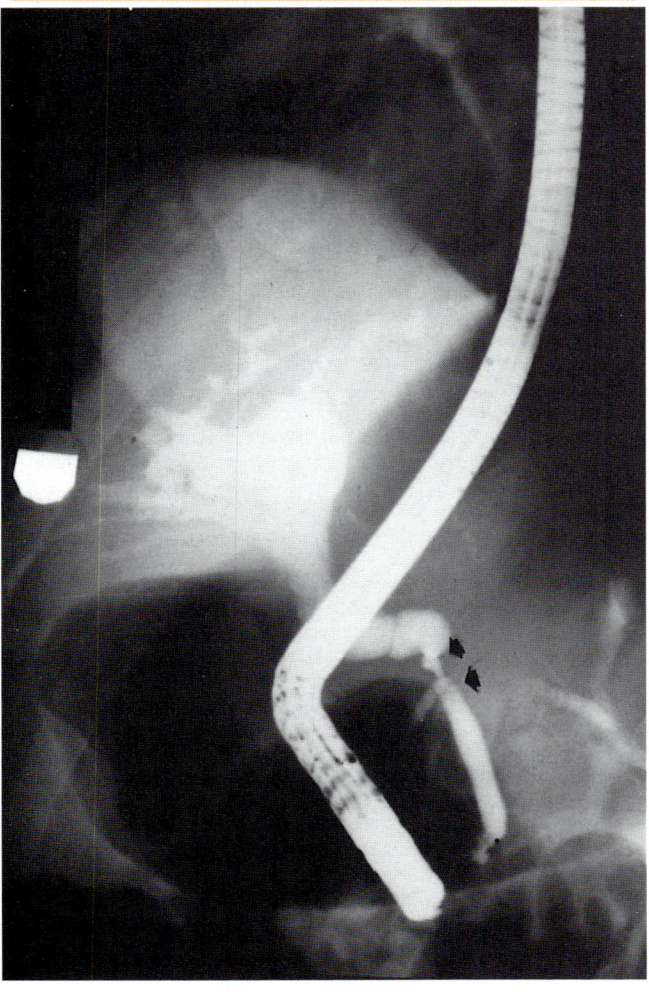

Figure 10.15 Pancreatic carcinoma: 'double duct' sign. There is stricture of both the MPD and the contiguous portion of the intrapancreatic CBD. The MPD is normal downstream from the stenosis and uniformly dilated upstream of the neoplastic area.

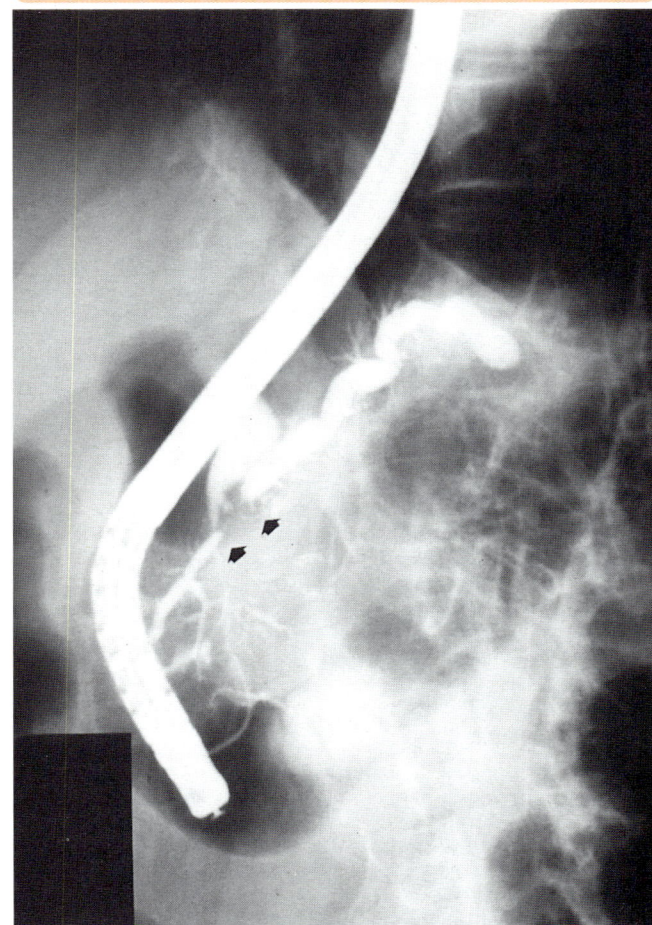

obstruction is seen in both the ducts (Figure 10.16) a neo-plastic disease should be strongly suspected.

Brush cytology and biopsy are needed to establish the diagnosis. The distance between the two ducts in patients with a double duct sign is of some diagnostic value. In malignancy, the two ducts generally remain close to each other – at a distance of less than 10mm[54]. In benign disease this distance may increase to > 20mm.

CONCLUSION

CT scanning and ERCP are, at present, the main means of correctly diagnosing pancreatic neoplasia. Between the two imaging modalities, however, ductography represents the gold standard – even if radiographic images should be supported, when possible, by cytologic or bioptic validations.

This invasive diagnostic approach, still considered by many clinicians to be a prerequisite to surgical intervention, is losing value for two main reasons. The first reason is that some surgeons believe that the results of ERCP rarely alter the mangement of the patient when a CT scan reveals a pancreatic mass [55–57]. It follows that ERCP should be reserved for a small subset of patients with a doubtful CT scan or when the clinical presentation is suggestive of pancreatic neoplasia but the CT scan is normal. The second reason, which could lead to a restricted use of ductography, is related to the development of MRI. As the use of MRI eventually leads to a precise staging of neoplasia based on this technique [11,58], together with accurate diagnosis, ERCP could remain in use as a means of palliative treatment of inoperable tumours.

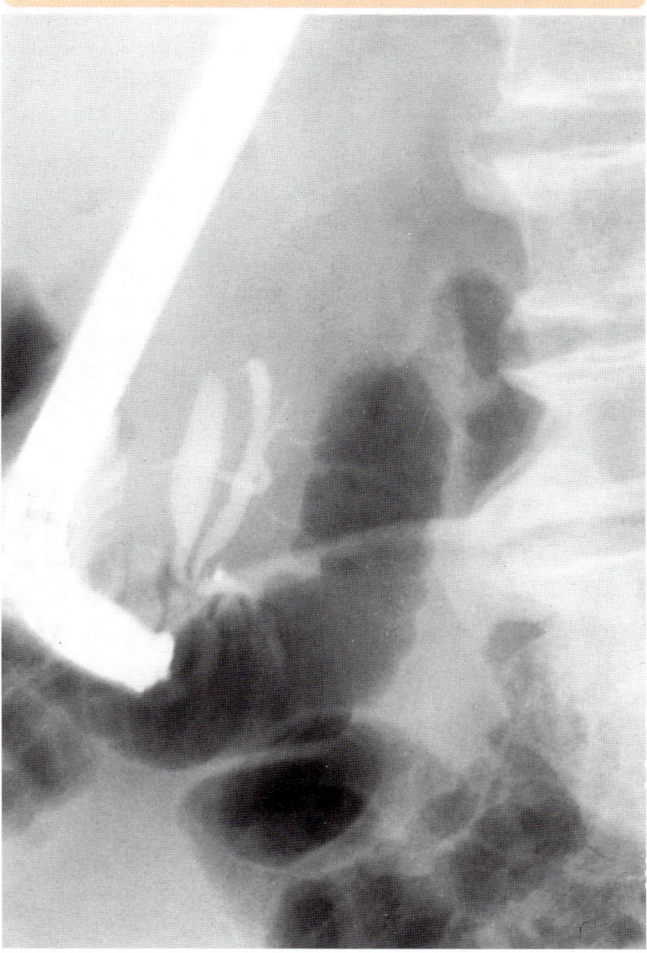

Figure 10.16 Pancreatic carcinoma: 'double duct sign'. There is complete obstruction of both the CBD and MPD.

References

1. Niederau C, Grendell JH. Diagnosis of pancreatic carcinoma. Imaging techniques and tumor markers. *Pancreas* 1992; 7:66–86.
2. Rosch T, Reinhard L, Braig C et al. Endoscopic ultrasound in pancreatic tumor diagnosis. *Gastrointest Endosc* 1991; 37:347–52.
3. Snady H, Cooperman A, Siegel J. Endoscopic ultrasonography compared with computed tomography with ERCP in patients with obstructive jaundice or small periampullary mass. *Gastrointest Endosc* 1992; 38:27–34.
4. Muller M, Meyerberger C, Bertshinger P, Scheer R, Marineck B. Pancreatic tumors: evaluation with endoscopic US, CT, and MR imaging. *Radiology* 1994; 190:745–51.
5. Morimoto K, Shimoi M, Shirakawa T et al. Biliary obstruction: evaluation with three-dimensional MR cholangiography. *Radiology* 1992; 183:578–80.
6. Hall-Craggs MA, Allen CM, Owens CM et al. MR cholangiography: clinical evaluation in 40 cases. *Radiology* 1993; 189:423–7.
7. Yshizaki Y, Wakayama T, Okada Y, Kobayashi T. Magnetic resonance cholangiography for evaluation of obstructive jaundice. *Am J Gastroenterol* 1993; 88:2072–7.
8. McKee J, Chuttani R, Barish M et al. Magnetic resonance cholangiopancreatography (MRCP): a noninvasive test for pancreas divisum. *Gastrointest Endosc* 1996; 43:410.
9. McAndrew P, Maniatis A, Jowell P et al. A comparison of magnetic resonance cholangiopancreatography (MRCP) and ERCP in the evaluation of chronic pancreatitis. *Gastrointest Endosc* 1996; 43:388.
10. Takasu A, Arakura T, Shinoregawa T. Application of magnetic resonance cholangiopancreatography to pancreatic disease. *Digestion* 1996; 57:269.
11. Soto JA, Barish M, Yucel EK et al. Magnetic resonance cholangiography: comparison with endoscopic retrograde cholangiopancreatography. *Gastroenterology* 1996; 110:589–97.
12. Staib L, Gaurange F, Stollfuss J et al. Pancreatic cancer or pancreatitis? Diagnostic value of positron-emission-tomography. *Digestion* 1995; 56:322.
13. Kawai K, Yasuda K, Nakajima M. Endoscopic diagnosis of cancer of the pancreas. In *Gastroenterologic Endoscopy*. Edited by MV Sivak Jr. WB Saunders, Philadelphia. 1987; 821–38.
14. Freeny P, Lawson T. *Radiology of the Pancreas*. Springer-Verlag, New York. 1982.
15. Silvis S, Rohrmann C, Vennes J. Diagnostic accuracy of endoscopic retrograde cholangiopancreatography in hepatic biliary and pancreatic malignancy. *Ann Intern Med* 1976; 84:438–40.
16. Freeny P, Ball T. Endoscopic retrograde cholangiopancreatography (ERCP) and percutaneous transhepatic cholangiography (PTC) in the evaluation of suspected pancreatic carcinoma. Diagnostic limitations and contemporary roles. *Cancer* 1981; 47:1666–78.
17. Stewart E, Vennes J, Geenen J. *Atlas of Endoscopic Retrograde Cholangiopancreatography*. Mosby, St Louis. 1977.
18. Haseman J, Lehman GA, Howes R, Sherman S. The sensitivity of ERCP in the diagnosis of pancreatic adenocarcinoma. *Gastrointest Endosc* 1993; 39:317 (abstract).

19. Lehman GA. Application of ERCP and endoscopic tissue sampling techniques in the detection of pancreatic neoplasms. *Int J Pancreatol* 1994; 16:264–8.
20. Tsuchiya R, Noda T, Harada N *et al*. Collective review of small carcinomas of the pancreas. *Ann Surg* 1986; 205:77–81.
21. Ariyama J, Suyama M, Satoh K. Role of endoscopy in the diagnosis of small pancreatic ductal adenocarcinoma. *Dig Endosc* 1994; 6:371–8.
22. Kawanishi H, Pallard M. Endoscopic evaluation of cancer of pancreas. *Semin Oncol* 1979; 6:309–17.
23. Nix G, Van Overbeeke I, Wilson J, Ten Kate F. ERCP diagnosis of tumors in the region of the head of the pancreas. Analysis of criteria and computer-aided diagnosis. *Dig Dis Sci* 1988; 33:577–86.
24. Calleja G, Barkin JS. Neoplastic conditions of the pancreatic ducts. In *Text and Atlas of ERCP*. Edited by S Silvis, C Rohrmann, HJ Ansel. Igaku-Shoin, Tokyo. 1994; 361-83.
25. Stadelmann O, Safrany L, Loffler A *et al*. Endoscopic retrograde cholangiopancreatography in the diagnosis of pancreatic cancer. *Endoscopy* 1974; 6:84–93.
26. Tsuchiya R, Hemmi T, Kouda N *et al*. Endoscopic aspiration biopsy of the pancreas. *Gastroenterology* 1977; 73:1050–3.
27. Anacker H, Weiss HD, Kramann B. The ERCP in lesions of the pancreas and the papilla duodeni. In *Endoscopic Retrograde Pancreatico-Cholangiography (ERCP)*. Edited by H Anacker, HD Weiss, B Kramann. Springer-Verlag, Berlin. 1977; 56–96.
28. Ogoshi K. Diseases of the pancreas and the biliary system. In *Endoscopic Retrograde Cholangiopancreatography*. Edited by T Takemoto, T Kasugai. Igaku-Shoin, Tokyo. 1979; 159–76.
29. Testoni PA, Tittobello A. Colangiopancreatografia retrograda (ERCP). Criteri radiologici di diagnostica differenziale. In *Il Cancro del Pancreas Esocrino*. Officine Grafiche Garzanti, Milano. 1989; 85–104.
30. Huibregtse K, Tytgat GNJ. Endoscopic retrograde cholangiopancreatography (ERCP). In *Hepatobiliary and Pancreatic Malignancies. Diagnosis, Medical and Surgical Management*. Edited by NJ Lygidakis, GNJ Tytgat. Georg Thieme Verlag, Stuttgart. 1989; 100–14.
31. May G, Gardiner R. *Clinical Imaging of the Pancreas*. Raven Press, New York. 1987.
32. Shah S, Movson J, Ransil B, Waxman I. ERCP findings correlate with tumor size in patients with resectable pancreatic cancer. *Am J Gastroenterol* 1995; 90:1612 (abstract).
33. Kowdley K, Variyam E, Sivak M. Obstructive jaundice caused by pancreatic carcinoma in the setting of a normal pancreatogram. *Gastrointest Endosc* 1995; 41:158–60.
34. Fink A, Ayale V, Chapman M, Cotton PB. Radiologic pitfalls in endoscopic retrograde pancreatography. *Pancreas* 1986; 1:180–7.
35. Lough LR, Vincent LM, Rohrmann CA. Distortion of pancreatic anatomy during ERCP. Effect of patient position and endoscopic manipulation. *Am J Gastroenterol* 1989; 84:1122.
36. Liguory C, Lefebvre JF. Retrograde pancreatography. Technical tips and spectrum of pathology. *Gastrointest Endosc Clin N Am* 1995; 5:81–104.
37. Kruse A, Thommesen P, Frederiksen P. Endoscopic retrograde cholangio-pancreatography in pancreatic cancer and chronic pancreatitis. Differences in morphologic changes in the pancreatic duct and the bile duct. *Scand J Gastroenterol* 1978; 13:513–17.
38. Reuben A, Cotton PB. Endoscopic retrograde cholangiopancreatography in carcinoma of the pancreas. *Surg Gynecol Obstet* 1979; 148:179–84.
39. Taylor AJ, Carmody TJ, Schmalz MJ *et al*. Filling defects in the pancreatic duct on endoscopic retrograde pancreatography. *Am J Radiol* 1992; 159:1203.
40. Jowell PS. Assessment of pancreatic duct strictures. *Gastrointest Endosc Clin N Am* 1995; 5:125–43.
41. Kaufman A, Sivak M, Ferguson R. Endoscopic retrograde cholangiopancreatography in pancreatic islet cell tumors. *Gastrointest Endosc* 1988; 34:47–52.
42. Hodgkinson D, Remine W, Weiland L. Pancreatic cyst adenoma: a clinicopathologic study of 45 cases. *Arch Surg* 1978; 113:512–19.
43. Yamaguchi K, Enjoji M. Cystic neoplasms of the pancreas. *Gastroenterology* 1987; 92:1934–43.
44. Warshaw A, Ruthedge P. Cystic tumors mistaken with pancreatic pseudocysts. *Ann Surg* 1987; 205:393–8.
45. Warshaw A. Mucinous cystic tumors and mucinous ductal ectasia of the pancreas. *Gastrointest Endosc* 1991; 37:199–200.
46. Delcenserie R, Dupas J, Joly J *et al*. Microcystic adenoma of the pancreas demonstrated by endoscopic retrograde pancreatography. *Gastrointest Endosc* 1988; 34:52–4.
47. Itai Y, Ohhashi K, Nagai H *et al*. Ductatatic mucinous cystoadenoma and cystoadenocarcinoma of the pancreas. *Radiology* 1986; 161:697–700.
48. Sessa F, Solcia E, Capella C *et al*. intraductal papillary-mucinous tumors represent a distinct group of pancreatic neoplasms: an investigation of tumour cell differentiation n K-ras, p53 and c-erb B-2 abnormalities in 26 patients. *Virschows Arch* 1994; 425:357-367.
49. Loftus E, Olivares-Pakzad B, Batts K *et al*. Intraductal papillary-mucinous tumors of the pancreas: clinico-pathologic features, outcome, and nomenclature. *Gastroenterology* 1996; 110:1909–18.
50. Nickl N, Lawson M, Cotton PB. Mucinous pancreatic tumors: ERCP findings. *Gastrointest Endosc* 1991; 37:133–8.
51. Bastid C, Bernard J, Sarles H, Payan M, Sahel J. Mucinous ductal criteria of the pancreas: a premalignant disease and a cause of obstructive pancreatitis. *Pancreas* 1991; 6:15–22.
52. Dabezies M, Campana T, Friedman A. ERCP in the diagnosis of ductectatic mucinous cystadenocarcinoma of the pancreas. *Gastrointest Endosc* 1990; 36:410–11.
53. Freeny P, Bilbao M, Katon R. Blind evaluation of endoscopic retrograde cholangiopancreatography (ERCP) in the diagnosis of pancreatic carcinoma: the "double duct" and other signs. *Radiology* 1976; 119:271–4.
54. Plumley TF, Rohrmann CA, Freeny PC, Silverstein FE, Ball TJ. Double duct sign: reassessed significance in ERCP. *Am J Radiol* 1982; 138:31–5.
55. Alvarez C, Livingston EH, Ashley SW, Schwarz M, Reber HA. Cost-benefit analysis of the work-up for pancreatic cancer. *Am J Surg* 1993; 165:53–60.
56. Tmedum T, Sarr M, Douglas M, Farnell M. An argument against routine percutaneous biopsy ERCP, or biliary stent placement in patients with clinically resectable periampullary masses: a surgical perspective. *Pancreas* 1995; 11:283–8.
57. Chang AC, Kovacs BJ, McCracken JD, Walter MH, Chen YK. How good is ERCP in the diagnosis of pancreatic cancer with normal or atypical CT findings? *Am J Gastroenterol* 1995; 90:188 (abstract).
58. Di Magno E. Preoperative staging of pancreatic ductal cancer in USA. *Int J Pancreatol* 1994; 16:112–14.

Cystic neoplasms

Khay G. Yeoh & Robert H. Hawes

INTRODUCTION

Cystic neoplasms comprise approximately 10% of all cystic lesions of the pancreas[1–3], while an estimated 90% are benign pseudocysts and other types of cyst are uncommon [4] (Figure 11.1). These estimates are based on the literature and do not reflect the diagnostic impact of new technologies that have improved the quality of pancreatic imaging, including spiral (helical) computed tomography (CT), magnetic resonance imaging (MRI), endoscopic retrograde cholangiopancreatography (ERCP) and endoscopic ultrasonography (EUS). Neoplastic cysts are not infrequently misdiagnosed as pseudocysts[5–7], however, the differentiation is important because management is radically different. The treatment for symptomatic pseudocysts is drainage whereas neoplastic cysts generally require resection. Experience with these new technologies has provided some useful pointers helpful in differentiating neoplastic cysts from benign pseudocysts. The importance of an early and accurate diagnosis of cystic neoplasm lies in the fact that resection can be curative if performed before local invasion or metastasis has occurred [8].

TYPES OF CYSTIC NEOPLASM

Cystic neoplasms of the pancreas are true cysts and are lined by epithelium, in contrast to pseudocysts, which are cystic cavities lacking an epithelial lining. Pseudocysts are filled with amylase-rich fluid and are surrounded by a fibrous encapsulating wall, whereas cystic tumours contain amylase-poor fluid and are lined by epithelium. The main types of cystic tumour of the pancreas are mucinous cystic neoplasms, serous cystadenoma and mucinous ductal ectasia.

Mucinous cystic neoplasms

Mucinous cystic neoplasms (MCNs) are the commonest type of cystic tumour of the pancreas [1], ranging from benign (cystadenoma) to malignant (cystadenocarcinoma) lesions. They are usually large tumours with reported sizes ranging from 2–26cm in diameter, and occur mainly in the body and tail of the pancreas [1]. Cystadenocarcinomas are usually larger than cystadenomas. On cut section, they are seen to consist of multilocular cysts filled with thick haemorrhagic or mucous fluid. The cysts are lined with a mucin-producing columnar epithelium. Foci of calcification are often present in the tumour wall, and may be detected radiologically. They occur most frequently in women aged 40–60 years and often present as an abdominal mass with associated pain. There is a strong female preponderance, with a sex ratio of 6:1 in one large series [9]. Cystadenomas are premalignant lesions; biopsies are unreliable in differentiating malignant from benign

Figure 11.1 Cystic lesions of the pancreas.

Benign	Neoplastic
Congenital cysts	Mucinous cystadenoma and cystadenocarcinoma
Single cysts	Serous cystadenoma
Polycystic disease	Mucinous ductal ectasia
Acquired cysts	Papillary cystic epithelial neoplasm
Pseudocysts	Cystic islet cell tumor
	Hemangioma
	Lymphangioma
	Other cystic tumors

lesions because of the frequent concurrence of benign and malignant epithelium in the same tumour and the possibility of sampling error [6,10,11].

Therefore the treatment for all mucinous cystic neoplasms consists of total resection; good cure rates are achieved in the absence of spread.

Serous cystadenoma

Also called microcystic adenoma, serous cystadenoma (SCA) is the second commonest type of cystic tumour of the pancreas. SCAs are benign [4], large (mean diameter 10cm in a large series [12]) tumours composed of multiple tiny cysts with a sponge-like appearance on cross-section. There is often an irregular central stellate scar within the tumour that may contain calcification in a characteristic 'sunburst' pattern that could be a helpful radiological feature. SCAs have a profuse blood supply, which allows demonstration by angiography. The cysts are lined by cuboidal cells containing glycogen in the cytoplasm but little or no mucin. Tumours are found in elderly patients with a mean age of occurrence in the seventh decade and there is a slight female preponderance [4]. In an autopsy series of 34 cases, one third of individuals had been asymptomatic [12]. The most common symptom was abdominal pain or discomfort. A third of patients had tumours in the head of the pancreas and some presented with obstructive jaundice. Lewandrowski *et al.* described five cases of macrocystic SCA with simple cuboidal epithelium, and suggested that the term 'serous cystadenoma' be used instead of microcystic adenoma [13].

Mucinous ductal ectasia

Also known as intraductal papillary mucinous tumour, mucinous ductal ectasia (MDE) is an intraductal tumour [14,15] that

Figure 11.2   Clinical and ERP features in MDE.

Author (Ref)	n	Clinical characteristics			Predominant involvement				ERP features			
		Mean age (range) Sex M : F	Abd pain*	Amylase raised*	D	H	B	T	Gaping papilla	Mucin visible	Dilated MPD or SB	Filling defects
Itai et al. 1986 (53)	5	67 (57–72) 3:2	4 (80)	3 (60)	–	5	0	0	ND	ND	3 (60)	4 (80)
Loftus et al. 1996 (19)	15	68 (53–90) 11:4	11 (73)	5 (33)	6	6	1	2	2/10 (20)	2/10 (20)	10/10 (100)	7/10 (70)
Obara et al. 1991 (54)	9	68 (61–87) 6:3	5 (56)	4 (44)	–	6	2	1	8 (89)	3 (37)	9 (100)	9 (100)
Ohta et al. 1992 (18)	7	66 (54–71) 5:2	5 (71)	5 (71)	–	2	3	2	ND	ND	6 (86)	5 (71)
Rickaert et al. 1991 (15)	8	62 (47–85) 5:3	7 (88)	5 (63)	–	6	1	1	5 (63)	5 (63)	8 (100)	6 (75)
MUSC **	9	63 (39–85) 5:4	8 (89)	6 (67)	1	7	1	0	8 (89)	8 (89)	9 (100)	9 (100)

D = diffuse; H = head; B = body; T = tail; MPD = main pancreatic duct; SB = side-branch; ND = Not described
* Number, % in parentheses
** Digestive Disease Center, Medical University of South Carolina, unpublished data

has previously sometimes been confused with MCN [16]. More than 100 cases have been reported in the literature but its true prevalence is unknown because limited awareness and misdiagnosis as chronic pancreatitis or MCN has led to under-reporting [17]. We have seen nine cases from 1618 ERCPs performed in the past 2 years at our institution (Figure 11. 2). MDE is characterized by dilation and filling of the main pancreatic duct (MPD) or side branches with thick mucin, leading to obstruction and recurrent acute pancreatitis. Histology shows hyperplastic columnar epithelium in papillary arrangements that project into the duct. The epithelium may appear normal, or may exhibit atypia or frank carcinoma. MDE most frequently occurs in the head of the pancreas, predominantly in men in the sixth to seventh decade [14,18]. A history of intermittent episodes of abdominal pain or relapsing pancreatitis is common. Serum amylase levels may be raised [18]. MDE is regarded as a premalignant tumour [19] and therefore the recommended treatment is complete surgical resection of the lesion.

Other cystic tumours of the pancreas

Papillary cystic epithelial neoplasms are rare tumours, that occur in young women [20,21]. The tumours tend to be large, cystic and often haemorrhagic [22]. Histologically, tumour cells are arranged in either solid sheets or in papillae with fibrovascular cores projecting into cystic spaces. Mucin production is not prominent. The tumour usually presents as a progressively enlarging upper abdominal mass. It is usually slow growing and curable, but metastases and recurrence have been reported [4, 22].

Cystic degeneration may occur in pancreatic tumours that are normally solid. In a series of 130 cystic tumours of the pancreas, two were islet cell neoplasms [1]. Ductal adenocarcinomas may also undergo necrosis and cystic degeneration, and accounted for 6 of 50 cystic tumours in a series reported by Talamini et al. [23].

DIAGNOSIS AND DIFFERENTIATION FROM PSEUDOCYSTS

Differentiation of pseudocysts from cystic neoplasms (Figure 11.3) is critical because the management is radically different. While pseudocysts are usually treated using drainage and conservative measures, cystic neoplasms require resection, which carries a high rate of cure in the absence of invasion or metastases. Fernandez-del Castillo and Warshaw have summarized pointers useful in differentiating these lesions [1].

Clinical presentation

Patients with benign pseudocysts virtually always have a history consistent with acute or chronic relapsing pancreatitis. There is a male predominance and often a history of chronic alcohol abuse. Most cystic neoplasms occur in females with no history of alcoholic excess and no history of acute or chronic pancreatitis or trauma [2,5], with the exception of patients with MDE, who can present with acute or relapsing pancreatitis. Cystic neoplasms usually present with vague abdominal pain, weight loss and a palpable mass [2,11,23,24]. Serum amylase levels are elevated in 50–75% of patients with symptomatic pseudocysts but are usually normal in patients with cystic neoplasms, with the exception of MDE in which they may be intermittently elevated. Aspiration of cystic fluid may provide useful information (Figure 11.4). Pseudocyst contents are of low viscosity, rich in amylase and low in tumour markers, while fluid from MCNs is of high viscosity and has low amylase and high levels of carcinoembryonic antigen (CEA) [25,26]. CA 15-3 and CA 72-4 levels may be useful for differentiation of mucinous cystadenocarcinomas from benign neoplasms [27,28]. Cystic fluid cytology is useful in differentiating mucinous from non-mucinous pancreatic cysts and may provide evidence of malignancy [29]. An inflammatory smear without epithelial cells suggests a pseudocyst, but may also occur when a cystic neoplasm undergoes degenerative changes [29].

Figure 11.3 Differentiation of pseudocysts from cystic neoplasms of the pancreas.

	Pseudocysts	Cystic neoplasms
Demography	More frequent in males	More frequent in females (except MDE)
History of acute or chronic pancreatitis	Antecedent acute or chronic pancreatitis or trauma History of alcohol	No antecedent factors
Serum amylase	Elevated in majority	Normal, except with MDE
Cystic fluid	Fluid clear in SCA, mucoid in MCN	Fluid is opalescent, or may contain blood and necrotic debris
	High amylase content	Low amylase content
	Tumour markers low	Tumour markers may be elevated
	Cytology inflammatory	Cytology often positive
Imaging	Usually single cyst	Frequently multicystic
	No solid components in cyst	Solid components, septae, loculations are characteristic
	Calcification may be diffuse in CP	Focal calcification in tumor
ERCP *Communication with PD*	Communication in majority	No communication with ducts, except for MDE
Ductal system	Features of CP	No CP
Surgical findings	Thick wall with abnormal pancreas	Epithelial lining (may be discontinuous) Adjacent normal pancreas

MCN = mucinous cystic neoplasm; SCA = serous cystadenoma;
MDE = mucinous ductal ectasia; CP = chronic pancreatitis

Imaging

Plain radiographs may show an upper abdominal soft tissue mass and sometimes the presence of calcification within the tumour. Calcification is more frequent in SCA, in which it occurs centrally, often in a 'sunburst' pattern, whereas MCNs exhibit peripheral calcification.

Ultrasonography (US) findings of multiple cysts, internal septae or solid components within the cyst suggest a diagnosis of cystic neoplasm [30,31]. US of SCA usually shows a polycystic lobulated mass with a central hyperechoic zone. MCNs are large multilocular cystic masses, with internal septae and irregular cyst walls [21]. MDE is characterized by a markedly dilated MPD, that is often associated with parenchymal atrophy.

CT (Figure 11.5) is able to demonstrate calcification, the tumour wall and vascularity. In cystic neoplasms, the wall of the lesion may be calcified while the rest of the pancreas is normal; this is in contrast to pseudocysts, which may be accompanied by diffuse intraductal calcification associated with chronic pancreatitis. SCA are hypodense, encapsulated and lobulated masses that exhibit contrast enhancement. A central scar and sunburst calcification is characteristic but only seen in a minority of cases. MCN presents as a well encapsulated mass with large areas of low density. Dynamic scanning shows contrast enhancement of the cyst wall. The presence of solid tissue excrescences on CT correlated with a pathological diagnosis of cystadenocarcinoma in Friedman *et al.*'s series [32]. Warshaw reported that CT was useful in detection of cysts and in showing rim calcification but was not reliable in differentiating neoplasms from pseudocysts, serous tumours from mucinous tumours, or benign tumours from malignant tumours [6]. Johnson *et al.* suggested that the number of cysts within the tumour (more than six cysts in microcystic adenomas and six or fewer in MCN) and the diameter of the majority of cysts within the tumour (2cm for microcystic adenomas and >2cm for MCN) were useful criteria in distinguishing between microcystic adenoma and MCN [33].

MRI was considered by Minami *et al.* to be equal or slightly superior to CT in the diagnosis of pancreatic cystic neoplasms, with good demonstration of cystic content, septae, shape and wall thickness but not calcification [34]. MDE has also been demonstrated on MRI [35].

Angiography of cystic tumours may show hypervascularity, enlarged feeding arteries, tumour blush and neovascularity. SCA are characteristically hypervascular [20,21,32] but not invariably so [6]. Mucinous cystadenoma is usually hypovascular but cystadenocarcinoma may be hypervascular [6]. Angiography of pseudocysts shows avascularity and displacement of vessels without neovascularity or tumour blush [5,30.] In general, arteriography may be useful in the preoperative assessment of pancreatic resections but is generally not very useful in the differential diagnosis of the type of cystic tumour [6].

Cystic lesion	Viscosity	CEA	CA 15-3	CA 72-4	Amylase	Cytology
Pseudocyst	Low	Low	Low	Low	High	Inflammatory
Serous cystadenoma	Low	Low	Low	Low	Usually low	50% positive
Benign mucinous cystic neoplasm	Usually high	High	High	Low	Usually low	Usually positive
Mucinous cystadenocarcinoma	High	High	High	High	Usually low	Usually positive

Figure 11. 4 Cystic fluid markers useful in differential diagnosis.
Adapted from Fernandez-del Castillo and Warshaw [1] (with permission).

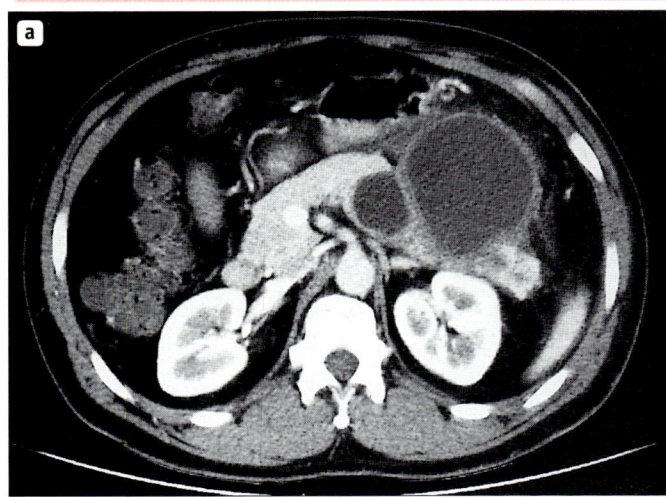
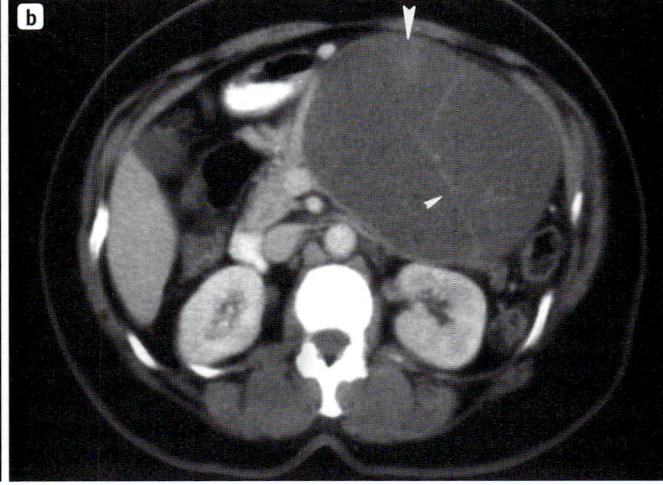

ERCP

ERCP is sensitive and accurate in diagnosing pancreatic disease and pancreatic malignancy [36–39] and is useful in the diagnosis of cystic neoplasm [40–43]. Because the pancreatogram reveals the presence of abnormalities in almost all patients with pseudocysts [44–46], pancreatography may help to differentiate pseudocysts from neoplastic cysts (Figure 11.6). In particular, ERCP is the best modality for diagnosing MDE, which has characteristic endoscopic and pancreatographic features.

MPD abnormalities

Cystic neoplasms may cause ductal abnormalities adjacent to the lesion, including occlusion (Figure 11.7), stenosis, and displacement of the duct. Duct obstruction and stenoses are more frequent with malignant cystic neoplasms [6,40], while duct displacement reflects the size of the cystic mass and may occur with either malignant or benign lesions. These ductal abnormalities may also be caused by pseudocysts and therefore differentiation of the diagnoses is helped by findings remote from the lesion such as ductal changes of chronic pancreatitis which are highly associated with pseudocysts (Figure 11.8). A

Figure 11.6 ERCP features in pseudocysts and cystic neoplasms.

	Pseudocyst	Cystic neoplasm
Cyst **Cyst-duct communication**	Demonstrable in majority	Absent
Mass effect (draping or displacement)	Occurs with large lesions	Occurs in large tumours
Main pancreatic duct abnormalities	Features of chronic pancreatitis: occlusion, irregularity, ectasia, stenosis, calculi	Duct changes in proximity to lesion
		Absence of ductal changes of chronic pancreatitis
Rest of pancreas	Features of chronic pancreatitis	Normal
Duct branches	Irregular, non-filling	Normal
Calcification	Diffuse calcification away from the lesion	Focal calcification adjacent to tumor

Figure 11. 7 ERCP image showing occlusion of the main pancreatic duct. This sign may be seen in chronic pancreatitis or neoplastic disease. In the context of cystic neoplasms, it occurs more commonly with malignant lesions than with benign lesions.

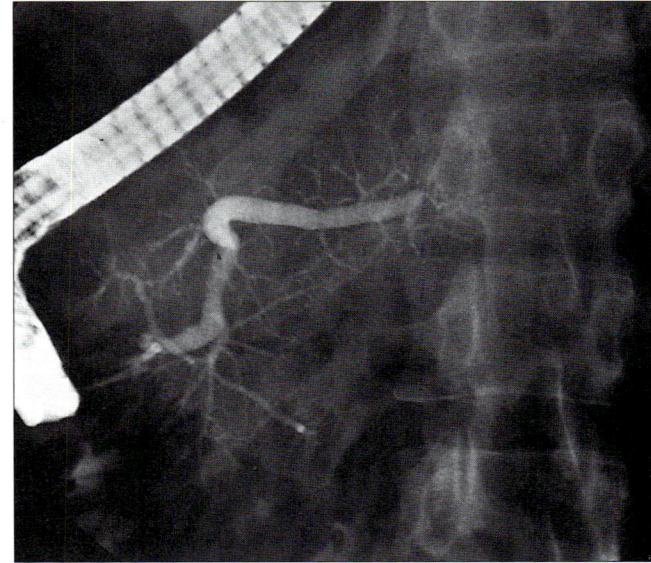

Figure 11.8 Relative frequencies of pancreatogram abnormalities in pseudocyst and cystic neoplasms.

Author (Ref)	Type of lesion	Number of patients	Endoscopic retrograde pancreatography features No. of patients (%)					
			Normal	Draping	Stenosis	Communi- cation	Occlusion	Chr panc
O'Connor *et al.* 1986(44)	PC	37	0 (0)	4 (11)	NE	24 (65)	11 (30)	18 (49)
Silvis *et al.* 1974 (45)	PC	16	0 (0)	3 (19)	0 (0)	12 (75)	12 (75)	most
Sugawa *et al.* 1979 (46)	PC	76	0 (0)	3 (4)	NE	61 (80)	3 (4)	76 (100)
Combined	PC	129	0 (0)	10 (8)	0 (0)	97 (75)	26 (20)	94/113 (83)
Warshaw *et al.*1990 (6)	CN	37*	50%	13 (35)	3 (8)**	0 (0)	4 (11)**	0 (0)
Gazelle *et al.* 1993 (40)	CN	38	9 (24)	14 (37)***		5 (13)	10 (26)	0 (0)
Pinson *et al.* 1990 (42)	CN	11	0 (0)	1 (9)	2 (18)	0 (0)	8 (73)	0 (0)

PC = Pseudocyst
CN = Cystic neoplasm

NE = not evaluated or uncertain from presented data
* figure excludes two cases of mucinous ductal ectasia
** all cases of occlusion and stenosis occurred in mucinous cystadenocarcinoma
*** figure given is for draping or narrowing

normal pancreatogram was reported in 35% of 23 patients with benign cystic neoplasms but in only one (7%) of 15 patients with malignant tumours [40].

Ductal communication with cyst

A cyst–duct communication (Figure 11.9) is seen in 63–80% of patients with pseudocysts [36,44,45,47] but is usually absent in neoplastic cysts [5,8,37,40] with the exception of MDE [18]. In the case of a pseudocyst, filling of the cavity may occur directly from the MPD, from a perforation of the pancreatic duct wall, or by rupture of a ductule [46]. Although demonstration of a cyst–duct communication strongly favours the diagnosis of pseudocyst, it is not entirely specific because there have been anecdotal reports of mucinous cystic neoplasms communicating with the ductal system [7,31,41,48–50], presumably by tumour fistulization.

Chronic pancreatitis

Typical findings of chronic pancreatitis such as MPD or side branch irregularities and ectasia or calcification of the pan-creas away from the cystic lesion occur in the majority of patients with pseudocysts [44–46] whereas these changes are not seen in patients with cystic neoplasms [5].

Calcification

Calcification in a diffuse pattern is pathognomonic for chronic pancreatitis whereas focal calcification may be a feature of cystic neoplasms.

Cholangiographic abnormalities

Cystic neoplasms or pseudocysts that involve the head of the pancreas may produce secondary changes in the bile duct, including displacement, effacement, stenosis, obstruction and fistula formation.

Pseudocyst versus cystic neoplasms

As explained above, the diagnosis of neoplastic cyst on pan-creatographic findings is favoured by the absence of features of chronic pancreatitis and absence of cyst–duct communication.

Benign versus malignant cystic neoplasms

Malignant neoplasms are almost always abnormal on pan-creatography, although up to a third of benign cystic neo-plasms may have normal pancreatograms [40]. Obstruction of the MPD is a strong indicator of malignancy (Figure 11.10). In 38 patients with cystic neoplasms, obstruction of the MPD was seen in only one (SCA) of 23 patients (4%) with benign neoplasms and in 9 of 15 patients (60%) with malignant neo-plasms [40]. Other signs, such as stenosis, draping and com-munication, occurred in both benign and malignant neoplasms and hence were not useful for differentiation. In a review of 67 patients with cystic neoplasms, including 27 cases of mucinous cystadenocarcinoma, Warshaw *et al.* found that stenosis occurred in 18% of cancers and obstruc-tion in 24% and that neither sign occurred in benign cystic neoplasms [6].

Figure 11.9 ERCP image demonstrating communication between the MPD and a pancreatic pseudocyst.

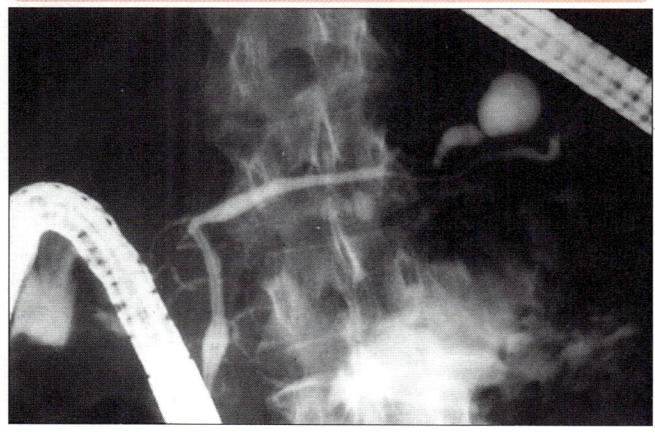

Figure 11.10 ERCP image showing occlusion of the MPD in the head of the pancreas with a fistula into the distal common bile duct, in a patient with mucinous cystadenocarcinoma.

Figure 11.11 Duodenoscopic view of the main papilla in a patient with MDE showing a gaping orifice exuding mucin.

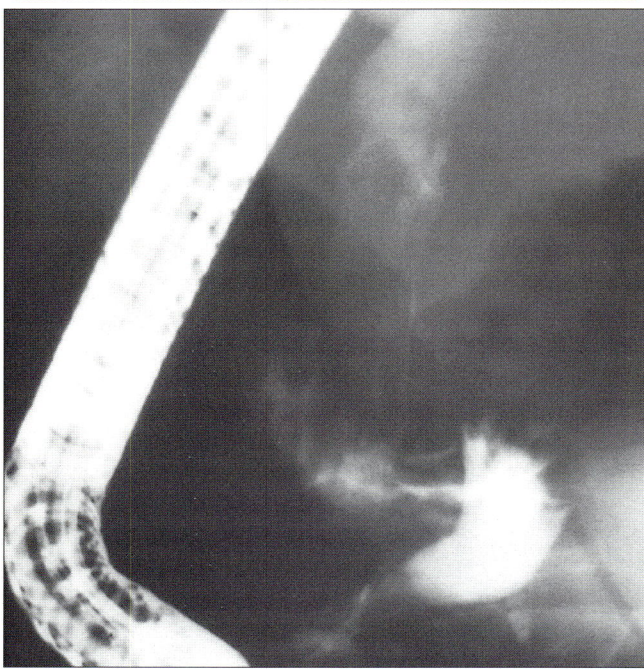

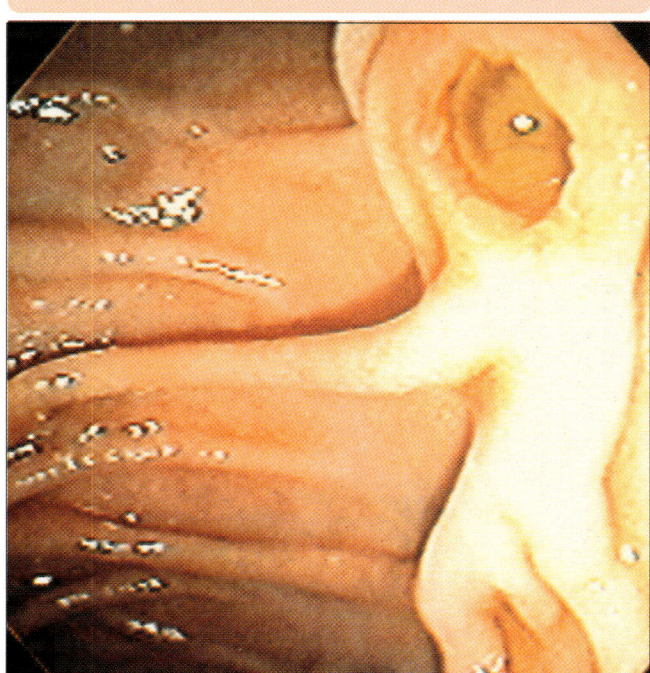

Mucinous ductal ectasia

The ERCP appearance of MDE is pathognomonic. The pancreatic orifice is widely patent and mucin is often seen exuding from it [15,19,51] (Figure 11.11). On pancreatography the MPD is typically seen to be grossly dilated, either diffusely or segmentally [52]. The cystic dilation is due to mucin hypersecretion leading to obstruction of the duct. Involvement and dilation of side branches gives an appearance of grape-like clusters of contrast material [53,54]. Amorphous radiolucent filling defects within the ductal system are seen (Figure 11.12) which correspond to globules of mucin causing ductal obstruction [18,19,55]. Specimens for histology may be obtained by aspiration or brush cytology or by pancreatic biopsy (Figure 11.13). Pancreatoscopy may be helpful in MDE [56–59] since it can easily visualize the papillary tumours which have a frond-like or finger-like appearance (Figure 11.14), can obtain biopsies and can aid in planning the extent of pancreatic resection.

Figure 11.12 ERCP image in MDE showing (a) filling defects within the MPD caused by mucin globules and (b) a markedly dilated MPD with filling defects representing mucin plugs and an intraductal papillary tumour.

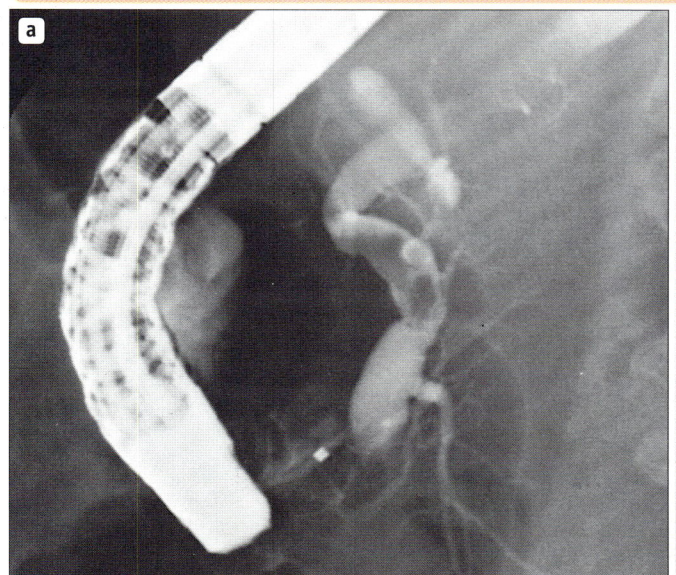

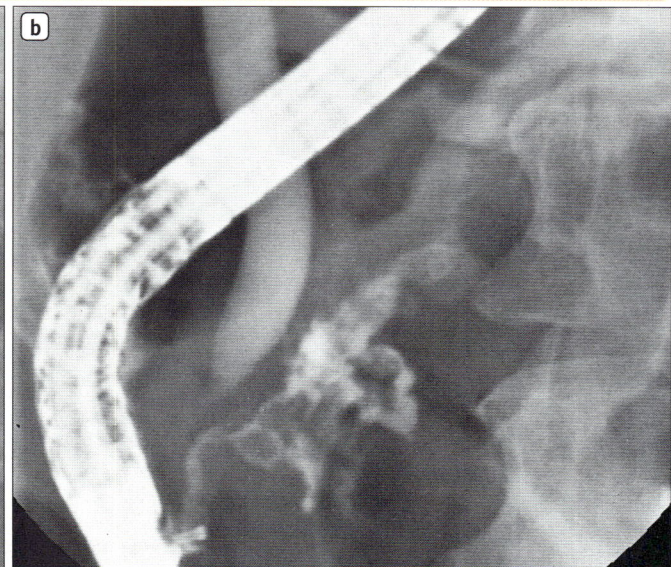

Figure 11.13 Biopsy forceps introduced into the dilated MPD to obtain tissue specimens in a patient with MDE of the pancreas.

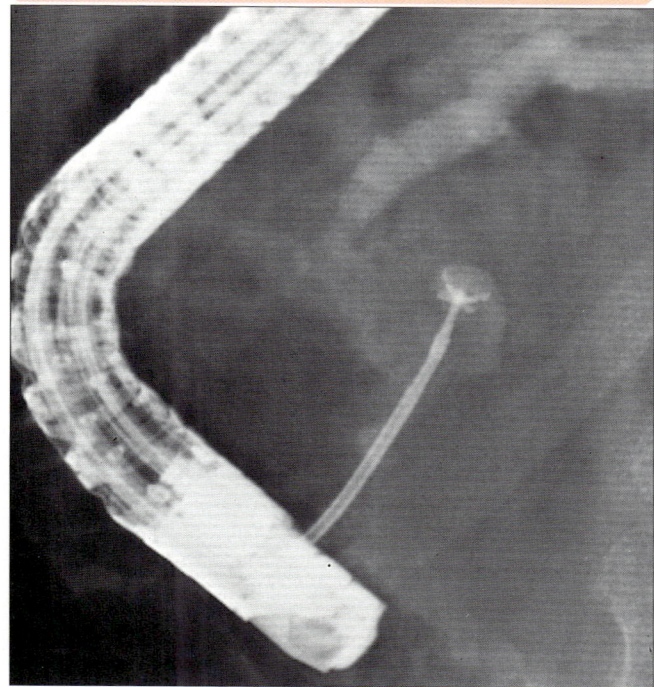

Usefulness of preoperative ERCP for cystic lesions

Preoperative ERCP has a well established role in the management of pseudocysts. Pancreatography is successful in 84–92% of cases of pseudocyst [44,46] and has a sensitivity of 80% in diagnosing pseudocyst [46]. Filling of the cavity with contrast medium unequivocally demonstrates the cyst. ERCP has been documented to be safe and the incidence of post-procedure clinical sepsis has been reported to be 4% [44]. The procedure is helpful in defining the anatomical relationship of the pseudocyst to pancreatic and common bile ducts and is useful in the planning of the appropriate operation. ERCP

is also useful in demonstrating the site of leak in pancreatic ascites, pleural effusions and into viscus. O'Connor reported [44] that ERCP influenced the choice of operation in 19 of 39 cases (49%).

In an analogous manner, ERCP has been shown to be useful in the management of cystic neoplasms. Pinson *et al.* reported that ERCP significantly affected the treatment plan by changing the clinical impression to neoplasia in 8 of 11 patients (73%) presenting with cystic lesions, and helped confirm the diagnosis in the other cases [42]. ERCP results obviated further investigations, hastened surgical intervention and helped in planning the surgery [42]. The risk of post-ERCP sepsis might be lower for cystic neoplasms than for pseudocysts because of the absence of ductal communication in the majority of cases, presumably reducing the theoretical risk of introducing infection into the cyst. ERCP gives additional information on the site of the cyst in relation to the pancreatic and biliary ducts, thereby aiding in planning the surgical approach.

EUS and future trends

EUS is excellent at showing the internal architecture of the cystic lesion, being superior to CT and extracorporeal US in this respect. Fine-needle aspiration biopsy can be performed using a linear array echo-endoscope. The use of EUS in the diagnosis of cystic neoplasms has been described [60,61]. EUS is able to visualize internal septations and solid tissue within the cystic lesion (Figure 11.15) which, if present, suggest a neoplastic aetiology. MDE (Figure 11.16) has been demonstrated on EUS [56] and papillary projections are visible in 93% of cases [62]. In large tumour masses, the EUS penetration depth may not permit complete visualization of the tumour and its margins. EUS also assists in local staging by providing information on infiltration into the gastric or duodenal wall, common bile duct, portal venous system and coeliac axis.

Magnetic resonance cholangiopancreatography (MRCP) is a relatively new imaging technique with the advantage of obtaining images of the biliary and pancreatic systems non-invasively and without use of any oral or intravenous contrast agent. Early reports on its sensitivity and accuracy are encour-

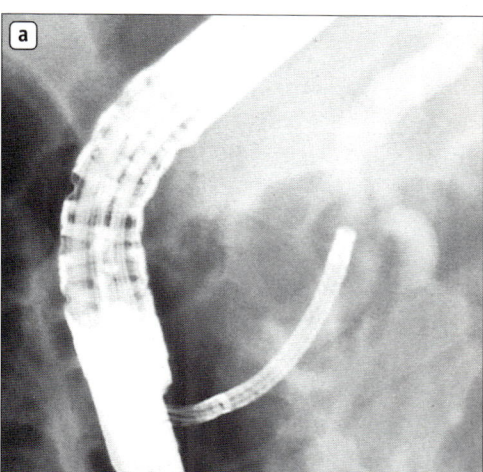

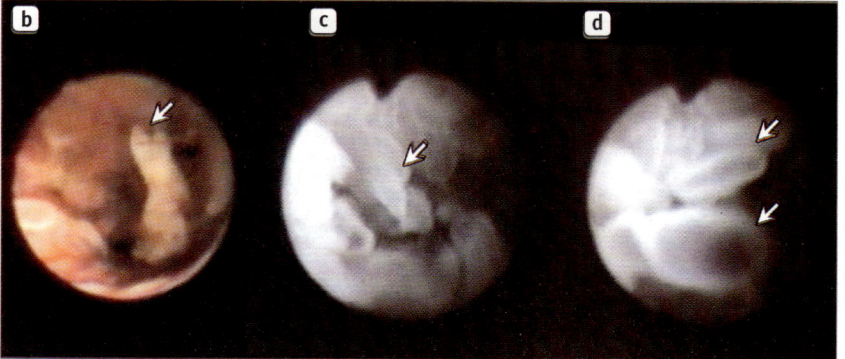

Figures 11.14 Pancreatoscopy with miniscope in MDE. (a) Insertion of Olympus XCHF BP 30 miniscope into the MPD. (b) Pancreatic ductoscopy demonstrating frond-like, and (c),(d) finger-like projections of an intraductal tumour.

Figure 11.15 Linear scanning EUS image showing (a) a neoplastic cyst in the body of the pancreas with thick septations and echogenic mass within the cyst representing a tumour; (b) fine-needle aspiration biopsy of the same lesion. Pathology showed mucinous cystadenoma.

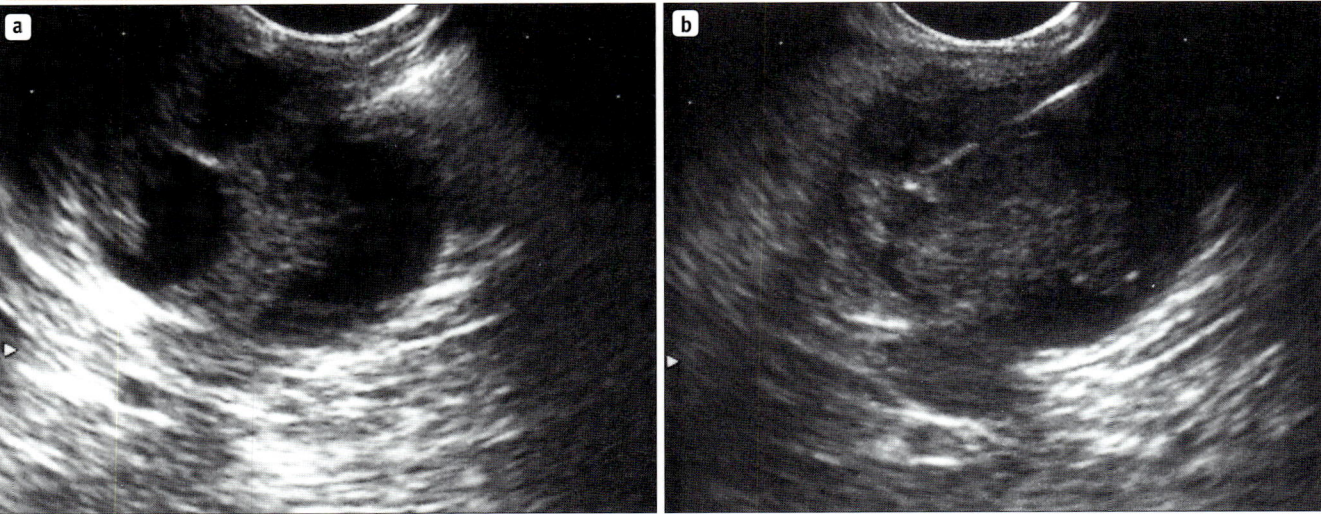

aging. Takehara et al. [63] compared findings from MRCP imaging of the pancreatic duct in patients with chronic pancreatitis against ERCP findings, and reported agreement between the two modalities in 83–92% of cases of ductal dilation, 70–92% in cases of ductal narrowing, and 92–100% in cases of filling defects. Barish et al. [64] reported a respiratory-triggered, three-dimensional, multi-slab turbo spin-echo technique for MRCP with impressive results. Respiratory triggering reduces respiratory motion artefacts and three-dimensional acquisition improves the signal-to-noise ratio and spatial resolution. Diagnostic MRI images were obtained in 29/30 patients, with agreement with ERCP findings in 88% of patients with diseases of the pancreatic duct. While there are no published series on the use of MRCP for diagnosis of cystic neoplasms, several authors have reported that the combination of CT and ERCP provides the most accurate and complete evaluation of pancreatic neoplasms [36,42]. MRCP essentially combines information on both parenchymal and ductal disease in one investigation, and we predict its increasing use in the investigation of pancreatic cystic lesions.

Cystic lesions of the pancreas are increasingly being diagnosed, as the result of greater use of imaging modalities such as ultrasonography and CT scanning. Although cystic neoplasms constitute the minority of pancreatic cysts, differentiation from the more common pseudocysts is critical because of the difference in treatment. Accurate diagnosis is rewarded by the good potential for cure if resection is performed before either invasion or metastasis has occurred. The present diagnostic algorithm for cystic lesions of the pancreas consists of

Figure 11.16 Radial scanning EUS view of the head of the pancreas with cystic areas representing dilated ectactic ducts filled with mucin, in a patient with MDE.

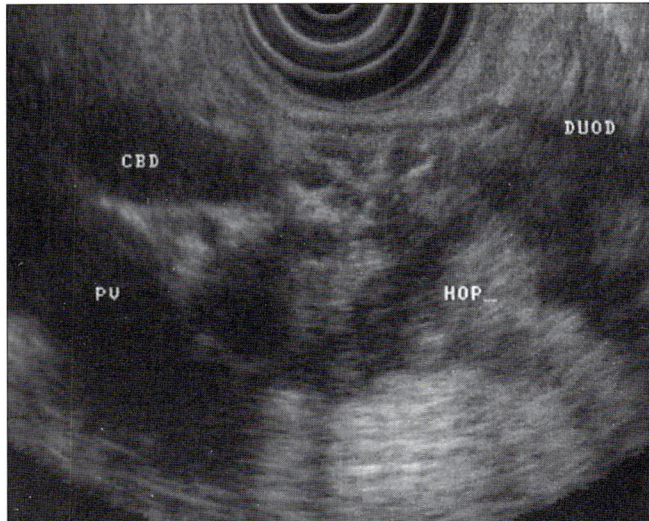

CT scan, ERCP and EUS (if available). The endoscopic techniques allow tissue specimens to be obtained to assist in diagnosis. Cyst fluid analysis may also be helpful when the diagnosis is unclear. Further experience with the newer technologies, such as EUS and MRCP, will clarify their value in the diagnostic algorithm.

References

1. Fernandez-del Castillo C, Warshaw AL. Cystic tumors of the pancreas. *Surg Clin N Am* 1995; 75(5):1001–16.

2. Warren KW, Athanassiades S, Frederick P, Kune GA. Surgical treatment of pancreatic cysts: review of 183 cases. *Ann Surg* 1966; 163:886–91.

3. Becker WF, Welsh RA, Pratt HS. Cystadenoma and cystadenocarcinoma of the pancreas. *Ann Surg* 1965; 161:845–60.

4. Howard JM. Cystic neoplasms and true cysts of the pancreas. *Surg Clin N Am* 1989; 69(3):651–65.

5. Warshaw AL, Rutledge PL. Cystic tumors mistaken for pancreatic pseudocysts. *Ann Surg* 1987; 205:(4)393–7.

6. Warshaw AL, Compton CC, Lewandrowski KB, Cardenosa G, Mueller PR. Cystic tumors of the pancreas: new clinical, radiologic, and pathologic observations in 67 patients. *Ann Surg* 1990; 212:(4)432–45.

7. Lumsden A, Bradley EL III. Pseudocyst or cystic neoplasm: differential diagnosis and initial management of cystic pancreatic lesions. *Hepatogastroenterol* 1989; 36:462–6.

8. Declore R, Thomas JH, Forster J, Hermreck AS. Characteristics of cystic neoplasms of the pancreas and results of aggressive surgical treatment. *Am J Surg* 1992; 164:437–42.

9. Compagno J, Oertel JE. Mucinous cystic neoplasms of the pancreas with overt and latent malignancy (cystadenocarcinoma and cystadenoma): a clinicopathologic study of 41 cases. *Am J Clin Pathol* 1978; 69:573–80.

10. Yamaguchi K, Enjoji M. Cystic neoplasms of the pancreas. *Gastroenterology* 1987; 92:1934–43.

11. Hodgkinson DJ, ReMine WH, Weiland LH. A clinicopathologic study of 21 cases of pancreatic cystadenocarcinoma. *Ann Surg* 1978; 188:679–84.

12. Compagno J, Oertel JE. Microcystic adenomas of the pancreas (glycogen-rich cystadenomas): a clinicopathologic study of 34 cases. *Am J Clin Pathol* 1978; 69:289–98.

13. Lewandrowski KB, Warshaw AL, Compton CC. Macrocystic serous cystadenoma of the pancreas: a morphologic variant differing from microcystic adenoma. *Human Pathol* 1992; 23:(8)871–5.

14. Yamada M, Kozuka S, Yamao K, Nakazawa S, Naitoh Y, Tsukamoto Y. Mucin-producing tumor of the pancreas. *Cancer* 1991; 68:159–68.

15. Rickaert F, Cremer M, Deviere J, Tavares L, Lambilliotte JP, Schroder S, et al. Intraductal mucin-hypersecreting neoplasms of the pancreas: a clinical study of eight patients. *Gastroenterology* 1991; 101:512–19.

16. Warshaw AL. Mucinous cystic tumors and mucinous ductal ectasia of the pancreas. *Gastrointest Endosc* 1991; 37:(2)199–201. (editorial)

17. Lichtenstein DR, Carr-Locke DL. Mucin-secreting tumors of the pancreas. *Gastrointest Endosc Clin N Am* 1995; 5:(1)237–58.

18. Ohta T, Nagakawa T, Akiyama T, Fukushima W, Ueno K, Miyazaki I, et al. The "duct-ectatic" variant of mucinous cystic neoplasm of the pancreas: Clinical and radiologic studies of seven cases. *Am J Gastroenterol* 1992; 87:300–4.

19. Loftus EV, Olivares-Pakzad BA, Batts KP, Adkins MC, Stephens DH, Sarr MG et al. Intraductal papillary-mucinous tumors of the pancreas: Clinicopathologic features, outcome, and nomenclature. *Gastroenterology* 1996; 110:(6)1909–18.

20. Howard JM. Cysts of the pancreas. In *Surgical Diseases of the Pancreas*. Edited by JM Howard, GL Jordan Jr, HA Reber. Lea & Febiger, Philadelphia. 1987:539–63.

21. Mathieu D, Guigui B, Valette PJ, Dao T-H, Bruneton JN, Bruel JM, et al. Pancreatic cystic neoplasms. *Radiol Clin N Am* 1989; 27:163–76.

22. Zinner MJ, Shurbaji MS, Cameron JL. Solid and papillary epithelial neoplasms of the pancreas. *Surgery* 1990; 108:475–80.

23. Talamini MA, Pitt HA, Hruban RH, Boitnott JK, Coleman J, Cameron JL. Spectrum of cystic tumors of the pancreas. *Am J Surg* 1992; 163:117–24.

24. Hodgkinson DJ, ReMine WH, Weiland LH. Pancreatic cystadenoma: a clinicopathologic study of 45 cases. *Arch Surg* 1978; 113:512–19.

25. Lewandrowski KB, Southern JF, Pins MR, Compton CC, Warshaw AL. Cyst fluid analysis in the differential diagnosis of pancreatic cysts. A comparison of pseudocysts, serous cystadenomas, mucinous cystic neoplasms, and mucinous cystadenocarcinoma. *Ann Surg* 1993; 217:(1)41–7.

26. Lewandrowski KB, Lee J, Southern JF, Centeno B, Warshaw AL. Cyst fluid analysis in the differential diagnosis of pancreatic cysts: a new approach to the preoperative assessment of pancreatic cystic lesions. *Am J Radiol* 1995; 164:815–19.

27. Alles AJ, Warshaw AL, Southern JF, Compton CC, Lewandrowski KB. Expression of CA 72-4 (TAG-72) in the fluid contents of pancreatic cysts. A new marker to distinguish malignant pancreatic cystic tumors from benign neoplasms and pseudocysts. *Ann Surg* 1994; 219:(2)131–4.

28. Rubin D, Warshaw AL, Southern JF, Pins M, Compton CC, Lewandrowski KB. Expression of CA 15.3 protein in the cyst contents distinguishes benign from malignant pancreatic mucinous cystic neoplasms. *Surgery* 1994; 115:(1)52–5.

29. Centeno BA, Lewandrowski KB, Warshaw AL, Compton CC, Southern JF. Cyst fluid cytologic analysis in the differential diagnosis of pancreatic cystic lesions. *Am J Clin Pathol* 1994; 101:(4)483–7.

30. Freeny PC, Weinstein CJ, Taft DA, Allen FH. Cystic neoplasms of the pancreas: New angiographic and ultrasonographic findings. *Am J Radiol* 1978; 131:795–802.

31. Yamaguchi K, Hirakata R, Kitamura K. Mucinous cystic neoplasm of the pancreas: Estimation of grade of malignancy with imaging techniques and its surgical implications. *Acta Chir Scand* 1990; 156:553–64.

32. Friedman AC, Lichtenstein JE, Dachman AH. Cystic neoplasms of the pancreas. Radiological-pathological correlation. *Radiology* 1983; 149:45–50.

33. Johnson CD, Stephens DH, Charboneau JW, Carpenter HA, Welch TJ. Cystic pancreatic tumors: CT and sonographic assessment. *Am J Radiol* 1988; 151:1133–8.

34. Minami M, Itai Y, Ohtomo K, Yoshida H, Yoshikawa K, Iio M. Cystic neoplasms of the pancreas: comparison of MR imaging with CT. *Radiology* 1989; 171:53–6.

35. Lee M-G, Auh YH, Cho KS, Chung YH, Han DJ, Yu ES. Mucinous ductal ectasia of the pancreas: MRI. *J Comput Assist Tomogr* 1992; 16:495–6.

36. Foley WD, Stewart ET, Lawson TL, Geenan J, Loguidice J, Maher L, et al. Computed tomography, ultrasonography, and endoscopic retrograde cholangiopancreatography in the diagnosis of pancreatic disease: a comparative study. *Gastrointest Radiol* 1980; 5:29–35.

37. Kawai K, Yasuda K, Nakajima M. Endoscopic diagnosis of cancer of the pancreas. In *Gastroenterologic Endoscopy*. Edited by MV Sivak. WB Saunders, Philadelphia. 1987:821–38.

38. Silvis SE, Rohrmann CA, Vennes JA. Diagnostic accuracy of endoscopic retrograde cholangiopancreatography in hepatic, biliary, and pancreatic malignancy. *Ann Intern Med* 1976; 84:438–40.

39. DiMagno EP, Malagelada JR, Taylor WF, Go VLW. A prospective comparison of current diagnostic tests for pancreatic cancer. *New Engl J Med* 1977; 297:737–42.

40. Gazelle GS, Mueller PR, Raafat N, Halpern EF, Cardenosa G, Warshaw AL. Cystic neoplasms of the pancreas: evaluation with endoscopic retrograde pancreatography. *Radiology* 1993; 188:(3)633–6.

41. Herrera L, Glassman CI, Komins JI. Mucinous cystic neoplasm of the pancreas demonstrated by ultrasound and endoscopic retrograde pancreatography. *Am J Gastroenterol* 1980; 73:512–15.

42. Pinson CW, Munson JL, Deveney CW. Endoscopic retrograde cholangiopancreatography in the preoperative diagnosis of pancreatic neoplasms associated with cysts. *Am J Surg* 1990; 159:510–13.

43. Cross MR. Mucinous cystadenoma of the pancreas: endoscopy as an aid to diagnosis. *Gastroenterology* 1980; 79:944–7.

44. O'Connor M, Kolars J, Ansel H, Silvis S, Vennes J. Preoperative endoscopic retrograde cholangiopancreatography in the surgical management of pancreatic pseudocysts. *Am J Surg* 1986; 151:18–24.

45. Silvis SE, Vennes JA, Rohrmann CA. Endoscopic pancreatography in the evaluation of patients with suspected pancreatic pseudocysts. *Am J Gastroenterol* 1974; 61:452–9.

46. Sugawa C, Walt AJ. Endoscopic retrograde pancreatography in the surgery of pancreatic pseudocysts. *Surgery* 1979; 86:639–47.

47. Silvis SE, Rohrmann CA, Vennes JA. Diagnostic criteria for the evaluation of the endoscopic pancreatogram. *Gastrointest Endosc* 1973; 20:51–5.

48. Delcenserie R, Dupas JL, Joly JP, Descombes P, Mortier F, Capron JP. Microcystic adenoma of the pancreas demonstrated by endoscopic retrograde pancreatography. *Gastrointest Endosc* 1988; 34:52–4.

49. Sachs JR, Deren JJ, Sohn M, Nusbaum M. Mucinous cystadenoma: pitfalls of differential diagnosis. *Am J Gastroenterol* 1989; 84:811–16.

50. Calan LD, Levard H, Hennet H, Fingerhut A. Pancreatic cystadenoma and cystadenocarcinoma: diagnostic value of preoperative morphological investigations. *Eur J Surg* 1995; 161:35–40.

51. Block KP, Mahvi D, Voytovich M, Watkins JL, Mosley R, Reichelderfer M. Mucinous ductal ectasia in an octogenarian: successful treatment with the Whipple procedure. *Am J Gastroenterol* 1996; 91:(2)388–90.

52. Obara T, Maguchi H, Saitoh Y, Itoh A, Arisato S, Ashida T, *et al.* Mucin–producing tumor of the pancreas: natural history and serial pancreatogram changes. *Am J Gastroenterol* 1993; 88:564–9.

53. Itai Y, Ohhashi K, Nagai H, Murakami Y, Kokubo T, Makita K, *et al.* "Ductectatic" mucinous cystadenoma and cystadenocarcinoma of the pancreas. *Radiology* 1986; 161:697–700.

54. Obara T, Maguchi H, Saitoh Y, Ura H, Koike Y, Kitazawa S, *et al.* Mucin-producing tumor of the pancreas: a unique clinical entity. *Am J Gastroenterol* 1991; 86:1619–25.

55. Dabezies MA, Campana T, Friedman AC. ERCP in the diagnosis of ductectatic mucinous cystadenocarcinoma of the pancreas. *Gastrointest Endosc* 1990; 36:(4)410–11.

56. Nickl NJ, Lawson JM, Cotton PB. Mucinous pancreatic tumors: ERCP findings. *Gastrointest Endosc* 1991; 37:(2)133–8.

57. Riemann JF, Kohler B. Endoscopy of the pancreatic duct: value of different endoscope types. *Gastrointest Endosc* 1993; 39:367–70.

58. Kohler B, Kohler G, Riemann JF. Pancreoscopic diagnosis of intra-ductal cystadenoma of the pancreas. *Dig Dis Sci* 1990; 35:382–4.

59. Kozarek RA. Direct pancreatoscopy. *Gastrointest Endosc Clin N Am* 1995; 5:(1)259–67.

60. Rosch T, Classen M. Pancreatic carcinoma. In *Gastroenterologic Endosonography*. Edited by D Elder. New York: Thieme, New York. 1992:114–33.

61. Rosch T, Lorenz R, Braig C, Feuerbach S, Siewert JR, Schusdziarra V, *et al.* Endoscopic ultrasound in pancreatic tumor diagnosis. *Gastrointest Endosc* 1991; 37:347–52.

62. Kobayashi G, Fujita N, Lee S, Kimura K, Watanabe H, Mochizuki F. Correlation between ultrasonographic findings and pathological diagnosis of mucin producing tumor of the pancreas. *Nippon Shokakibyo Zasshi* 1990; 87:235–42.

63. Takehara Y, Ichijo K, Tooyama N, Kodaira N, Yamamoto H, Tatami M, *et al.* Breath-hold MR cholangiopancreatography with a long-echo-train fast spin-echo sequence and a surface coil in chronic pancreatitis. *Radiology* 1994; 192:73–8.

64. Barish MA, Yucel EK, Soto JA, Chuttani R, Ferrucci JT. MR cholangiopancreatography: efficacy of three-dimensional turbo spin-echo technique. *Am J Radiol* 1995; 165:295–300

Therapy **4**

12

Chronic pancreatitis

Michel Cremer & Jacques Devière

INTRODUCTION

Chronic pancreatitis (CP) has an incidence of between 2 and 10 new cases per 100 000 people per year in Western countries. It leads ultimately to irreversible damage of the pancreas with exocrine and endocrine insufficiency. Pain is the major clinical debilitating symptom, and this presents early in the course of the disease in the majority of cases[1–3].

With the exception of the very rare hereditary CP, of which the gene has been identified on chromosome 7[4,5], the aetiology of CP has not yet been demonstrated. Chronic alcoholism is a precipitating factor but the disease can develop in non-alcoholic subjects and is then qualified as 'idiopathic' CP.

Although the pathophysiology of CP is still discussed in terms of 'stone theory' (in which the primary abnormality is the formation of protein plugs caused by a congenital lack of lithostatine[6]) and the 'necrosis fibrosis theory' (in which fibrosis and ductal stricture are the result of focal inflammation and necrosis[7–9], pain is most often associated with interstitial hypertension and repeated episodes of ischaemia that results from both ductal hypertension and a lack of compliance in the diseased pancreas[10]. It is also probable that, when CP is established, these repeated episodes of ischaemia contribute to the irreversible process of fibrosis.

Until recently, ERCP findings have been the gold standard for the morphological diagnosis of CP. The main features of ductal abnormalities that have been observed are described in various classifications using ERCP findings as a criteria of severity[11–13]. These classifications are useful not only in the differential diagnosis of CP but also as a guide to management.

Magnetic resonance cholangiopancreatography (MRCP) is a major advance in the demonstration of the ductal anatomy of the pancreas. This technique gives satisfactory pancreatograms in most cases of CP without the need for any ductal or intravenous contrast medium injection or irradiation[14].

Furthermore, the development of dynamic secretin magnetic resonance pancreatography (DSMRP) has improved the quality of the morphological information available, especially for patients with no abnormalities on computerized tomography (CT) or ultrasound scans[15]. DSMRP can also detect anatomical variations and a dominant dorsal duct, the presence of which dictates the approach to the minor papilla if a stricture is found and endotherapy required. DSMRP also enables the clinician to decide if endotherapy is needed without the morbidity related to the diagnostic procedure itself. This information could become an important tool in identifying, before ERCP is performed, those patients with painful pancreatitis who could benefit from drainage procedures.

Despite these sophisticated improvements in imaging techniques, a plain film of the pancreatic area remains mandatory for detecting small or large calcified calculi responsible for the obstruction of the main pancreatic duct (MPD). For diagnostic purposes, the detection and location of tiny areas of calcification is only possible using CT scanning without contrast injection. In patients with a normal pancreatogram, the presence of tiny areas of calcification on the 'CT scan plain film' is the best criterion for distinguishing between acute pancreatitis and chronic pancreatitis at the early stage.

This chapter discusses endotherapy techniques in chronic pancreatitis. It is important to note that these drainage procedures are indicated for patients with pain and marked morphological changes of CP[12,13] (Figure. 12.1) and not for patients with anatomical variants or mild pancreatitis with no

Figure 12.1 Morphological classification of chronic pancreatitis.

Types

I.   Mild and moderate changes (Cambridge classification)

II.   Focal changes in the head

      Segmental changes in the tail

III.   Diffuse changes (chain of lakes)

IV.   Segmental changes in the head

V.   Complete obstructive stricture in the head

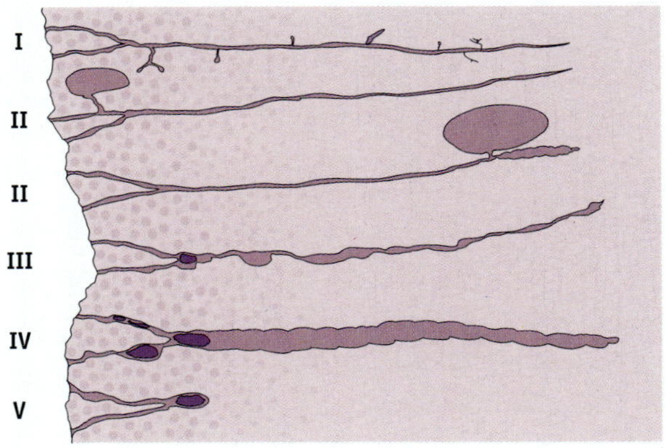

Types II to IV represent severe changes in the Cambridge classification

stones or strictures in the MPD. In patients with morphological evidence of MPD obstruction, improving MPD drainage gives the best chance of improving the pain syndrome. In the other cases, it is likely that papillary dysfunction will be the only abnormality and that the MPD is normal. In these cases, not only is the risk of damaging normal ducts by manipulation higher but the results of these manipulations are largely inconsistent[16] and the implantation of material in the normal MPD could precipitate the development of morphological lesions of CP[17]. Therefore, in the absence of demonstrable MPD stones or strictures, endoscopic manipulation of the pancreas remains largely experimental.

ENDOTHERAPY FOR CHRONIC PANCREATITIS

Pain management

The aim of endotherapy in painful CP is to decompress the MPD, just as it is with the surgical drainage procedures that have been performed for many years.

Other possible goals of MPD drainage are slowing of the evolution of atrophy and pancreatic insufficiency by decreasing the chronic ischaemia of the pancreas, and improving steatorrhoea by restoring the residual flow of pancreatic juice to the duodenum.

The rationale for proposing the endoscopic approach as first-line treatment before surgery includes the fact that ductal decompression is able to ensure pain control, that it is possible by this means to avoid resection, and that it is possible to produce simultaneous delivery of pancreatic juice and bile into the duodenum (Figure 12.2).

The world-wide development of endotherapy as a treatment for CP has been much slower than that of endotherapy for biliary diseases for several reasons, including the rarity of the disease, the heterogeneity of its morphological presentation, the technical requirements (lithotriptor with precise X-ray focusing, experienced medical, surgical, and radiological teams, sophisticated accessories), and perhaps also the medicosocial approach to patients with alcohol-related diseases.

Although the authors performed the first endoscopic pancreatic sphincterotomy 20 years ago[18] for a patient presenting with chronic pancreatitis and an impacted calcified stone at the level of the papilla, most developments of endotherapy for CP started only 10 years ago[10,19,20] with the availability of extra-corporeal shock wave lithotripsy (ESWL). ESWL produces disintegration of calcified calculi into fragments of a few millimetres' diameter in nearly all cases, thereby facilitating their extraction. Many centres are presently involved in the endoscopic management of CP, with good immediate technical results, though data are not available for a comparison of long-term follow-up with that of surgical series[21-26] (Figure 12.3).

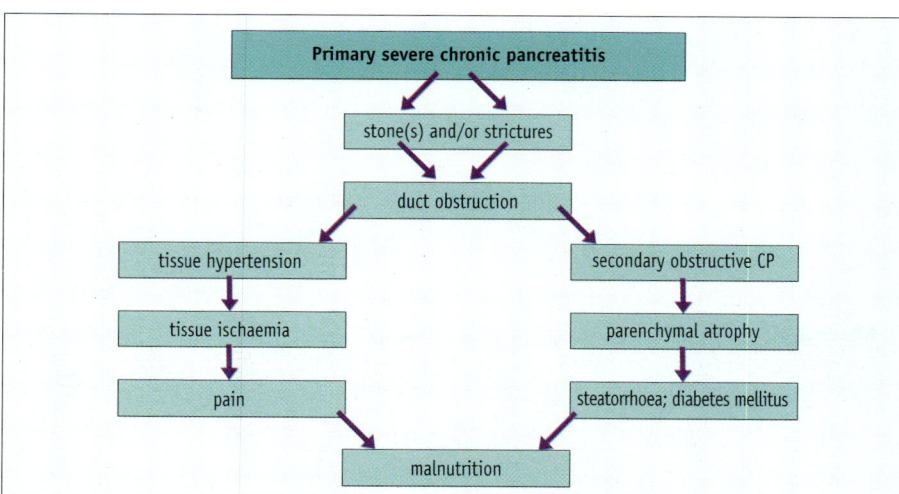

Figure 12.2 Rationale for pancreatic endotherapy.

Figure 12. 3 Endotherapy for severe chronic pancreatitis – technical results and complications.

Author (ref)	Patients (n)	Complete stone clearance (%)	Adequate MPD drainage (%)	Complications (%)
Cremer M et al. (10)	76	ND	94	5
Delhaye M et al. (20)	123	59	90	9
Sauerbruch T et al. (19)	24	42	94	8
Binmoeller KF et al. (35)	93	ND	88	6
Smits ME et al. (22)	51	70	ND	18
Ponchon T et al. (23)	33	ND	85	30
Dumonceau JM et al. (25)	70	50	ND	13
Bittencourt PL et al. (24)	119	82	91	4
Total	**589**	**65**	**90**	**9**

ND – not defined.

Endotherapy methodology

The endoscopic treatment of CP has to be guided by the morphological information obtained prior to ERCP by various imaging techniques (plain film, MRCP or spiral CT).

In mild or moderate CP in the Cambridge classification (type I in our classification) (see Figure 12.1), it is open to question whether decompression would be beneficial to the patient presenting with acute relapsing clinical attacks of pancreatitis. Only control trials will give the answer to the long-term effectiveness of pancreatic sphincterotomy as the treatment for the earliest stage of primary CP.

For patients with type II CP – pseudocyst without gross abnormality of the MPD – one must be prepared to perform a cyst duodenostomy or a cyst gastrostomy after having recognized the bulging of the cyst against the upper gastrointestinal tract. If the cyst is of a suitable size (< 5cm diameter) and communicates with the MPD, a pancreatic endoscopic sphincterotomy (EPS) combined with nasopancreatic drain placement is often sufficient to achieve cyst resolution.

Extra-corporeal shock wave lithotripsy (ESWL)

Since most of the patients referred with severe chronic pancreatitis of types III, IV, and V have embedded calculi obstructing the MPD, the principle in these cases is to remove the stones and to treat strictures if necessary. If calcified stones are present, ESWL may be performed before sphincterotomy. Good-quality plain films of the pancreatic area taken in left and right oblique positions are necessary for deciding on this preliminary treatment (Figure 12.4). Without previous ESWL, the deep cannulation of the MPD fails in 50% of these patients. On the other hand, ESWL is usually not necessary for patients with radiolucent stones. These 'protein plugs' are usually friable and can be extracted immediately after sphincterotomy[27].

It is very important to use a lithotriptor with a focusing system with two X-ray generators. Localization of stones by ultrasound lacks precision and efficacy. The high quality of the fluoroscopy obtained in two axes at 45° angulation (Lithostar; Siemens, Erlangen, Germany) is mandatory for small calculi and for less densely calcified stones. This is the key point for reaching a 99% success of disintegration. Analgesia using Midazolam and Meperidim is usually sufficient to perform the procedure but general anaesthesia is sometimes necessary for less compliant patients and, in these cases, ESWL and therapeutic ERCP may be performed consecutively.

During ESWL, hundreds of shock waves per minute are delivered at 19kV. Each session lasts about 30 minutes, and there is a mean required number of 1500 shock waves for each stone. The quality of fragmentation is evaluated by fluoroscopic control. Multiple or very large stones sometimes require repeated ESWL sessions.

Recently, a Japanese group[28] applied ESWL without subsequent endoscopic approach in 32 patients with stones in the MPD. Complete disintegration was obtained in all cases, and there was further ductal clearance in 24 patients, without the need for endoscopic extraction. Pain relief was obtained

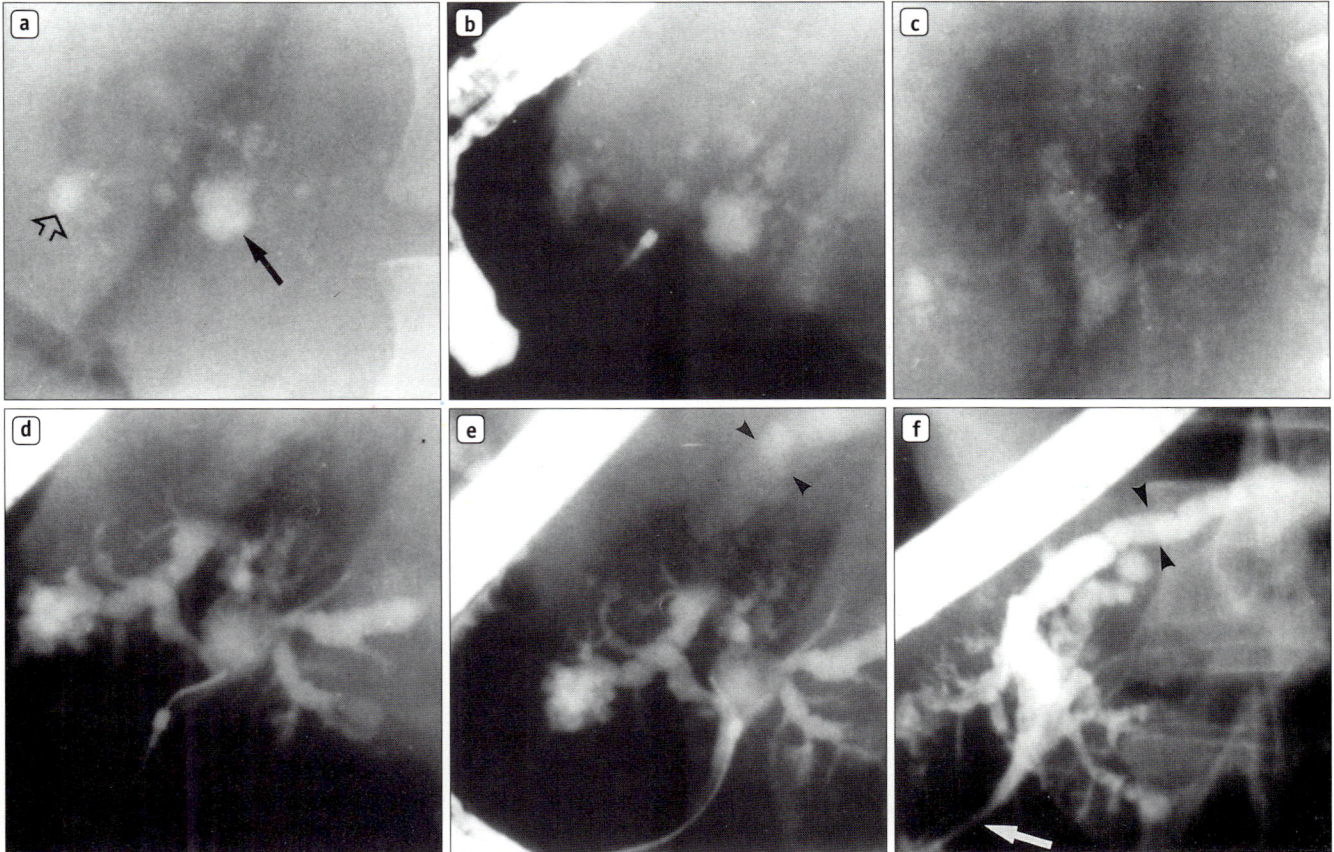

Figure 12.4 Successive aspects of pancreatic stones visualized by plain films before and after ESWL (a,b,c). Corresponding pancreatography (d,e,f).

in 79% of the patients after a mean period of 44 months. Although this option is probably limited to patients without associated stricture, it deserves further investigation as a first-line treatment for such patients.

Endoscopic pancreatic sphincterotomy (EPS)

EPS is the cornerstone of pancreatic endoscopy and the technique that finally provides access to the MPD[29]. EPS in chronic pancreatitis not only decreases the pancreatic duct pressure but also, and most importantly, facilitates the extraction of calculi. EPS is performed at the major papilla in most patients, but at the minor papilla in patients with pancreas divisum and in those with a 'dominant' dorsal duct, in whom therapeutic access to the MPD is much easier through the accessory papilla.

Pancreatic sphincterotomy may be done directly by inserting a papillotome (most often over a guide wire) into the pancreatic duct and directing the cut (using pure cutting current to avoid further fibrosis) between the 10 and 11 o'clock positions. This has the potential limitation of difficult access to the bile duct and, mainly, of difficult evaluation of the extent of the pancreatic cut. Therefore, EPS is usually performed in two steps: first, biliary papillotomy and then pancreatic septotomy. Endoscopic biliary sphincterotomy (EBS) as the first approach may also have the advantage of avoiding the rare biliary complications that can occur after primary EPS – the day after EPS some patients have presented with jaundice, probably caused by oedema at the level of the biliary sphincter. After biliary sphincterotomy, the pancreatic orifice is usually seen at the 5 o'clock position on the margins of the sphincterotomy. The orifice can often be better visualized by gently sucking air into the duodenum, thereby producing transient opening. When deep cannulation of the MPD has been achieved, pancreatic sphincterotomy or 'septotomy' is performed using pure cutting current. The cut is done with the distal part of the cutting wire, at the 12 o'clock position, over a length of 5–8cm (depending on the diameter of the MPD) to create the largest possible access.

For minor papilla sphincterotomy, a similar technique is used. The access to the duct is, however, sometimes more difficult, requiring the use of a special cannula or needle-tip catheter (Wilson–Cook) or the help of a hydrophilic guide wire (Terumo). In very difficult cases, the technique of pancreatic rendezvous can also be used[30].

EPS is sometimes the only endoscopic technique required in cases of pancreatic stones impacted at the papilla or of relatively small floating stones or protein plugs in the MPD that can pass spontaneously to the duodenum. However, these cases are unusual and sphincterotomy usually has to be followed by removal of stone fragments, by stenting, or by both.

Extraction of calculi

The ability to remove a stone is related to its size, the degree of impaction, and the presence of downstream stricture. Stones are usually very hard and impacted into the MPD wall or the outlets of secondary ducts. Therefore, ESWL is often necessary before any attempt at extraction can be made. ESWL fragments the stones into small particles, making the extraction much easier.

Figure 12.5 Removal of stone fragments using an opened dormia basket with minimal contrast medium injection.

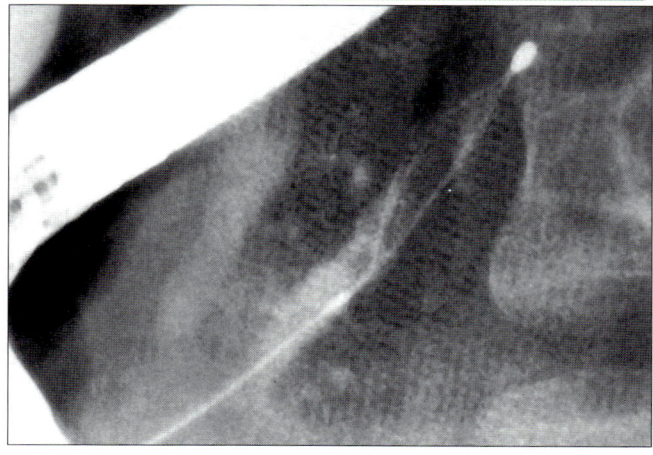

In order to extract these stone fragments, the authors usually begin with a small dormia basket. The open basket is passed into the pancreatic duct. When the stones are visible on the plain film, a good trick is to introduce the dormia basket without contrast medium injection (Figure 12.5). The localization of the residual fragments is easier and the basket can be 'fiddled' at the level of the stones to trap them. Another trick is to pass the open basket into the duct, turn it on its axis in the sheet, and perfuse the sheet with saline – we call this 'rotation perfusion', and it is useful for elimination of small fragments. Finally, slightly inflated balloon catheters can be used in some cases, but they are of limited help in the pancreas.

If multiple sessions of endoscopy are necessary, a nasopancreatic catheter is left in place between sessions, and this is either perfused with saline or drained, depending on whether or not there is an associated stenosis. This procedure can also be used as a clinical indication of the need for further pancreatic stenting. Indeed, if a patient tolerates, without pain, perfusion via a nasopancreatic catheter, this strongly suggests the absence of significant stricture. On the other hand, if perfusion via the nasopancreatic catheter is painful it has to be placed for drainage, and further stone extraction and/or stenting must be considered[29].

PANCREATIC STENTING

Pancreatic stenting will ultimately be required in about 60% of patients with advanced chronic pancreatitis. Stent implantation is decided on clinical (see above) and morphological grounds. The relevant morphological grounds are the presence of an MPD stricture with upwards dilatation in the head of the pancreas. The methods of insertion of the stent include EPS followed by bougienage (up to 11 F.). If dilatation is difficult, a nasopancreatic catheter can be left in place for 24 hours, which makes further dilatation easier. Only large calibre (10 F.) stents are used in these cases, since their design is adapted to the anatomy of the pancreatic duct (Figure 12.6). After stenting, the disappearance of pain, which is observed in the large majority of cases, usually correlates with a reduction in the size of the MPD (Figure 12.7).

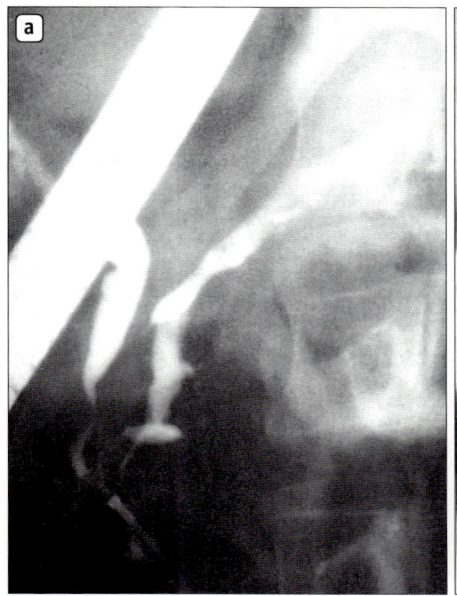
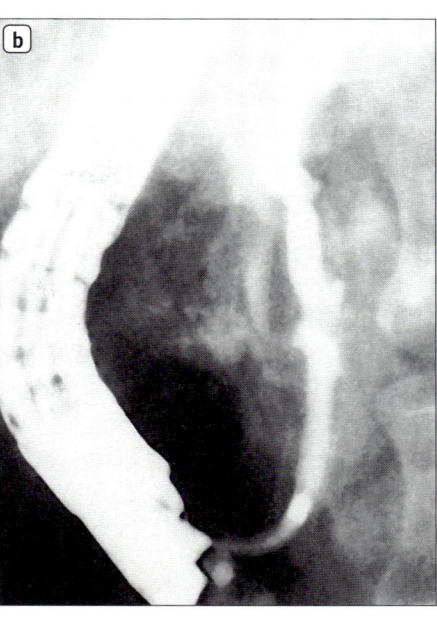

Figure 12.6 Type IV chronic pancreatitis with distal MPD stricture requiring the placement of a 10 F. stent.

Author (ref)	Patients (n)	Immediate pain relief (%)	→Late pain relief (%)	Years	Surgery (%)
Cremer M et al. (21)	76→64	94	94	3.1	15
Delhaye M et al. (20)	107→88	100	85	1.2	8
Binmoeller KF et al. (35)	93→69	74	87	4.9	26
Smits ME et al. (22)	51→49	ND	82	2.8	12
Ponchon T et al. (23)	33→23	74	52	1.0	14
Bittencourt PL et al. (24)	119→69	91	86	5.3	14
Total	**479→362**	**89**	**85**	**3.2**	**15**

ND – not defined.

Figure 12.7 Pain relief after ESWL + EPS ± stenting.

Figure 12.8 ESWL + EPS (stenting excluded) for patients without significant MPD stricture at first treatment.

Author	Patients (n)	Immediate pain relief (%)	Patients (n)	Late pain relief (%)	Years follow-up	Surgery (%)
Sauerbruch T et al. (19)	24	N	24	50	2	8
Dumonceau JM et al. (25)	70	95	46	54	5	5

* pain relapses were treated by a single endoscopic session in two thirds of the patients.

However, if plastic stents are able to relieve MPD stricture and to induce symptomatic improvement, their ability to maintain duct patency and keep the patient free of symptoms after their removal is observed in only a minority of cases after prolonged stenting. Therefore, stenting requires careful follow-up, and stents have to be changed either systematically (every 6–12 months) or 'on demand' in compliant patients when pain recurs. This can be done on an ambulatory basis. However, it is necessary to discuss with the patient the choice between elective surgical drainage of the MPD and repeated stent exchanges. In those patients who require stenting, a randomized trial would be the ideal method for determining the best long-term therapy[31], also taking into account the evolution of exocrine and endocrine

functions. However, such a trial would be difficult to achieve not only because of the low frequency of the disease but also because physicians refer patients to highly specialized centres specifically for endoscopic treatment and are not willing to consider random surgical decompression as a first attempt at pain relief.

Currently, it seems established that in severe chronic pancreatitis, endoscopic MPD drainage can provide long-term pain relief with a minimal complication rate (Figure 12.8), especially as far as major complications are concerned. Endoscopic MPD could be considered as a first approach to painful severe pancreatitis, and further studies will better define those patients who could benefit from elective surgery after initial endotherapy.

Figure 12. 9 (a) A large pseudocyst bulging against the gastric wall. (b) Pancreatography showing complete disruption with extravasation of contrast medium. A pancreatic sphincterotomy will be performed. (c) Cyst gastrostomy to drain the cyst into the stomach.

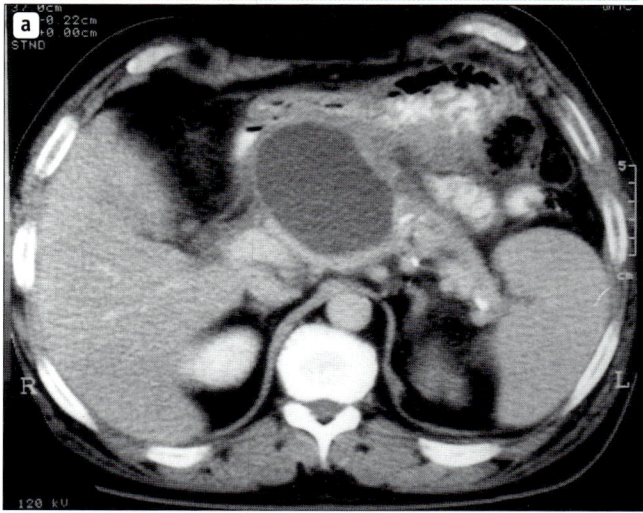

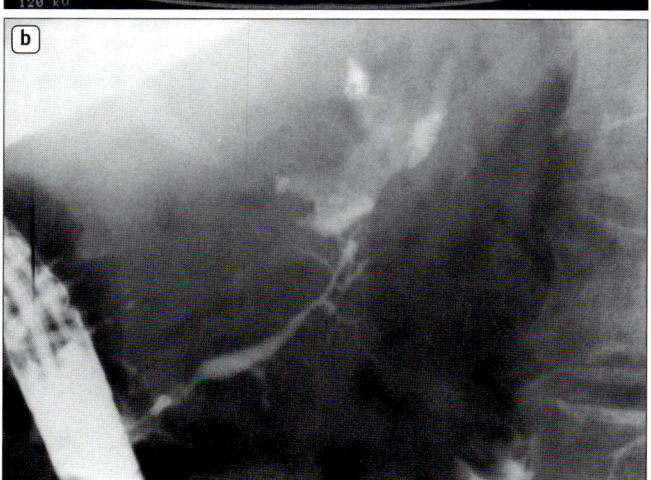

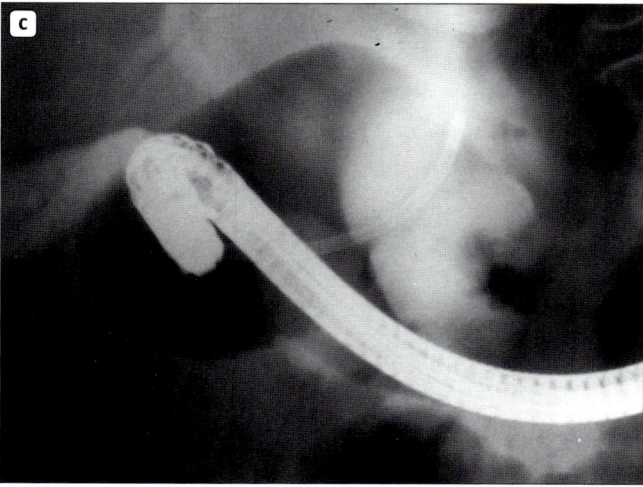

ENDOSCOPIC CYSTOENTEROSTOMY

Endoscopic cystoenterostomy must be considered as a part of the general management of severe chronic pancreatitis[32–34] and must be performed with ductal decompression if required. There is increasing experience with endoscopic drainage of cysts complicating chronic pancreatitis, and longer follow-up data are available. The drainage can be transmural or transpapillary if the cyst is communicating with the pancreatic duct and not clearly adjacent to the stomach or duodenum[35,36]. It has been suggested[37,38] that, when the cyst is accessible by the transpapillary route, this approach has to be considered as first-line treatment. This seems reasonable except in the presence of ductal disruption in the setting of severe chronic pancreatitis[39], where both transmural drainage (to drain the residual secretion of the proximal pancreas) and transpapillary MPD decompression (to avoid relapse of the collection) are often required (Figure 12.9). It appears from these cumulative data that endoscopic approaches can be considered as first-line treatment for pseudocysts that are adjacent to the upper gastrointestinal tract and for those that communicate with the MPD – this offers a definitive treatment in 65–93% of cases.

CONCLUSION

The indications for endoscopic management of chronic pancreatitis are strictly limited to severe types of pancreatitis in which a ductal obstruction is demonstrated morphologically. This technique has been successful over recent years, it has minimal complications, and it allows the avoidance or postponement of surgery. The indications might well become better defined in the future, enabling a more careful selection of patients. Endotherapy has the major advantage of being able to be repeated without an increase in morbidity. It can be proposed relatively early in the course of the disease when pain is present and when morphological lesions of the MPD can be demonstrated. It can be considered as a repeatable treatment that can be adapted to successive problems in the course of a chronic disease. It is highly probable that, with the development of non-invasive techniques such as MRCP, ERCP will stop being useful and even become unethical when used solely for the purpose of imaging the biliary and pancreatic ducts, and that pancreatic endotherapy will become the main means of gaining endoscopic access to the pancreas.

References

1. Amman RW, Akovbiantza A, Largiader F *et al.* Course and outcome of chronic pancreatitis. *Gastroenterology* 1984; 86:820-8.

2. Sahel J, Sarles H. Chronic calcifying pancreatitis and obstructive pancreatitis – two entities. In *Pancreatitis, Concepts and Classification*. Edited by KE Gyr, MV Singer, H Sarles. Excerpta Medica, Amsterdam; 1984; 47–9.

3. Worning H. Incidence and prevalence of chronic pancreatitis. In *Chronic Pancreatitis*. Edited by H Beger, M Buchler, H Ditschuneit. Springer-Verlag, Berlin; 1990:8–14.

4. Le Bodic L, Bignon JD, Raguenes O *et al.* The hereditary pancreatitis gene maps to long arm of chromosome 7. *Hum Mol Genet* 1996; 5:549–54.

5. Whitcomb DC, Preston RA, Aston CE *et al.* A gene for hereditary pancreatitis maps to chromosome 7q35. *Gastroenterology* 1996; 110:1975–80.

6. Multigner L, Sarles H, Lombardo D *et al.* Pancreatic stone protein II. Implication in stone formation during the course of chronic alcoholic pancreatitis. *Gastroenterology* 1985; 89:387–91.

7. Klöppel G. Focal necrosis: primary event in the pathogenesis of chronic pancreatitis? In *Chronic Pancreatitis*. Edited by H Beger, M Buchler, H Ditschuneit. Springer-Verlag, Berlin; 1990:71–6.

8. Van Laethem JL, Robberecht P, Resibois A *et al.* Transforming growth factor beta promotes development of fibrosis after repeated courses of acute pancreatitis in mice. *Gastroenterology* 1996; 110:576–82.

9. Amman RW, Heitz PU, Klöppel G. Course of alcoholic chronic pancreatitis. A prospective clinico-morphological long-term study. *Gastroenterology* 1996; 111:224–31.

10. Cremer M, Devière J, Delhaye M, *et al.* Non-surgical management of severe chronic pancreatitis. *Scand J Gastroenterol* 1990; 25(Suppl 175):77–84.

11. Kasugai T, Kuno N, Kizu M. Endoscopic pancreatocholangiography. II. The pathological endoscopic pancreatocholangiogram. *Gastroenterology* 1972; 63:227–34.

12. Cremer M, Toussaint J, Hermanus A *et al.* Les pancréatites primitives : classification sur base de la pancréatographie endoscopique. *Acta Gastroenterol Belg* 1976; 39:522–46.

13. Axon ATR, Classen M, Cotton P *et al.* Pancreatography in chronic pancreatitis: international definition. *Gut* 1984; 25:1107–12.

14. Reinhold C, Bret PM. Current status of MR cholangiopancreatography. *Am J Roentgenol* 1996; 166:1285–95.

15. Matos C, Metens Th, Devière J *et al.* Pancreatic duct: morphological and functional evaluation dynamic secretin magnetic resonance pancreatography. *Radiology* 1997; in press.

16. Lehman G, Sherman S. Pancreas divisum. Diagnosis, clinical significance and management alternatives. *Gastrointest Endosc Clin North Am* 1995; 5:145–70.

17. Smith MT, Sherman S, Ikenberry SO *et al.* Alterations in pancreatic ductal morphology following polyethylene pancreatic stent therapy. *Gastrointest Endosc* 1996; 44:268–75.

18. Cremer M. Abstract of the Third International Symposium on Endoscopy. Brussels, February 1977.

19. Sauerbruch T, Holl J, Sackmann M *et al.* Extracorporeal shock wave lithotripsy for pancreatic duct stones. *Gut* 1989; 30:1406–40.

20. Delhaye M, Vandermeeren A, Baize M *et al.* Extracorporeal shock wave lithotripsy of pancreatic calculi. *Gastroenterology* 1992; 102:610–20.

21. Cremer M, Devière J, Delhaye M *et al.* Stenting in severe chronic pancreatitis: results of medium term follow-up in seventy-six patients. *Endoscopy* 1991; 23:171–6.

22. Smits ME, Rauws EAJ, Tytgat GNJ *et al.* Endoscopic treatment of pancreatic stones in patients with chronic pancreatitis. *Gastrointest Endosc* 1996; 43:556–60.

23. Ponchon T, Bory RH, Hedelius F *et al.* Endoscopic stenting for pain relief in chronic pancreatitis: results of a standardized protocol. *Gastrointest Endosc* 1995; 42:452–6.

24. Bittencourt PL, Delhaye M, Devière J *et al.* Immediate and long-term results of pancreatic ductal drainage in severe painful chronic pancreatitis. *Gut* 1996; 39:A99.

25. Dumonceau JM, Devière J, Le Moine O *et al.* Endoscopic drainage in chronic pancreatitis associated with ductal stones: long-term results. *Gastrointest Endosc* 1996; 43:547–55.

26. Costamagna G, Gabbrielli A, Multimagni M *et al.* Endoscopic pancreatic sphincterotomy (EPS): is this a safe procedure? Results in 128 EPS. *Gastroenterology* 1996; 110:A383.

27. Schneider MU, Lux G. Floating pancreatic duct concrements in chronic pancreatitis. Pain relief by endoscopic removal. *Endoscopy* 1985; 17:8–10.

28. Sohara H, Hoshino M, Hayakawa T *et al.* Single application extracorporeal shock wave lithotripsy is the first choice for patients with pancreatic duct stones. *Am J Gastroenterol* 1996; 91:1388–94.

29. Devière J, Cremer M. *Techniques of ERCP*. Universa Press, Wetteren, Belgium; 1996.

30. Ghattas G, Devière J, Blancas JM *et al.* Pancreatic rendez-vous. *Gastrointest Endosc* 1992; 38:590–4.

31. Lehman GA, Sherman S. Pancreatic stones: to treat or not to treat? *Gastrointest Endosc* 1996; 43:625–6.

32. Cremer M, Devière J, Engelholm J. Endoscopic management of cysts and pseudocysts in chronic pancreatitis. A 7 years experience. *Gastrointest Endosc* 1989; 35:1–9.

33. Kozarek RA, Brayko CM, Harlan J *et al.* Endoscopic drainage of pancreatic pseudocyst. *Gastrointest Endosc* 1985; 31:322–5.

34. Grimm HT, Meyer WH, Nam V *et al.* New modalities for treating chronic pancreatitis. *Endoscopy* 1989; 21:70–4.

35. Binmoeller KF, Seifert H, Walter A *et al.* Transpapillary and transmural drainage of pancreatic pseudocysts. *Gastrointest Endosc* 1995; 42:219–24.

36. Smits ME, Rauws EA, Tytgat GN *et al.* The efficacy of endoscopic treatment of pancreatic pseudocysts. *Gastrointest Endosc* 1995; 42:202–7.

37. Catalano MF, Geenen JE, Schmalz MJ *et al.* Treatment of pancreatic pseudocysts with ductal communications by transpapillary pancreatic duct endoprosthesis. *Gastrointest Endosc* 1995; 42:214–18.

38. Barthet M, Sahel J, Bodiou-Bertei C *et al.* Endoscopic transpapillary drainage of pancreatic pseudocysts. *Gastrointest Endosc* 1995; 42:208–13.

39. Devière J, Bueso H, Baize M *et al.* Complete disruption of the main pancreatic duct: endoscopic management. *Gastrointest Endosc* 1995; 42:445–51.

13

Pancreatic pseudocysts

Kees Huibregtse & Chi Pong Kwan

INTRODUCTION

Pancreatic pseudocysts are localized collections of pancreatic secretions without an epithelial lining, resulting from pancreatic inflammation or damage. They were once thought to be an unusual complication of pancreatitis but with modern imaging techniques an incidence of 16–50% is found in the course of acute pancreatitis and 20–40% in chronic pancreatitis[1]. Chronic alcoholism is the underlying cause in 69–90% of cases and gallstones in 10–30%[2]. Occasionally, trauma to the pancreatic duct from external force or from an accident during surgery can result in the formation of pseudocysts.

The pathogenesis of pseudocyst formation and the timing of therapeutic intervention differs between acute and chronic pseudocysts[1]. Acute pseudocysts may develop as a consequence of an acute exacerbation of pancreatitis and may contain necrotic debris. Chronic pseudocysts may develop by rupture of a side branch of the pancreatic duct, allowing the gradual escape of pancreatic secretions into the surrounding tissue. Rupture of a side branch may occur if obstruction of a major branch of the pancreatic duct is present caused by stones, protein plugs or strictures, which are frequently found in patients with chronic pancreatitis.

A more expectant policy is pursued in patients with acute pseudocysts as opposed to chronic pseudocysts. Acute pseudocysts will often resolve spontaneously. So, provided the patient is asymptomatic, an initial 4–6-week period of observation is justified. Additionally, a minimum of 4–6 weeks from the time of diagnosis is required for the wall to become sufficiently mature for safe internal drainage. After the 4–6-week period, small pseudocysts (< 4–6cm diameter) can be safely left under observation, but larger lesions should be treated by internal drainage, especially when they cause symptoms.

Symptomatic chronic pseudocysts larger than 4–6cm in diameter should be drained soon after the diagnosis has been made, as the risk of serious complications increases with time.

Until recently, surgery was the standard treatment of pancreatic pseudocysts. Surgical options are internal drainage via the stomach, duodenum or jejunum (Roux-Y anastomosis) and/or partial pancreas resection. The choice of operation depends on the anatomy and size of the pseudocysts, the extent of the underlying disease and the surgeon's preference. Surgical internal drainage is associated with a morbidity and mortality of 30–40% and 2–10%, respectively, and a recurrence rate of 0–15%[3–5]. The most severe complication of partial pancreas resection is the development of exocrine and endocrine insufficiency.

The development of percutaneous and endoscopic interventional techniques to treat biliary and pancreatic disease has changed the scene and the treatment of these diseases is no longer only the realm of surgeons. The effectiveness and duration of percutaneous drainage are related to the presence of communication between the pseudocyst and the pancreatic duct. Morbidity and mortality after percutaneous catheter drainage are 0–30% and 0–10%, respectively[2,6,7]. The recurrence rate varies between 0 and 30% and depends mainly on the presence of communication between the pancreatic duct and the pseudocyst.

DIAGNOSIS

There is a wide range of differential diagnoses for cystic lesions in the pancreas and it is important to review the history, physical findings and investigations carefully before making a definitive diagnosis of pancreatic pseudocyst. Any aetiology, including neoplastic (e.g. mucinous and serous cystadenoma as well as cystadenocarcinoma), inflammatory, congenital and traumatic, can be implicated. The first step is to differentiate benign from malignant lesions as their plans of management are different, but unfortunately misdiagnoses are well documented[8,9]. In general, a history of pancreatitis, the presence of a solitary cyst (shown by imaging) and raised serum amylase support the diagnosis of pancreatic pseudocyst. On the other hand, multiple cysts without other pancreatic or peripancreatic inflammatory changes and the presence of an eccentric solid component within the wall of the cystic mass strongly favour the diagnosis of cystic neoplasm.

It has recently been recommended that the mucinous entity of cystic neoplasms should be resected because of the high malignant potential whereas serous cystic tumours, which are almost always benign, should be left alone. Aspiration of cystic fluid, and determination of viscosity, glycogen, amylase, cytology, and tumour antigens may be helpful to differentiate pancreatic pseudocysts from various cystic neoplasms[10] (Figure 13.1).

Role of diagnostic ERCP

Diagnostic endoscopic retrograde cholangiopancreatography (ERCP) can provide information on the pancreatic duct and its connection, if any, with the pseudocyst. Compression of the bile duct due to the pseudocyst may also be shown. Preoperative ERCP has been reported to change the management plan of surgery in 58% of cases[11]. The significance of the connection between the pseudocyst and the pancreatic duct in deciding between surgical and non-surgical drainage is controversial[6,12].

Figure 13.1 Cystic fluid indices used to differentiate pancreatic pseudocysts from cystic neoplasms.

Diagnosis	Viscosity	Glycogen	Amylase	CA (ng/ml)	CA15.3	CA72-4	Cytology
Pseudocyst	Low	–	+	Low (<25)	Low (<30)	Low	–
Serous cystadenoma	Low	+	–	Low (<25)	Low (<30)	Low	50% +
Mucinous cystadenoma	Usually high	–	Freq +	High (>25)	Low(<30)	Intermediate	+ usually
Mucinous cystadenocarcinoma	High	–	Freq +	High (>25)	High (>30)	High	+ usually

Freq = Frequently; +: Positive; –: Negative; CEA: Carcinoembryonic antigen

Figure 13.2 Endoscopic view of a typical bulge in the stomach, caused by a pancreatic pseudocyst. A needle-knife papillotome is ready to make the perforation.

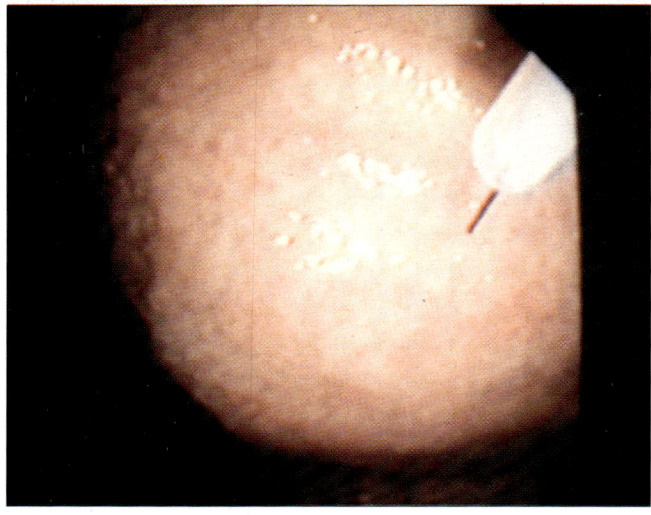

Figure 13.3 Endoscopic view of a needle-knife that has perforated the gastric wall.

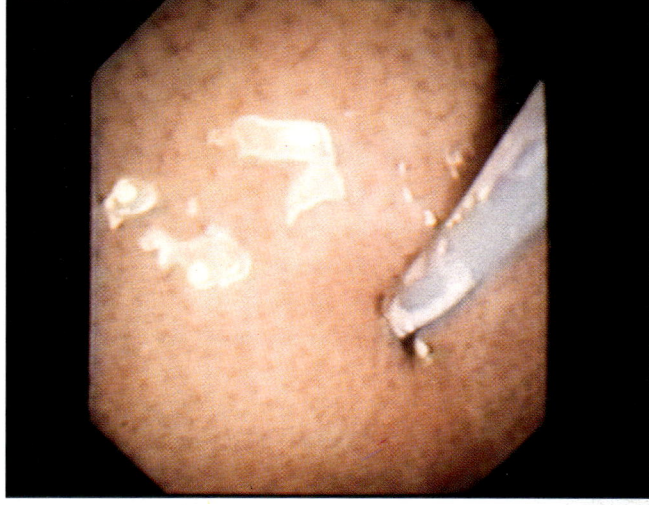

ENDOSCOPIC MANAGEMENT

Method

The aim of endoscopic treatment is to create a communication between the pseudocyst and the gut lumen so that drainage can occur. The net effect is similar to the principle of surgical construction of an internal fistula. The commonly used routes include cystoduodenostomy, cystogastrostomy and drainage via the pancreatic duct. For cystoduodenostomy and cystogastrostomy an obvious bulge should be seen during endoscopy (Figure 13.2) and the distance between the pseudocyst and the bowel wall should not exceed 1cm as measured by computed tomography (CT) scan, ultrasonography and preferably endosonography[13,14]. A diathermic needle-knife papillotome can be used to perform the transgastric or transduodenal puncture (Figure 13.3). Once the sheath of the needle-knife is in the cyst, the needle can be removed. Cystic fluid can be collected through the sheath. This fluid is sent for culture, cytology, biochemistry and tumour antigen determination. X-ray contrast medium is then injected for visualization of the cyst (Figures 13.4–13.10). A guide wire is advanced through the sheath and the sheath can be removed, leaving the guide wire in place. A dilating catheter or balloon catheter is then inserted to enlarge the puncture site before insertion of the stent

Figure 13.4 A large pseudocyst is filled with contrast medium via the sheath of a needle-knife papillotome.

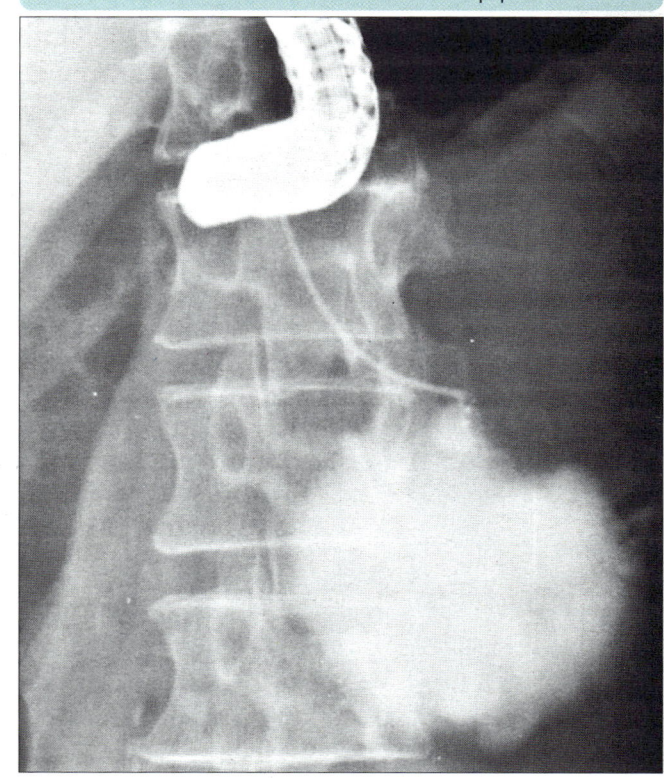

Figure 13.5 A 6 Fr. catheter is advanced far into the cyst for insertion of a stent via the gastric wall.

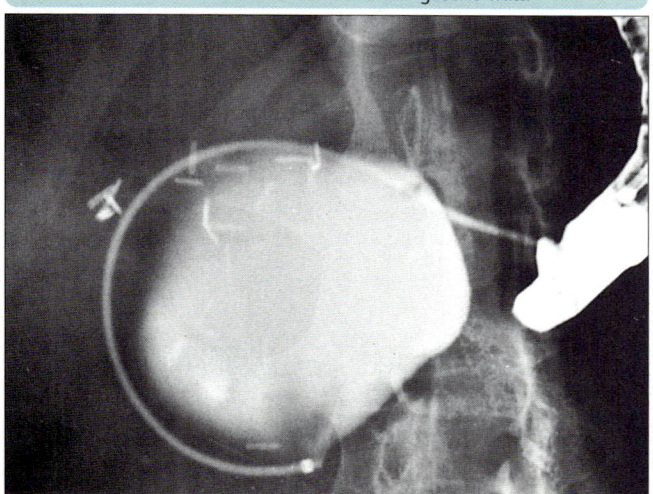

Figure 13.6 A straight 10 Fr. endoprosthesis is inserted into a pseudocyst via the gastric wall.

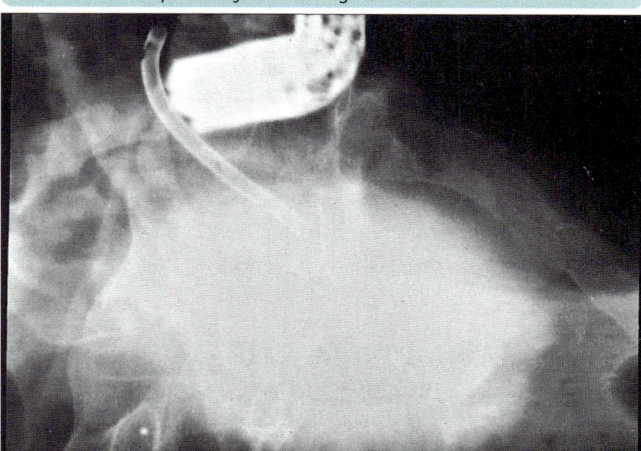

Figure 13.7 The sheath of a needle-knife papillotome is advanced far into a pseudocyst via the duodenal wall.

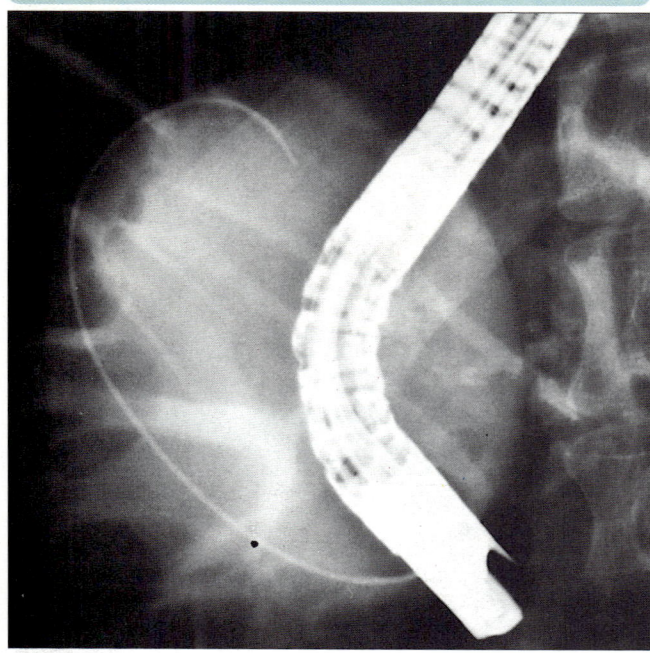

Figure 13.8 A nasocystic catheter is placed in a pseudocyst via the duodenal wall.

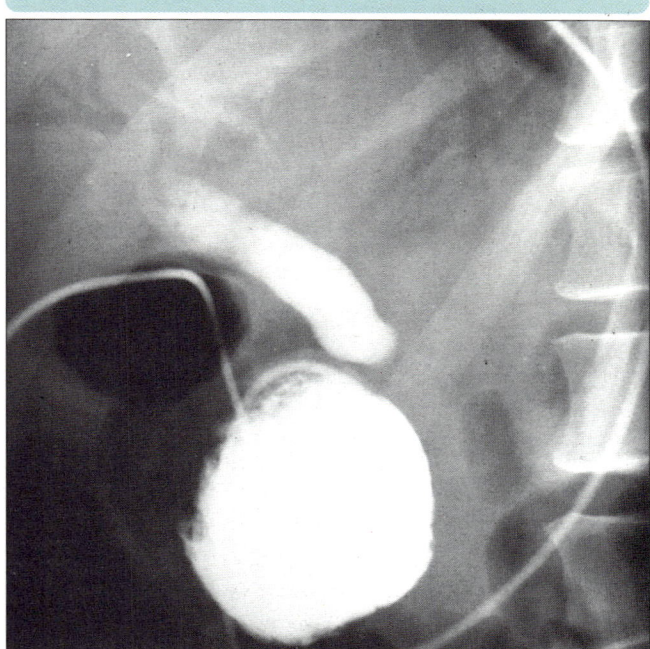

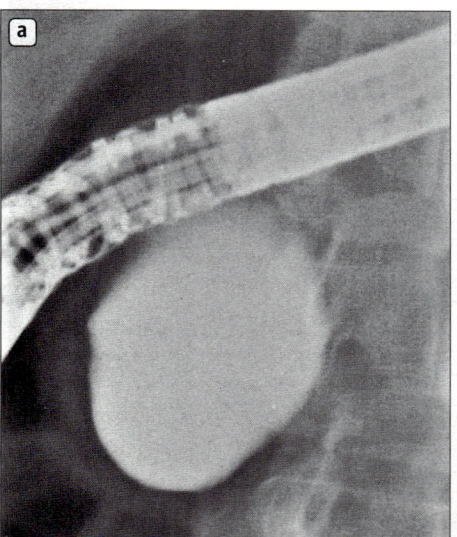

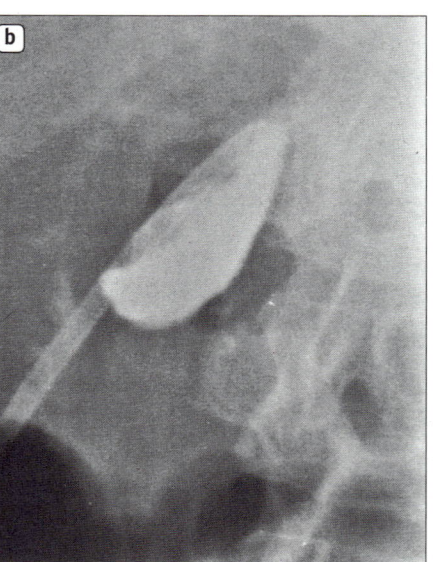

Figure 13.9 (a) A large pseudocyst is punctured via the duodenal wall. (b) After stent placement there is ready emptying of the pseudocyst.

Figure 13.10 The pancreatic duct is cannulated with a diagnostic catheter. There is filling of the pseudocyst, which drains via an endoprosthesis into the duodenum.

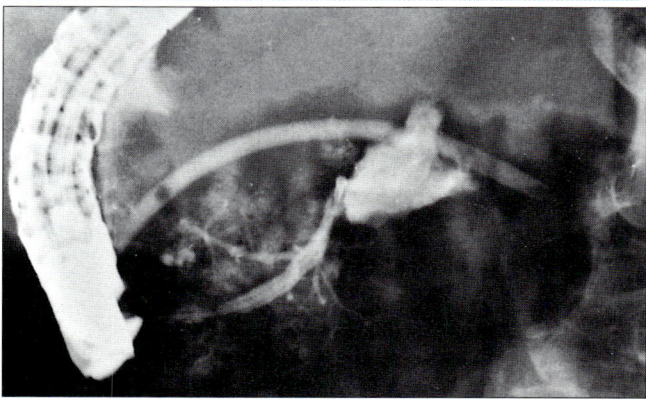

Figure 13.11 Endoscopic view of an endoprothesis inserted in a pseudocyst via the gastric wall, with abundant flow of clear fluid.

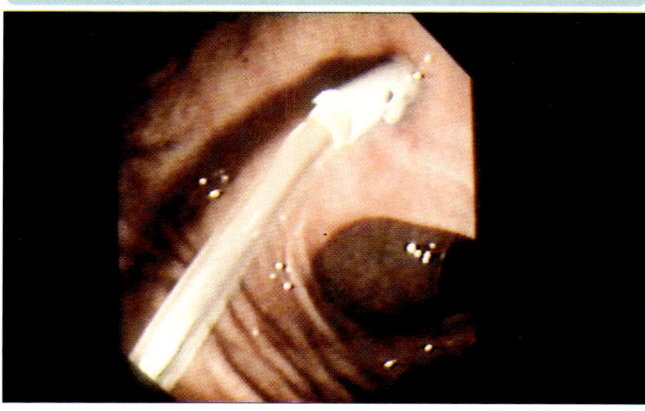

Figure 13.12 A large pseudocyst with debris and fistula. An endoprosthesis and nasocystic drain have been inserted via the stomach wall. Filling with contrast medium via the nasocystic drain results in flow of contrast medium via the endoprosthesis into the stomach.

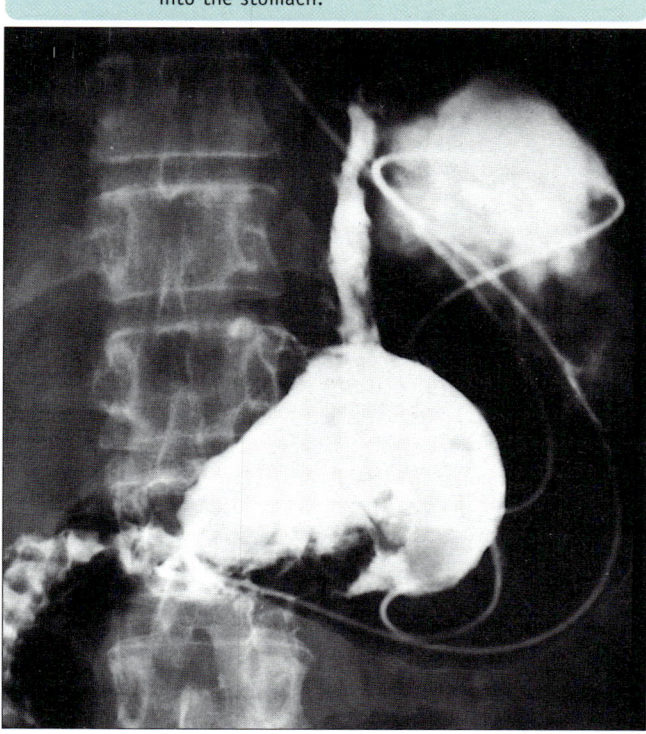

Figure 13.13 (a) A pseudocyst in the uncinate process. (b) An endoprosthesis was inserted in this pseudocyst via the papilla of Vater.

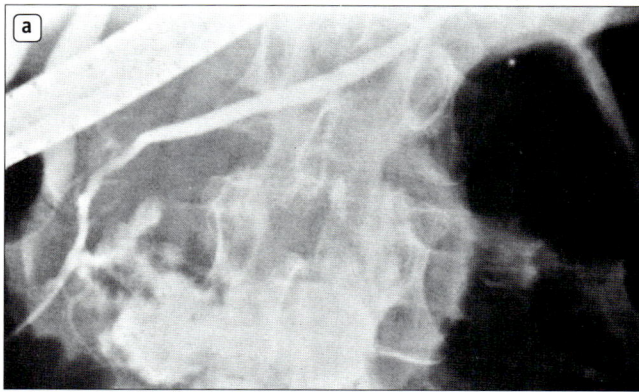

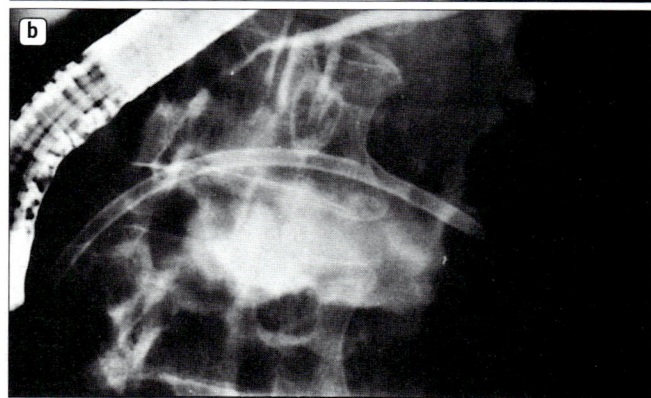

or nasocystic catheter. Double pigtail as well as straight Amsterdam-type stents can be used (Figure 13.11). An additional nasocystic drain is inserted in the cyst for flushing, when the cystic fluid is not clear and contains debris or pus (Figure 13.12). It is essential that cannulation is maintained with the help of guide wires from the time of initial puncture until the insertion of the endoprosthesis. Knecht and Kozarek have therefore developed a double-channel fistulotome that allows immediate placement of a guide wire into the cyst[15]. Cremer *et al.* have also developed a device that facilitates insertion of a stent into pseudocysts[16]. Another route for drainage is created by the insertion of a stent or nasobiliary drain via the papilla of Vater during ERCP (Figure

13.13). The approach depends on the anatomy of the pancreatic duct shown during ERCP and the presence of communication between the pseudocyst and the main pancreatic duct. A stent or nasobiliary drain via the papilla of Vater is introduced, following standard techniques, across the site of ductal disruption or into the pseudocyst[17,18]. Additional pancreatic sphincterotomy, dilatation of strictures, or stone removal, may be necessary[19]. The risks of puncturing the bowel wall are avoided but the procedure is technically more difficult. The procedure is much more difficult for cysts in the corpus and tail of the pancreas; catheters and guide wires must be advanced through an often tortuous pancreatic duct[13].

Results of endoscopic treatment

The results of endoscopic treatment in about 300 patients have been reported in the literature (Figure 13.14)[18,20–27]. The majority of patients had an endoscopic cystenterostomy. Successful cystenterostomy was achieved in 92–100% of patients and long-term success was reported in 70–80% of patients with chronic pseudocysts. Results of endoscopic retrograde pancreatic drainage (ERPD) were less consistent, with long-term success rates ranging from 33% to 61%.

Complications

Bleeding and perforation are the major hazards of cystenterostomy procedures and are reported in 0–25% of patients, with associated mortality of 0–8% (Figure 13.14). Endosonography can accurately measure the distance between the pseudocyst and the bowel wall enabling the best site for puncture to be selected. In addition, the presence of major vessels secondary to chronic pancreatitis-induced segmental portal hypertension can be excluded. The routine use of endosonography before cystenterostomy seems to be extremely useful and can probably prevent major bleeding and perforation[14]. Recently Grimm et al. reported direct puncture of a pseudocyst under endosonographic guidance[28]. They used a linear sector scan that permitted visualization of the needle and the pseudocyst in the same plane, improving the safety of the puncture. This method will also allow endoscopic treatment of pseudocysts that do not bulge in the gastrointestinal lumen. Howell described the use of endoscopic needle aspiration in eight patients, in the search for the best site for the definitive puncture[29]. He injected contrast medium after puncturing the intestinal wall. The fluoroscopic findings of an intracystic or extracystic puncture could be easily differentiated and a larger perforation avoided. Entry into a vein could also be diagnosed and the need for further manipulation obviated.

Sepsis is another potentially hazardous problem, which fortunately has been uncommonly reported. The patients generally respond well to antibiotics, stent exchange, saline perfusion via a nasocystic drain, or additional percutaneous drainage. Sepsis secondary to stent occlusion may develop, in which case stent exchange should be performed. Prophylactic antibiotics before and after drainage procedures is recommended. The presence of pancreatic necrosis associated with the pseudocyst is a high risk factor for developing sepsis after non-operative interventions[30]. A nasocystic drain for flushing should be inserted alongside the endoprosthesis for proper clearance of the cyst lumen, when the cystic fluid is not clear.

Timing of intervention

Pancreatic pseudocysts that cause symptoms, lead to complications or enlarge during follow-up should be treated. Asymptomatic pseudocysts should initially be observed and closely monitored. Conservative treatment was successful in 35–57% of cases in several recent series of patients with pancreatic pseudocysts of mixed aetiology[3–5,31,32]. The 'million dollar question' concerns the correct timing of intervention in asymptomatic and persistent pseudocysts. Traditionally, intervention was recommended for pseudocysts greater than 5–6cm in diameter that persist longer than 6 weeks[33]. The rationale was based on the presumed high rate of occurrence (30–50%) of potentially fatal complications[3] and the markedly reduced chance of resolution after this period of time. These recommendations are challenged by recent research using CT scan to follow up the course of the pseudocysts. Complications only occurred in 11% of 75 patients after a mean follow-up period of one year in a retrospective study by Yeo[31]. Another retrospective study showed a complication rate of 9% in 68 patients followed for a mean period of 46 months[4]. Extension of the observation period to 12 or more weeks with close follow-up by modern imaging techniques has been suggested[34]. Even the once-accepted dictum that all persistent pancreatic pseudocysts require drainage has been challenged. The size of the cyst as an indication of operative treatment is also considered inappropriate, since 27% of pseudocysts larger than 10cm in diameter resolved spontaneously in Yeo's study[31]. The natural course of pancreatic pseudocysts is highly variable and it is difficult to predict the course and outcome of an individual case.

Figure 13.14 Results of endoscopic treatment of pseudocysts.

Author (ref)	Therapy	n	Initial success rate (%)	Definitive therapy (%)	Recurrence (%)	Early complications (%)	Mortality (%)	Mean follow-up time (mo)
Smits et al. (25)	All	37	92	70	5	16	0	21
Cremer et al. (20)	ECE	33	97	82	12	6	0	31
Froeschle et al. (2)	All	37	N/A	84	N/A	N/A	3	37
Dohmoto & Rupp (21)	All	21	81	76	0	0	0	5–40 (range)
Barthet et al. (23) chronic pancreatis	All	71	N/A	72	18	15	1	1–98 (range)
Barthet et al. (22) acute pancreatitis	All	12	N/A	58	N/A	25	8	N/A
Barthet et al. (24)	ERPD	30	100	86	23	13	0	15
Howell et al. (27)	All	64	N/A	94	11	24	N/A	10
Binmoeller et al. (26)	ERPD	53	94	94	23	11	0	22
Catalano et al. (35)	ERPD	21	100	80	31	4	0	37

ECE = Endoscopic cystenterostomy; ERPD = Endoscopic retrograde pseudocyst drainage; All = ECE and ERCD; N/A = Not available.
Initial success = achieve initial drainage; definitive therapy = reduction of pseudocyst size with pain improvement without further surgical intervention.

References

1. Grace PA, Williamson RCN. Modern management of pancreatic pseudocysts. *Br J Surg* 1993; 80:573–81.

2. Froeschle G, Peyer-Pannwitt U, Brueckner M *et al.* A comparison between surgical, endoscopic and percutaneous management of pancreatic pseudocysts: long term results. *Acta Chir Belg* 1993;102–6.

3. Williams KJ, Fabian TC. Pancreatic pseudocysts: recommendations for operative and non-operative management. *Am Surgeon* 1992; 58:199–205.

4. Vitas GJ, Sarr MS. Selected management of pancreatic pseudo-cysts: operative versus expectant management. *Surgery* 1992; 111:123–30.

5. Sanfey H, Aguilar A, Jones RS. Pseudocysts of the pancreas, a review of 97 cases. *Am Surgeon* 1994; 60:661–8.

6. Freeny PC. Percutaneous management of pancreatic fluid collections. *Balliere's Clin Gastroenterol* 1992; 6:259–72.

7. Criado E, De Stafano AA, Weiner TM *et al.* Long term results of percutaneous catheter drainage of pancreatic pseudocysts. *Surg Gynecol Obstet* 1992; 175:293–8.

8. Warshaw AL, Rutledge PL. Cystic tumours mistaken for pancreatic pseudocyst. *Ann Surg* 1987; 205:393–8.

9. Pyke CM, van Heerden JA, Colby TV *et al.* The spectrum of serous cystadenoma of the pancreas. *Ann Surg* 1992; 215:1132–9.

10. Rosenfield AT. The evaluation of pancreatic cysts: current concept. *J Clin Gastroenterol* 1995; 20:94–5.

11. Nelson WH, Townsend CM Jr, Thompson JC Preoperative endo-scopic retrograde cholangicpancreatography (ERCP) in patients with pancreatic pseudocysts associated with resolving acute and chronic pancreatitis. *Ann Surg* 1989; 209:532–40.

12. Ahearne PM, Baillie JM, Cotton PB *et al.* An endoscopic retrograde cholangiopancreatography (ERCP)-base algorithm for the manage-ment of pancreatic pseudocysts. *Am J Surg* 1992; 163:111–16.

13. Sahel J. Endoscopic drainage of pancreatic cysts. *Endoscopy* 1991; 23:181–4

14. Fockens P, Johnson TG, van Dullemen HM *et al.* Endosonography is a prerequisite before endoscopic drainage of pancreatic pseudo-cysts. *Gastrointest Endosc* 1996; 43:16A.

15. Knecht GL, Kozarek RA. Double-channel fistulotome for endoscopic drainage of pancreatic pseudocyst. *Gastrointest Endosc* 1991; 37:356–7.

16. Cremer M, Deviere J, Baize M *et al.* New device for endoscopic cystoenterostomy. *Endoscopy* 1990; 22:76–7.

17. Huibregtse K. *Endoscopic Biliary and Pancreatic Drainage.* Georg Thieme Verlag, Stuttgart, 1988. (Thesis)

18. Kozarek RA, Ball TJ, Patterson DJ *et al.* Endoscopic transpapillary therapy for disrupted pancreatic duct and peripancreatic fluid col-lections. *Gastroenterology* 1991; 100:1362–70.

19. Huibregtse K, Smits ME. Endoscopic management of diseases of the pancreas. *Am J Gastroenterol* 1994; 89:S66–77.

20. Cremer M, Deviere J, Engelholm L. Endoscopic management of cysts and pseudocysts in chronic pancreatitis: long term follow-up after 7 years of experience. *Gastrointest Endosc* 1989; 35:1–9.

21. Dohmoto M, Rupp KD. Endoscopic drainage of pancreatic pseudo-cysts. *Surg Endosc* 1992; 6:118–24.

22. Barthet M, Bugallo M, Moretra LS. Treatment of pseudocysts in acute pancreatitis: retrospective study of 45 patients. *Gastroenterol Clin Biol* 1992; 16:853–9.

23. Barthet M, Bugallo M, Moretra LS *et al.* J. Management of cysts and pseudocysts complicating chronic pancreatitis. *Gastroenterol Clin Biol* 1993; 17:270–6.

24. Barthet M, Sahel J, Bodiou-Bertel C *et al.* Endoscopic transpapillary drainage of pancreatic pseudocysts. *Gastrointest Endosc* 1995; 42:208–13.

25. Smits ME, Rauws EAJ, Tytgat GN *et al.* The efficacy of endoscopic treatment of pancreatic pseudocysts. *Gastrointest Endosc* 1995; 42:202–7.

26. Binmoeller K, Seifert H, Walter A *et al.* Transpapillary and transmural drainage of pancreatic pseudocysts. *Gastrointest Endosc* 1995; 42:219–24.

27. Howell DA, Lehman GA, Baron TH *et al.* Endoscopic treatment of pancreatic pseudocysts: a restrospective multicenter analysis. *Gastrointest Endosc* 1995; 41:424 (abstract).

28. Grimm H, Binmoeller FK, Soehendra N. Endosonography-guided drainage of a pancreatic pseudocyst. *Gastrointest Endosc* 1992; 38:170–1.

29. Howell DA, Holbrook RF, Bosco JJ *et al.* Endoscopic needle local-ization of pancreatic pseudocysts before transmural drainage. *Gastrointest Endosc* 1993; 39:693–8.

30. Hariri M, Slivka A, Carr-Locke DL *et al.* Pseudocysts drainage pre-disposes to infection when pancreatic necrosis is unrecognized. *Am J Gastroenterol* 1994; 89:1781–4.

31. Yeo CJ, Bastidas JA, Lynch-Nyhan A *et al.* The natural history of pancreatic pseudocysts documented by computed tomography. *Surg Gynecol Obstet* 1990; 170:411–17.

32. Yeo CJ, Sarr MG. Cystic and pseudocystic diseases of the pan-creas. *Curr Prob Surg* 1994; 3:165–252.

33. Bradley EL, Clements JL Jr, Gonzalez AC. The natural history of pancreatic pseudocysts: a unified concept of management. *Am J Surg* 1979; 137:135–41.

34. Shearer MG, Imrie CW. Spontaneous resolution of pancreatic pseudocysts. *Digestion* 1990; 46:177–8.

35. Catalano MF, Geenen JE, Schmalz MJ *et al.* Treatment of pancreatic pseudocysts with ductal communication by transpapillary pancreat-ic duct endoprosthesis. *Gastrointest Endosc* 1995; 24:214–18.

14

Acute pancreatitis: is there a role for endoscopic treatment?

Seth A. Cohen & Jerome H. Siegel

INTRODUCTION

Endoscopic retrograde cholangiopancreatography (ERCP) has been established as a key technique in the diagnosis and treatment of both pancreatic and biliary tract disease[1,2]. The role of ERCP in acute pancreatitis, in general, remains debated and studied. In specific conditions, however, such as gallstone pancreatitis, pancreas divisum and acute idiopathic recurrent pancreatitis, ERCP has been shown to be the technique of choice[3–6]. These topics are reviewed elsewhere in this book and will not be discussed further. In this chapter, we will focus on the role of ERCP in other forms of acute pancreatitis.

Historically, there has been a reluctance to perform ERCP in the setting of acute pancreatitis because of the perception that performing pancreatography would increase the risk of precipitating or exacerbating the inflammatory condition. Although there have been reports that performing ERCP does aggravate the patient's pancreatitis or contributes to superinfection of pancreatic necrosis leading to death[7–8], this, fortunately, has been rare.

Figure 14.1 Results of ERCP in 353 patients with acute pancreatitis. (Adapted from Dunham *et al.*[11])

	n
Failed pancreatography	32
Evidence of chronic pancreatitis	77
Cancer of pancreas	6
Normal pancreatogram	133
Ductal stricture	29
Microcysts	21
Extravasation and leak	22*
Non-filling of areas of parenchyma	4*
Cut-off of the pancreatic duct	4*
Dilated pancreatic duct	9
Minimal changes of duct	8
Pancreas divisum	9
Vertical pancreas	1
	355

* *Radiological sign of pancreatic necrosis*

ACUTE PANCREATITIS

Zimmon reported the findings of ERCP in patients presenting with pancreatitis in 1974[9]. Twenty-eight of 63 patients studied were admitted to hospital with acute pancreatitis, the majority due to excessive alcohol intake. Seven of these 28 patients (25%) had normal pancreatography and three had gallstones; 15 patients (54%) showed evidence of acute pancreatitis on pancreatography, i.e. localized filling of secondary ductules and/or an acinar blush; two patients had gallstones and another two had obstruction of the main pancreatic duct in the body or tail due to non-communicating pseudocysts. The remaining six patients (21%) who presented with their first clinical episode of pancreatitis demonstrated ductular changes of chronic pancreatitis.

The use of ERCP in acute pancreatitis to confirm the diagnosis of gallstone pancreatitis, when non-invasive studies have failed to reveal stone disease, has been studied[10] but very little has been written about the systematic use of ERCP in non-biliary acute pancreatitis. Pioneering work has been performed by Cremer's group in Brussels[11,12]. They performed ERCP in 353 consecutive patients presenting with acute pancreatitis of all aetiologies during the period 1973 to 1980. Patients also underwent ultrasonography (US), and in the later years computed tomography (CT) scans were performed. The period between presentation and pancreatography was 15 days (mean), although 40% of patients

underwent ERCP within the first 72 hours. Neither pseudocyst nor pancreatic necrosis was a contraindication to ERCP, and all common bile duct stones detected were removed after performing sphincterotomy. Pancreatography was successful in 323 patients (91%); the findings are listed in Figure 14.1. Seventy-seven of 323 patients (24%) had morphological evidence of chronic pancreatitis on pancreatography despite the clinical presentation of acute pancreatitis. Six patients (1.9%) had ductal findings consistent with carcinoma. Of the remaining 240 patients, 133 (55%) had normal pancreatograms, 28 (12%) had evidence of necrotic pancreatitis, and 79 (33%) had other non-specific findings as listed (Figures 14.2 and 14.3). There was evidence of gallstone disease on cholangiography in 164 patients, the biliary tree was normal in 98 patients, while cholangiography failed in 93 patients. Three episodes of infection of pseudocysts were the only complications reported. Anecdotally, none of the patients with oedematous pancreatitis converted to necrotic pancreatitis after ERCP, which had been their greatest fear.

The Brussels group concluded that: (a) ERCP in conjunction with US and/or CT scanning could establish an aetiology of pancreatitis in most patients, which aided in dictating their immediate management; (b) ERCP was beneficial in diagnosing and treating biliary pancreatitis; (c)

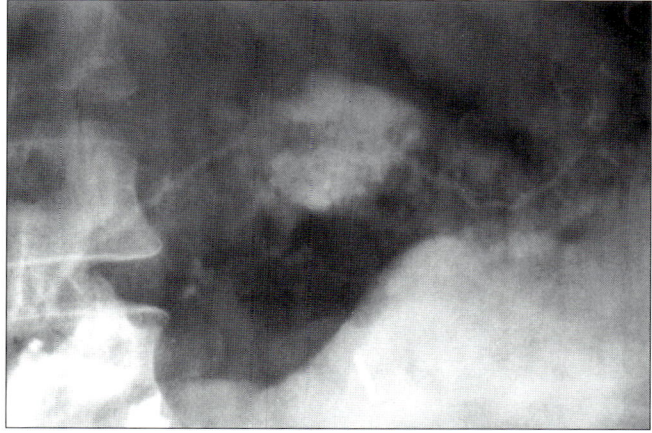

Figure 14.3 Endoscopic pancreatogram after an attack of acute pancreatitis. There is obstruction to the main duct.

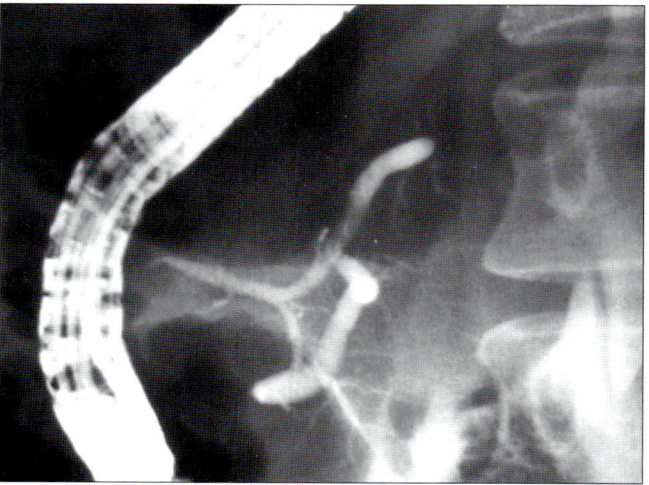

pancreatography also provided prognostic information – patients with normal ducts did not have severe disease and had a zero mortality, while 80% of patients with necrotic pancreatitis were identified and had higher rates of complications, mortality and need for surgery; and (d) pancreatography also identified the patients with underlying chronic pancreatitis and cancer although they had presented with acute pancreatitis, this was important as these patients were managed differently.

In another paper by the Brussels group, Gelin et al. retrospectively analysed the role of pancreatography as a prognostic indicator and a guide to surgical intervention[12]. They found that radiological abnormalities of the pancreatic duct increased in proportion to the severity of pancreatitis as judged by Ranson's criteria. Pancreatography offered prognostic information: there was no mortality with a normal study. In their opinion, ERCP predicted which patients would require surgical intervention. Endoscopic sphincterotomy, however, was not found to improve the outcome in established necrotic pancreatitis.

Thus, the Brussels group found the performance of ERCP to be safe in the setting of severe pancreatitis. Today, however, much of our morphological and prognostic information is obtained with dynamic CT scanning[13]; with the exception of gallstone pancreatitis, diagnostic pancreatography is performed electively after resolution of the acute attack.

The idea of using endoscopic pancreatography as a guide to surgical intervention was applied by another European group. After finding a disappointingly high reoperation rate after pancreatic necrosectomies, because of undetected pancreatic duct fistulae, Gebhardt and colleagues employed ERCP preoperatively in 10 patients with severe pancreatitis in order to guide surgical therapy[14]. Pancreatography was successful in 8 of 10 patients and the four patterns discerned are listed in Figure 14.4. If pancreatography demonstrated any fistula or area of necrosis this would guide the surgeon in dictating the extent of resection. Interestingly, Gebhardt et al. advocated non-operative treatment for necrotic cavities communicating with the duodenum, as these cavities drained and resolved spontaneously.

Hamilton et al. prospectively recorded the results of ERCP in patients who presented after one attack of acute pancreatitis[15]. Of 17 patients, pancreatography was successful in 11: seven were normal; one had gross chronic pancreatitis; and three showed 'minimal change' pancreatitis. Cholangiography was successful in 12 patients: seven were normal; two had previously known CBD stones confirmed; and three demonstrated previously undiagnosed cholelithiasis. After a median follow-up of 19 months, only two patients developed recurrent pancreatitis: one patient with minimal change pancreatitis and one in whom ERCP had failed. This group reinforced the notion of the utility of ERCP in diagnosing subclinical chronic pancreatitis.

Much of the literature involving ERCP and pancreatitis was written as the field of pancreaticobiliary endoscopy was evolving. Dynamic CT scanning is now preeminent in diagnosing and assessing the severity of pancreatitis. There are no contemporary reports in the English literature concerning the systematic use of ERCP in acute pancreatitis.

Figure 14.4 The four patterns found on ERCP in patients with severe necrotic pancreatitis. (Adapted from Gebhardt et al.[14])

1. Normal pancreatic duct with no signs of a fistula.

2. Isolated fistula (ductal disruption).

3. Normal duct system with segmental or diffuse parenchymal staining or extravasation.

4. Necrotic cavity in the head of the pancreas that has fistulized into the duodenum.

PERSISTENT PANCREATITIS

Geenen reported the use of ERCP in a small subgroup of patients who continued to manifest symptoms following an attack of acute pancreatitis[16,17]. These patients continued to have severe pain, particularly postprandially, and required total parenteral nutrition (TPN) and large doses of narcotics. In this cohort of patients there was no evidence of necrosis, pancreatic duct disruption or pseudocyst formation to explain the symptoms. The Milwaukee group reported the results of stenting the main pancreatic duct in six such patients following an acute attack of pancreatitis (a mean of 40 days). Short pancreatic duct stents , 5 and 7 French, were placed. Marked clinical improvement and resolution of abdominal pain was observed within 2–10 days (mean 4 days). All patients were weaned off TPN and narcotics and discharged within 2–7 days. This group postulated that pancreatic stent placement relieves functional obstruction of the pancreatic orifice that is due to either oedema or spasm[17].

PANCREATIC TRAUMA

Abdominal trauma – blunt abdominal trauma, deceleration injury or penetrating injury – can result, uncommonly, in traumatic pancreatitis and pancreatic duct disruption. The clinical diagnosis of pancreatic duct disruption is notoriously diffi-

cult[18], and morbidity and mortality increase when there is a > 24-hour delay in operative intervention. In 1980 Taxier *et al.* reported the elective preoperative use of ERCP to diagnose pancreatic duct injuries in patients who had sustained traumatic pancreatic injury in automobile accidents[19]. ERCP permitted accurate diagnosis of pancreatic duct disruption and also was used to direct surgical treatment in five patients, and to avoid an unnecessary laparotomy in one patient.

Barkin *et al.* prospectively investigated the safety and efficacy of urgent ERCP for suspected traumatic rupture of the pancreatic duct[20]. Fourteen patients (12 after blunt abdominal trauma and two with penetrating trauma) with epigastric tenderness and elevated serum amylase underwent ERCP (eight within 24 hours, three between 25 and 48 hours and three between 49 and 72 hours). The pancreatic duct was visualized in all patients although one patient required two ERCPs. In nine patients the pancreatic duct was normal, in four patients pancreatic duct disruption was demonstrated, and in one patient an irregularity of the duct was seen in the body of the gland (Figure 14.5).

Ductal disruption was confirmed at laparotomy in the four patients in whom it was seen on ERCP. Three patients underwent laparotomy on clinical grounds and after CT findings; none was found to have ductal disruptions, although one patient had a pancreatic capsular laceration that required debridement and drainage. The remaining seven patients had clinical resolution incompatible with significant pancreatic injury. Urgent ERCP was found to be safe and effective, with 100% sensitivity and specificity, and it was superior to CT scanning or peritoneal lavage.

STENTING FOR DUCTAL DISRUPTIONS

The application of therapeutic ERCP in the setting of acute pancreatitis has grown from diagnosing pancreatic ductal disruptions to treating them. Kozarek *et al.* reported the results of endoscopic treatment of 10 patients with pancreatic duct disruption and fluid collections associated with acute pancreatitis[21]. The aetiologies included three related to gallstone pancreatitis, three associated with pancreas divisum, two following motor vehicle accidents and one following ERCP; one patient's pancreatitis was idiopathic. All patients had previously failed to respond to medical management, and six had undergone percutaneous drainage that persisted to drain fluid without resolution (Figure 14.6). Endoscopic transpapillary nasopancreatic drains or pancreatic stents were placed, either across the ductal disruption or directly into the fluid/necrotic collection. Stents were left in place for a median of 6 weeks. Nine of 10 patients had resolution of the fluid collections as judged by CT scan, and 9 of 10 patients had resolution of symptoms. There were two acute complications: one episode of an infected fluid collection after the stent occluded, which resolved with further treatment; and one episode of mild pancreatitis after stent occlusion. Of note, 50% of the patients who underwent pancreatography at the time the stents were removed demonstrated stent-induced pancreatic ductal changes. Ultimately, three patients required surgery for pancreatic resection due to either recurrent or

Figure 14.5 Disrupted pancreatic duct after a gunshot wound. (a) CT scan after initial exploratory laparotomy: a swollen, inflamed pancreas is seen with an anteriorly placed drain. (b) ERCP (lateral view) demonstrates free extravasation of contrast medium into the peritoneum. Several surgical drains are present.

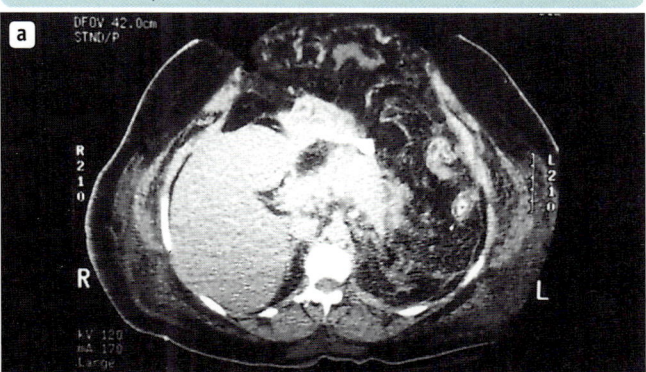

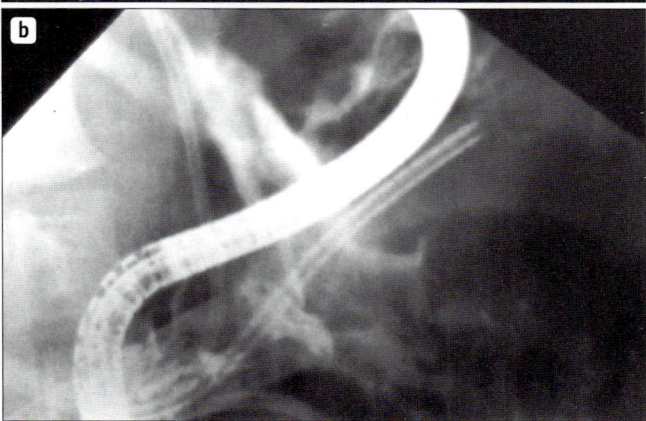

Figure 14.6 Obstructed pancreatic duct with a fluid collection in the tail after severe pancreatitis. There was persistent drainage after placement of a percutaneous catheter. (a) ERCP demonstrates obstruction of the pancreatic duct downstream of the fluid collection; the percutaneous catheter is seen on the right. (b) A guide wire and dilating catheter have traversed the obstruction, after which a stent has been placed. The percutaneous drainage ceased after several days.

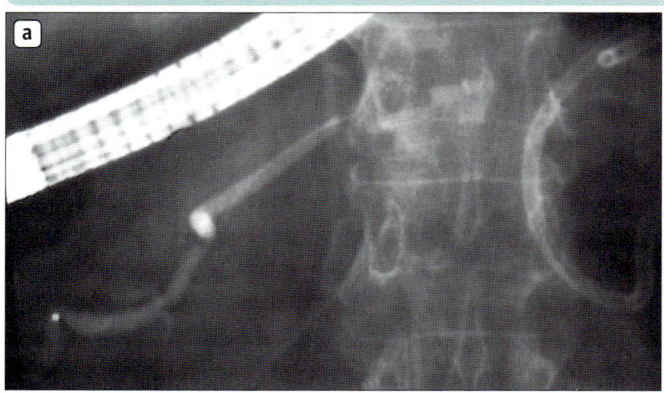
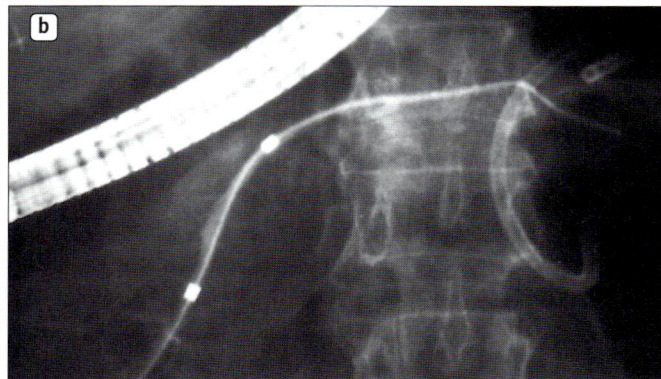

persistent disease. In Kozarek's series, endoscopic therapy was effective as definitive treatment in 7 of 10 patients while, in the other three patients, the treatment was palliative and permitted elective surgery at a subsequent date. There are other reports in which pancreatic stents were placed for pancreatic duct fistulae[22], but the majority of the

treated cases involve chronic pancreatitis[23,24].

Some investigators have suggested that ERCP should serve a primary role in the endoscopic drainage of pseudocysts, even in the setting of acute necrotic pancreatitis[25] but this is controversial[26]. Endoscopic drainage of pseudocysts is discussed in Chapter 13.

References

1. Siegel JH. *Endoscopic Retrograde Cholangiopancreatography; Technique, Diagnosis, Therapy*. Raven Press, New York. 1992.
2. Huibregtse K. *Endoscopic Biliary and Pancreatic Drainage*. Georg Thieme Verlag, Stuttgart. 1988.
3. Neoptolemos JP, Carr-Locke DL, London NJ et al. Controlled trial of urgent endoscopic retrograde cholangiopancreatography and endoscopic sphincterotomy vs. conservative treatment for acute pancreatitis due to gallstones. *Lancet* 1988; 2:979–83.
4. Lans JI, Geenen JE, Johnson JF, Hogan WJ. Endoscopic therapy in patients with pancreas divisum and acute pancreatitis: a prospective, randomized, controlled clinical trial. *Gastrointest Endosc* 1992; 38:430–4.
5. Siegel JH, Ben-Zvi JS, Pullano W, Cooperman A. Effectiveness of endoscopic drainage for pancreas divisum: endoscopic and surgical results in 31 patients. *Endoscopy* 1990; 22:129–33.
6. Venu RP, Geenen JE, Hogan W et al. Idiopathic recurrent pancreatitis; an approach to diagnosis and treatment. *Dig Dis Sci* 1989; 34:56–60.
7. Ammann RW, Deyhle P, Betikoffer E. Fatal necrotizing pancreatitis after peroral cholangiopancreatography. *Gastroenterology* 1973; 64:320–3.
8. Cotton PB, Lehman G, Vennes J et al. Endoscopic sphincterotomy complications and their management; an attempt at consensus. *Gastrointest Endosc* 1991; 37:383–93.
9. Zimmon DS, Falkenstein DB Abrams R et al. Endoscopic retrograde cholangiopancreatography in the diagnosis of pancreatic inflammatory disease. *Radiology* 1974; 113:287–92.
10. Goodman AJ, Neoptolemos JP, Carr-Locke DL et al. Detection of gallstones after acute pancreatitis. *Gut* 1985; 26:125–32.
11. Dunham F, De Toeuf J, Jeanty P et al. Complementarite et limites des differentes methodes d'investigation morphologique dans le diagnostic des pancreates aigues et de leurs complications. *Acta Chir Belg* 1981; 80:323–9.
12. Gelin M, Dunham F, Engelholm L et al. Apport de l'etude morphologique biliopancreatique dans le traitement des pancreatites aigues. *Acta Chir Belg* 1981; 80:357–62.
13. Balthazar EJ, Robinson DL, Megibow AJ. Acute pancreatitis: the value of CT in establishing prognosis. *Radiology* 1990; 174:331–6.
14. Gebhardt C, Riemann JF, Lux G. The importance of ERCP for the surgical tactic in haemorrhagic necrotizing pancreatitis. *Endoscopy* 1993; 15:55–8.
15. Hamilton I, Bradley P, Lintott DJ et al. Endoscopic retrograde cholangiopancreatography in the investigation and management of patients after acute pancreatitis. *Br J Surg* 1982; 69:504–6.
16. Geenen JE. ASGE distinguished lecture. Endoscopic therapy of pancreatic disease: a new horizon. *Gastrointest Endosc* 1988; 34:386–9.
17. Kaikaus RM, Jacob L, Geenan JE et al. "Smoldering pancreatitis" rapid resolution with pancreatic duct stent therapy. *Gastrointest Endosc* 1995; 41:425. (Abstract.)
18. Lukas C. Diagnosis and treatment of pancreatic and duodenal injury. *Surg Clin N Am* 1977; 57:49–65.
19. Taxier M, Sivak MV Jr, Cooperman A, Sullivan BH Jr. Endoscopic retrograde pancreatography in the evaluation of trauma to the pancreas. *Surg Gyn Obs* 1980; 150:65–8.
20. Barkin JS, Ferstenberg RM, Panullo W et al. Endoscopic retrograde cholangiopancreatography and pancreatic trauma. *Gastrointest Endosc* 1988; 34:102–5.
21. Kozarek RA, Ball TJ, Paterson DJ et al. Endoscopic transpapillary therapy for disrupted pancreatic duct and peripancreatic fluid collections. *Gastroenterology* 1991; 100:1362–70.
22. Saeed ZA, Ramirez FC, Hepps KS. Endoscopic stent placement for internal pancreatic fistulas. *Gastroenterology* 1993; 105:1213–17.
23. Kozarek RA, Paterson DJ, Ball TJ, Traverso LW. Endoscopic placement of pancreatic stent drains in the management of pancreatitis. *Ann Surg* 1989; 209:261–6.
24. Kozarek RA, Giranek GC, Traverso LW. Endoscopic treatment of pancreatic ascites. *Am J Surg* 1994; 68:223–5.
25. Howell DA, Baron TH, Lehman GA et al. Endoscopic drainage of pancreatic pseudocysts in the setting of necrotizing pancreatitis: a multicenter analysis. *Gastrointest Endosc* 1995; 41:423. (Abstract.)
26. Hariri M, Slivka A, Carr-Locke DL, Banks PA. Pseudocyst drainage predisposing to infection with pancreatic necrosis is unrecognized. *Am J Gastroenterol* 1994; 89:1781–4.

15

Acute biliary pancreatitis

Paul G. Wilson, James D. Evans,
Ogunju Ogunbiyi, & John P. Neoptolemos

INTRODUCTION

In 1901 Eugene Opie[1] suggested that an impacted stone at the ampulla of Vater caused acute pancreatitis by allowing bile to reflux into the pancreatic duct via a common channel that was formed by the union of the main bile duct (MBD) and the main pancreatic duct (MPD). This theory was based on a postmortem observation in one patient with acute haemorrhagic pancreatitis and though there is no doubt that gallstones and biliary sludge[2] are the commonest causes of pancreatitis in the Western world, the scenario described by Opie of an impacted stone is a very much less common cause of pancreatitis[3,4] than is migration of a stone from the MBD into the duodenum[5]. Indeed, Opie himself subsequently realized that gallstone passage could lead to attacks of acute pancreatitis[6]. There is still some considerable debate about how gallstones actually cause acute pancreatitis and because of this there has been ongoing speculation as to the best way to manage cholelithiasis in this setting. Over the last few years a number of useful studies have been undertaken that are helping to define the answers to these questions more clearly.

AETIOLOGY

Figure 15.1 lists the causes of acute biliary pancreatitis.

Cholelithiasis

Between 3% and 8% of patients with symptomatic gallstones will develop acute pancreatitis[7,8] though in those patients with microlithiasis (stones < 3mm in diameter) this figure may rise as high as 20–30%[9,10]. The incidence and fre-

quency of gallstone-associated acute pancreatitis varies with the prevalence of gallstones but in the Midlands region of England the incidence is of the order of 350 per million of population. The relative incidence tends to vary with alcohol consumption and susceptibility to the effects of alcohol but again in the Midlands the relative incidence is over 60%[4] (Figure 15.2).

Cholesterol gallstones are seen more commonly with increasing age, in females, in the obese, with certain drugs (e.g. clofibrate) and in gastrointestinal diseases such as Crohn's disease. Furthermore, conditions that predispose to the formation of pigment gallstones, such as chronic haemolysis, put individuals at an increased risk of pancreatitis and this has been demonstrated in children and teenagers[11]. Interestingly, though gallstones are much more common in females the percentage of male patients with symptomatic gallstones who suffer attacks of acute pancreatitis is higher[12]. Following treatment of gallstones with extracorporeal shockwave lithotripsy (ESWL), which breaks the stones into much smaller fragments, there is an incidence of 1.4% of attacks of acute pancreatitis[13].

Biliary sludge and crystals

Biliary sludge consists of bile supersaturated with cholesterol, cholesterol monohydrate crystals, mucin, glycoprotein, calcium bilirubinate crystals, cell debris and proteinaceous material[14]. Sludge in the gall bladder can be detected by ultrasonography (US) and is associated with any condition that reduces gall bladder contractility. The presence of biliary sludge within the gall bladder is a risk factor for progression to the formation of gall bladder stones[15].

The presence of cholesterol crystals on bile microscopy likewise indicates that the bile is capable of forming cholesterol stones within the biliary tree and the discovery of such crystals permits the diagnosis of 'gallstone' pancreatitis in those who have previously been labelled 'idiopathic' because of normal radiology[16,17]. When these patients undergo cholecystectomy the excised gall bladder frequently demonstrates microlithiasis in association with chronic inflammation.

It is, however, unclear whether the presence of biliary sludge without cholesterol crystals or bilirubinate granules on biliary microscopy is a risk factor for the development of acute pancreatitis. In 1991 a study by Ros et al.[18] found that of 51 patients with so-called idiopathic pancreatitis 50 had microscopic bile abnormalities and/or gallstones on follow-up US. Only one patient had an isolated finding of biliary sludge on US. A further study of 31 patients with acute pancreatitis[19] found that 23 patients (74%) had sludge on US and/or abnormal microscopic changes but two of these patients were excluded due to MBD obstruction. Of the

Figure 15.1 Aetiology of 'biliary' acute pancreatitis.	
Gallstones	Periampullary diverticulum
Cholesterolosis	Intraluminal diverticulum
Sludge (?)	Choledochocoele
ESWL for gallstones	Choledochal cyst
Complications of ERCP and ES	AUPBD
Surgery of the biliary tract	Parasitic infestation
Ampullary tumours	Sclerosing cholangitis
Cholangiocarcinoma	Sphincter dysfunction

ERCP = endoscopic retrograde cholangiopancreatography
ES = endoscopic sphincterotomy
AUPBD = anomalous union of the pancreatic and biliary ducts
ESWL = extracorporeal shockwave lithotripsy

Aetiology	Number	Median age (range) in years	Women	Predicted[b] severe	Clinically[c] severe
Gallstones	258 (62%)	63 (22–96)	159 (62%)	85 (34%)	71 (28%)
Alcohol	104 (25%)	41 (14–74)	17 (16%)	10 (10%)	25 (24%)
Miscellaneous	55[a] (13%)	58 (28–87)	26 (47%)	17 (31%)	15 (26%)
Total	417 (100%)	58 (28–87)	202 (48%)	112 (27%)	111 (27%)

[a] Idiopathic = 45, hyperlipidaemia = 5, hyperparathyroidism = 3, collagen disorders = 2.
[b] Based on a modified Imrie score 3.
[c] Based on actual clinical outcome.

Figure 15.2 Details of 258 patients with gallstone-associated acute pancreatitis compared to 159 patients with acute pancreatitis due to other causes. Data from Winslet et al. 1992[4].

remaining 21 patients, 11 were found to have sludge on US and 10 of these had calcium bilirubinate crystals on bile microscopy. It is known, however, that many healthy individuals have small amounts of calcium bilirubinate granules on microscopy[20] and unfortunately the authors did not quantify this, thus making the significance of their observation difficult to interpret. The remaining 10 patients did not have sludge on US: 8 had cholesterol crystals and 2 had calcium bilirubinate crystals. Furthermore, 3 of 14 patients with alcoholic pancreatitis had sludge detected on US but no microscopic abnormalities of the bile. It therefore seems possible that sludge formation is secondary to the pancreatitis rather than a cause and may have occurred due to the development of an ileus and reduced gall bladder contractility. Patients with sludge alone should be regarded as having 'idiopathic' pancreatitis until more data are available on this subject.

PATHOPHYSIOLOGY

Gallstone passage

It is now agreed that the passage of gallstones through the ampulla of Vater is the key event in the development of acute gallstone pancreatitis. The recognition that this was of major importance came with the observation that nearly all patients with gallstone pancreatitis have stones present in their faeces as compared to only 10% of those hospitalized for acute biliary colic but not having pancreatitis[5,21,22]. What continues to be of much more debate, however, is how the passage of a gallstone can bring about an attack of pancreatitis. At present the weight of evidence seems to be in favour of the common channel with bile reflux hypothesis, which was first put forward by Opie[1].

It is likely that a gallstone temporarily obstructing the ampulla allows bile to reflux into the pancreas if the appropriate anatomical situation arises. After the stone has passed, pancreatic juice drains freely from the MPD enabling the gland to release activated pancreatic enzymes and also allowing the enzymes to be inactivated by the antiproteases present. This would correlate with a mild attack of acute pancreatitis. However, if more stones were subsequently to migrate across the ampulla, leading to further episodes of temporary obstruction, then more activated enzymes would become trapped within the MPD and lead to more extensive pancreatic damage, ultimately progressing to a severe attack of pancreatitis.

The common channel

The common channel theory, as first proposed by Opie to explain the mechanism whereby gallstones induce acute pancreatitis, has been criticized as too simplistic since ampullary obstruction has been found in less than 5% of cases[4]. In addition, the terminal union of the MBD and MPD is too short to let the common channel situation arise in the majority of patients[23]. Despite doubts about the common channel theory, two patient studies[24,25] have demonstrated that a functional channel between the MBD and MPD can arise in gallstone-associated acute pancreatitis. In the larger of the two reports, 21 patients who had undergone open cholecystectomy and common bile duct exploration were studied[24]. All the patients had a T-tube in situ and they were divided into three groups: (a) those with gallstones alone; (b) those with gallstones and MBD stones; (c) those with acute gallstone pancreatitis. Patients were given a standard meal and the fluid from the T-tube collected and analysed for the presence of pancreatic enzymes. Patients with recent episodes of gallstone-induced acute pancreatitis were found to have a much higher (up to 100 times) resting and stimulated amylase activity in the T-tube fluid. None of the three groups of patients had any detectable duodenal enzymes in the fluid, which casts doubt on the duodenal reflux theory[26] as the cause of acute pancreatitis.

It is known, however, that the pressure in the MPD exceeds that in the MBD[27] and thus even if there were a common channel pancreatic juice would flow into the biliary tree rather than bile into the MPD. To counter this argument, however, high biliary pressures do occur in obstructive acute cholangitis[28] and such pressures could occur in acute pancreatitis if a stone temporarily obstructed the ampulla. In addition, contraction of the gall bladder in the face of biliary obstruction would also lead to a significant rise in pressure within the biliary tree, even if only for a short period of time. Oedema of the papilla following passage of a stone would also reduce the length of common channel required to allow biliopancreatic reflux to take place. Operative cholangiography has also shown that biliopancreatic reflux occurs more frequently in those patients who have had attacks of acute gallstone pancreatitis[7].

Pancreatic and bile duct dimensions

The sizes of the MPD and MBD increase with advancing age but patients with acute gallstone pancreatitis have a relatively greater increase in the size of these ducts[29]. This study of 120 patients showed that the 94 patients with gallstone pancreatitis had a mean MBD diameter of 9.2mm compared with a mean of 5.0mm in the 26 patients that had other causes of their pancreatitis. Those patients who had MBD stones present at the time of investigation had a greater MBD (12.5mm) and MPD (4.02mm) diameter than those whose MBD was clear but who had gall bladder stones (7.1mm and 3.45mm, respectively). Even when taking into account potentially confounding factors such as age and the presence of MBD stones those with gallstone pancreatitis still have larger diameters for the MBD and MPD[30]. In addition, patients who suffer acute pancreatitis also have larger cystic ducts[12] than those with gallstones alone. The larger the diameter of the biliary tree, the more likely is the passage of a stone sufficiently large to cause transient obstruction of the ampulla.

DIAGNOSIS OF CHOLELITHIASIS IN ACUTE PANCREATITIS

In order to confirm gallstones as the cause of an attack of acute pancreatitis, gallstones must be detectable and other aetiological factors excluded. US has an accuracy in excess of 95% for the detection of uncomplicated gallstones, but in acute pancreatitis this figure falls to around 70–80%[31,32]. This is because there is often an ileus with gas-filled loops of bowel thus obscuring the view for the ultrasonographer. Additionally there is a tendency for the smaller stones (diameter 3–7mm) to cause attacks of acute pancreatitis[5,33], which means that up to 30% of gallstones causing an attack will go undetected[31]. A way of increasing the sensitivity by 10–20% is to measure transaminases within 48 hours of an attack; an elevated level suggests that it is gallstones that are causing the acute pancreatitis[31,32].

Endoscopic retrograde cholangiopancreatography (ERCP) is the most accurate way of detecting gallstones in acute pancreatitis, with a sensitivity greater than 95%[29]. There is, however, an associated morbidity and mortality[34] with ERCP and it should not be undertaken in the acute situation unless there is indication and intention to perform some form of therapeutic intervention.

Evidence of cholelithiasis can arise during the convalescent phase of a patient's illness. This is usually following US but patients should not be labelled as having 'idiopathic' pancreatitis until an ERCP has been performed[35]. Even then a number of patients will be missed who have microlithiasis or who have passed all their stones into the duodenum. The diagnosis of microlithiasis can be made by sampling gall bladder bile and looking for cholesterol crystals with polarizing microscopy[16–18]. The presence of significant amounts of calcium bilirubinate crystals indicates the presence of pigment stones[17,36]. Gallstones or microlithiasis may ultimately only be discovered in a cholecystectomy specimen and therefore all patients with more than one attack of unexplained pancreatitis should have the gall bladder removed.

NATURAL HISTORY

Morbidity and mortality

Most attacks of gallstone-associated acute pancreatitis are mild and self-limiting. The complications are much the same as for any cause of acute pancreatitis, with the exception of acute cholangitis, which has a higher incidence of around 10%[4,37,38] (Figure 15.3). Patients with predicted mild attacks will have a median (range) hospital stay of 11 (4–27) days; patients who suffer a severe attack have a median length of

	Gallstones (n = 258)	Alcohol (n = 104)	Miscellaneous (n = 55)	Total (n = 417)
[a]**Systemic complications**				
Respiratory failure	18	15	6	39
Pleural effusion	7	6	1	14
Cardiac failure	5	0	2	7
Renal failure	3	1	2	6
Disseminated intravascular coagulation	1	0	0	1
Cerebrovascular accident	1	0	1	2
Pulmonary embolus	1	1	0	2
Multi-organ failure	7	3	3	13
[b]**Abdominal complications**				
Pancreatic necrosis	11	4	5	20
Pseudocyst	22	9	2	33
Pancreatic abscess	3	4	2	9
Duodenal obstruction	1	0	0	1
Gross ascites	3	2	4	9
Portal vein thrombosis	1	2	0	3
Acute cholangitis	25	0	1	26
Deaths	21(8.1%)	5(4.1%)	8(14.5%)	34(8.1%)

[a] *Despite adequate medical measures.*
[b] *Clinically significant complications, i.e. complications not based purely on imaging.*

Figure 15.3 Types and number of complications in 258 patients with gallstone-associated acute pancreatitis and 159 patients with acute pancreatitis due to other causes. Data from Winslet *et al.* 1992[4].

Type of study	Authors	Year	Number of patients	Number of deaths	Per cent mortality
Medical therapy	MRC Trial	1977	72	5	7.0%
Surgery	Stone et al. (3)	1981	31	1	3.0%
	Kelly and Wagner (42)	1988	82	2	2.4%
Endoscopic therapy	Neoptolemos et al. (39)	1988	53	3	5.7%
	Nowak et al. (52)	1990	94	9	10.4%
	Fan et al. (37)	1993	63	5	7.9%
	Fölsch et al. (38)	1995	112	6	5.4%
Total			**507**	**31**	**6.1%**

Figure 15.4 Mortality from gallstone-associated acute pancreatitis based on data from control arms of randomized trials.

stay of 17 (4–74) days (figures based on the conservative arm of an endoscopic intervention trial[39]).

Reported mortality for an attack of gallstone pancreatitis varies widely from zero[40] to as high as 20%[2]. This large variation in mortality rates results from the different population groups being studied, the proportion of severe cases within those groups, the different standards of medical care, and the types of specific interventions undertaken. To try and negate these confounding factors, probably the best indicator of 'natural' mortality due to acute pancreatitis is given by the conservative or 'placebo' arms of randomized treatments for acute pancreatitis. The overall mortality from the control arm of seven randomized trials (which ignores the severity of the attack) was 31 (6.1%) in 507 cases (Figure 15.4). Despite this, the true mortality is likely to be higher, as patients entered into trials usually have a lower mortality than non-trial patients.

Recurrent attacks

Patients who survive an attack of acute gallstone pancreatitis are at a 30–40% risk of a further attack[22,41] unless the gall bladder is removed. However, the timing of cholecystectomy is important, as early surgery in those with severe acute pancreatitis leads to an increase in morbidity and mortality[42,43], which is also the case for those patients undergoing laparoscopic cholecystectomy within one week of a severe attack[44]. The cumulative risk for a further attack of acute pancreatitis without surgery is not precisely known but the average time span between attacks in one study was 108 days[45]. The risk of death from a further attack of biliary acute pancreatitis is probably similar to that for a first attack but true figures are difficult to obtain because of biases in patient selection.

TREATMENT

General measures

As with any patient with acute pancreatitis, a detailed history and examination should be performed, the aetiology established and a predictive severity score calculated. The patient will require close monitoring and full supportive therapy including intravenous fluids, giving the patient nil by mouth, and the administration of parenteral analgesia as required. There is no evidence from any randomized clinical trials to date that any specific medical therapy is of benefit.

Rationale for pancreatic and biliary decompression

There is some experimental work in animals that suggests that decompression of the MBD and MPD improves outcome in acute pancreatitis. A study in the opossum compared the severity of pancreatitis after ligation of the MPD alone, the MPD and MBD separately (thus preventing reflux of bile into the MPD), and the common biliopancreatic duct[46]. Each animal group developed similarly severe acute pancreatitis and, consequently, it was concluded that the pressure in the MPD was the critical factor in the development of pancreatitis. However, earlier studies in the same animal model did not reach the same conclusions[47–49] as it was the combined MPD and MBD ligation that brought about the worst attack of pancreatitis.

It has been demonstrated in a rat model that repeated short-term obstruction of the pancreatic duct rather than a single episode of obstruction leads to a more severe attack of pancreatitis[50]. In addition, a further study from Steer's group demonstrated that, by relieving the obstruction to the MPD in the opossum, they could reduce the severity of an attack[51]. This experimental work suggests that relief of MPD and/or MBD obstruction is important.

Urgent versus delayed surgery

In the 1980s two randomized trials of early versus delayed surgery in acute gallstone pancreatitis were carried out in an attempt to decompress the biliary tree and pancreatic duct. In the first study[3], done by Stone, 65 patients were randomized to undergo either transduodenal sphincteroplasty and decompression within 73 hours of admission or delayed surgery once the patient was well. There was no significant difference between the two groups but there were no predictive criteria of severity used.

The second report[42] looked at 165 patients, who were randomized to either undergo surgery within 48 hours of presentation or have surgery delayed beyond this period of time. Those patients who were adjudged as severe by the Ranson criteria did worse with early surgery with a higher morbidity (83% vs 18%) and mortality (48% vs 12%) but those with predicted mild disease showed no difference between the two groups. The problem with this study is that patients in the active arm were operated on before a proper Ranson score could be obtained at 48 hours, which means that those who underwent early surgery were underscored for severity. In addition the patients in this study had only their biliary tree decompressed by means of a T-tube and did not have decompression of the MPD or have the MBD cleared of stones, which may explain some of the differences in outcome between this study and the earlier one by Stone[3].

Endoscopic decompression of MBD and MPD

To date there have been four randomized trials of urgent biliary decompression by endoscopic sphincterotomy, two of which have shown a clear benefit, the other two not showing such a clear advantage. The first study to be performed was done in Leicester in England[39] and randomized 121 patients with acute pancreatitis. Patients were prospectively stratified according to predictive severity using modified Glasgow criteria and then were randomized to undergo ERCP with or without endoscopic sphincterotomy (ES) or conservative treatment where patients were not permitted to have ERCP intervention. ES was performed if there were stones present in the bile duct. Overall, patients on whom early ES (within 72 hours) was performed did significantly better, with a morbidity of 12% and a mortality of 2%. This compared with a morbidity of 34% and a mortality of 8% in the conventionally managed group. In those patients with a predicted mild attack there was no difference in outcome in the two groups (morbidity 12%; mortality 0%) but there was significant improvement in those with predicted severe attacks (morbidity 24% vs 61%; mortality 1.7% vs 18%). In the severe group 63% of patients had urgent ES following ERCP for confirmed MBD stones.

The study has been criticized on the grounds that the observed improvement in outcome was due to the fact that it was relief of obstructive jaundice and concomitant cholangitis in the ES group that made the difference. However, if those with cholangitis are excluded from the analysis (six in the urgent ERCP group and five in the conservatively managed group) there is an even more pronounced benefit in the severe cases undergoing urgent ES (complication rate 15% vs 60%, p = 0.003). In addition, the median hospital stay in the severe group was reduced to 9.5 days for patients given urgent ERCP and ES compared to 17 days in the conservatively managed patients.

The second trial, from Katowice in Poland[52], studied 250 patients who had ERCP performed within 24 hours of admission. All of those with a bulging papilla suggesting the presence of an impacted stone (n = 62) had ES performed. The remaining 188 patients with normal appearances of the ampulla were then randomized to ES or conventional treatment, though they were not prospectively stratified before being randomized. Both morbidity and mortality were significantly reduced in the patients given ES (morbidity 14% vs 34%; mortality 1% vs 11%). It is interesting to note that most of the patients were tertiary referrals with a mean delay of 3.5 days between onset of symptoms and treatment, which suggests that even delayed ES can be of some benefit.

In the third trial, from Hong Kong[37], patients were randomized to ERCP, with or without ES, within 24 hours of admission. Control patients were permitted to undergo ERCP and ES only if they deteriorated. Overall there was a significant reduction in biliary sepsis in the urgent ES group (0% vs 12%) but no difference in morbidity or mortality. One of the major flaws with the study is that the method of severity assessment used was the Hong Kong system[53], which has subsequently been shown to be inadequate with a sensitivity of only 33% and specificity of 88%[54]. Although the Ranson system was also used, because it can only be fully ascertained at 48 hours, the groups cannot be compared because intervention in the active group took place within 24 hours. Furthermore, there were also 30 patients in whom the diagnosis was not gallstone-induced pancreatitis but, rather, the pancreatitis due to some other cause (alcohol, ascariasis, hyperlipidaemia and choledochal cyst). In addition there were 38 patients with 'idiopathic' pancreatitis. Once only those with gallstones are considered, the results are similar to those of the Leicester group (Figure 15.5).

The German Multicentre Study[38] collected 238 patients between 1989 and 1994 from 22 different hospitals. The

Severity of attack Treatment	City	n	Complications Local	Systemic	Deaths	Total
Mild ERCP/ES	Leicester	28	3	1	0	4
	Hong Kong	34	4	2	0	6
Total		**62**	**7(11%)**	**3(5%)**	**0**	**10(16%)**
Mild Conventional	Leicester	29	4	0	0	4
	Hong Kong	35	1	5[4][a]	0	6
Total		**64**	**5(8%)**	**5(8%)**	**0**	**10(16%)**
Severe ERCP/ES	Leicester	22	3	1	0	4
	Hong Kong	30	3	3	1	4
Total		**52**	**[b]6(12%)**	**[c]4(8%)**	**[d]1(2%)**	**[e]8(15%)**
Severe Conventional	Leicester	24	6	9	3	13
	Hong Kong	28	8	16[8]a	5	15
Total		**52**	**[b]14(27%)**	**[c]25(48%)**	**[d]8(15%)**	**[e]28(54%)**

[a] biliary sepsis; [b] p<0.05; [c] p<0.01; [d] p<0.05; [e] p<0.01.

Figure 15.5 Results of the Leicester[39] and Hong Kong[37] randomized trials of urgent ERCP and ES in patients with acute pancreatitis confirmed to be due to gallstones.

patients were randomized to undergo ERCP and ES within 72 hours or to be managed purely conservatively. All jaundiced patients were excluded from the study as they would undergo urgent ERCP and ES anyway, which is an important consideration, as it is patients with a serum bilirubin of > 40mol/l who are most likely to have MBD stones[55] and thus have the greatest benefit from urgent ERCP and ES. Although patients were stratified for severity there were some whose severity was 'undefined', which makes subsequent interpretation of the results more difficult. Another unusual feature of the study was that equal numbers of patients in each group (n = 11) developed cholangitis; it might be expected that if there had been adequate ES, and biliary drainage this would not have occurred, which suggests that at least in some of the centres the quality of ES was suspect. The difficulties highlighted above may explain why the study was unable to demonstrate a benefit in the urgent ERCP/ES group.

It is now generally agreed that any patient with even mild obstructive jaundice in association with gallstone acute pancreatitis should have an urgent ERCP and ES, and the argument for ES in those with concomitant cholangitis is even stronger (Figure 15.6). Mortality can be halved for those with cholangitis associated with acute pancreatitis by ES compared to other forms of surgical intervention, although it is still higher than in those with either condition in isolation[56]. The Leicester, Hong Kong and Katowice trials demonstrate that a significant reduction in local and systemic complications can be brought about by ES in patients with predicted severe attacks of pancreatitis due to gallstones. Urgent endoscopic intervention is not indicated for those with a predicted mild attack, unless there are signs of clinical deterioration. It should be remembered, however, that these procedures can potentially lead to life-threatening complications[57] and should only be performed by experts in those patients in whom there is a clear clinical indication.

Prevention of further attacks

It is now usually recommended that patients with an attack of gallstone-associated acute pancreatitis should undergo a cholecystectomy on the same admission, as there is a 30–40% risk of a further attack[22,41]. However, it is also agreed that the timing of surgery is important and that open[42,43] or laparoscopic[44] surgery should not be undertaken during the acute phase of an attack. Intraoperative cholangiography is essential to ensure that all stones are

Figure 15.6 Conventional treatment compared to endoscopic sphincterotomy in the treatment of acute cholangitis associated with acute pancreatitis.

Treatment	n	Deaths
Conventional		
Andrew and Johnson (62)	4	2
Ong et al. (63)	50	5
McMahon et al. (64)	7	3
Neoptolemos et al. (65)	9	3
Total	**70**	**13 (16%)**
Endoscopic sphincterotomy		
Neoptolemos et al. (65)	14	1 (7%)
Nowak et al. (56)	54	4 (8%)
Total	**68**	**5 (7.4%)**

cleared from the MBD, otherwise the patient still risks a further attack. Prior to laparoscopic cholecystectomy, many patients will undergo preoperative ERCP; this does not negate the need for intraoperative imaging as some gallstones could still have migrated in the time between the ERCP and surgery. Such stones can either be cleared at the time of surgery or with postoperative ERCP and ES.

It is now recommended by some authors that the most efficient way of handling the potential of persisting MBD stones is to select patients with a high probability of MBD stones for preoperative ERCP, done on the basis of clinical, biochemical and US findings[58,59]. Patients with a high probability of MBD stones being present at the time of surgery are those with cholangitis, obstructive jaundice, persistent hyperamylasaemia or with MBD stones on US. By the selective use of ERCP prior to surgery the unnecessary ERCP rate can be reduced to less than 10%[59].

ERCP and ES can be usefully employed in those patients who are at high risk for surgical procedures. A good sphincterotomy is a highly effective way of preventing recurrent attacks of acute biliary pancreatitis[60]. Most patients who suffer further attacks following this procedure are those in whom there is papillary stenosis, and they will benefit from repeated ES. There is, however, a significant complication rate of up to 20% for those patients in whom the gall bladder is left in situ[61] and thus all patients should undergo cholecystectomy where possible.

References

1. Opie EL. The etiology of acute haemorrhagic pancreatitis. *Bull Johns Hopkins Hosp* 1901; 121:182–8.

2. Corfield AP, Cooper MJ, Williamson RCN. Acute pancreatitis: a lethal disease of increasing incidence. *Gut* 1985; 26:724–9.

3. Stone HH, Fabian TC, Dunlop WE. Gallstone pancreatitis: biliary tract pathology in relation to time of operation. *Ann Surg* 1981; 194:305–10.

4. Winslet MC, Hall C, London NJM, Neoptolemos JP. Relationship of diagnostic serum amylase to aetiology and prognosis in acute pancreatitis. *Gut* 1992; 33:982–6.

5. Acosta JL, Ledesma CL. Gallstone migration as a cause for acute pancreatitis. *New Eng J Med* 1974; 190:484–7.

6. Opie EL. *Diseases of the pancreas. Its cause and nature.* Lippincott, Philadelphia. 1903.

7. Armstrong CP, Taylor TV, Jeacock J , Lucas, S. The biliary tract in patients with acute gallstone pancreatitis. *Br J Surg* 1985; 72:551–5.

8. Moreau JA, Zinsmeister AR, Melton LJ. Gallstone pancreatitis and the effect of cholecystectomy: a population-based cohort study. *Mayo Clin Proc* 1988; 63:466–73.

9. Houssin D, Castain GD, Lemoine J, Bismuth, H. Microlithiasis of the gallbladder. *Surg Gynecol Obstet* 1983; 157:20–40.

10. Farinon AM, Sianesi M, Zanella, E. Physiopathological role of microlithiasis in gallstone pancreatitis. *Surg Gynecol Obstet* 1987; 164:252–6.

11. Eichelberger MR, Hoelzer DJ, Koop CE. Acute pancreatitis: the difficulties of diagnosis and therapy. *J Ped Surg* 1982; 17:244–54.

12. Taylor TV, Rimmer, S, Holt, S, Jeacock J, Lucas, S. Sex differences in gallstone pancreatitis. *Ann Surg* 1991; 214:667–70.

13. Narwold DL. Gallstone lithotripsy. *Am J Surg* 1993; 165:431–4.

14. Lee SP, Nicholls JF. Nature and composition of biliary sludge. *Gastroenterology* 1986; 90:677–86.

15. Paumgartner G, Sauerbruch, T. Gallstones: pathogenesis. *Lancet* 1991; 338:1117–21.

16. Marks JE, Bonnoris, G. Intermittency of cholesterol crystals in duodenal bile from gallstone patients. *Gastroenterology* 1984; 87:622–7.

17. Neoptolemos JP, Davidson BR, Winder AF, Vallance, D. The role of duodenal bile crystal analysis in the investigation of "idiopathic" pancreatitis. *Br J Surg* 1988; 75:954-60.

18. Ros E, Navarro S, Bru C, Garcia–Puges A, Valderama R. Occult microlithiasis in 'idiopathic' acute pancreatitis: prevention of relapse by cholecystectomy or ursodeoxycholic acid therapy. *Gastroenterology* 1991; 101:1701–9.

19. Lee SP, Nicholls JF, Park HZ. Biliary sludge as a cause of acute pancreatitis. *New Eng J Med* 1992; 326:589–93.

20. Juniper K, Burson EN. Biliary tract studies II: the significance of biliary crystals. *Gastroenterology* 1957; 32:175–209.

21. Kelly TR. Gallstone pancreatitis: pathophysiology. *Surgery* 1976; 80:88–92.

22. Kelly TR. Gallstone pancreatitis: the timing of surgery. *Surgery* 1980; 88:345–9.

23. Elliot DW, Williams RD, Zollinger RM. Alterations in the pancreatic resistance to bile in the pathogenesis of acute pancreatitis. *Ann Surg* 1957; 146:669–82.

24. Hernandez CA, Lerch MM. Sphincter stenosis and gallstone migration through the biliary tract. *Lancet* 1993; 341:1371–3.

25. Lerch MM, Weidenbach H, Hernandez CA, Preclik G, Adler G. Pancreatic outflow obstruction as the critical event for human gallstone induced pancreatitis. *Gut* 1994; 35: 1501–3.

26. McCutcheon AD. Aetiological factors in pancreatitis. *Lancet* 1962;710–2.

27. Robinson TM, Dunphy JE. Continuous perfusion of bile protease through the pancreas. *J Am Med Assoc* 1963; 183:530–3.

28. Csendes A, Sepulveda A, Burdiles P *et al*. Common bile duct pressure in patients with common bile duct stones with or without suppurative cholangitis. *Arch Surg* 1988; 123:697–9.

29. Neoptolemos JP, Carr-Locke DL, London N, Bailey I, Fossard DP. ERCP findings and the role of endoscopic sphincterotomy in acute gallstone pancreatitis. *Br J Surg* 1988; 75:954–60.

30. Neoptolemos JP, Carr-Locke DL, Kelly K. Factors affecting the diameters of the common bile duct and pancreatic duct using endoscopic retrograde cholangiopancreatography. *Hepatogastroenterology* 1991; 38:243–7.

31. Neoptolemos JP, Hall A, Finlay DF, Berry JM, Carr-Locke DL, Fossard DP. The urgent diagnosis of gallstones in acute pancreatitis: a prospective study of the methods. *Br J Surg* 1984; 71:230–47.

32. Wang SS *et al*. Clinical significance of ultrasonography, computed tomography, and biochemical tests in the rapid diagnosis of gallstone-related pancreatitis: a prospective study. *Pancreas* 1988; 3:153–8.

33. Kelly TR. Gallstone pancreatitis. *Ann Surg* 1984; 200:479–85.

34. Ostroff JW, Shapiro HA. Complications of endoscopic sphincterotomy. In *ERCP: Diagnostic and Therapeutic Applications*. Edited by I Jacobsen. Elsevier, New York. 1989: 61–73.

35. Goodman AJ, Neoptolemos JP, Carr-Locke DL, Finlay DBL, Fossard DP. Detection of gallstones after acute pancreatitis. *Gut* 1985; 26:125–32.

36. Neoptolemos JP, Davidson BR, Vallence D, Winder AF. Bile-crystal analysis for the detection and type-identification of gallstones. *Biochem Soc Trans* 1987; 15:1912–13.

37. Fan ST, Lai CS, Mok FPT, Lo CM, Rheng SS, Wong J. Early treatment of acute biliary pancreatitis by endoscopic papillotomy. *New Eng J Med* 1993; 328:228–32.

38. Folsch UR *et al*. Controlled randomised multicentre trial of urgent endoscopic papillotomy for acute biliary pancreatitis. *Gastroenterology* 1995; 108S:A353.

39. Neoptolemos JP, London NJ, James D, Carr-Locke DL, Bailey IA, Fossard DP. Controlled trial of urgent endoscopic retrograde cholangiopancreatography and endoscopic sphincterotomy versus conservative treatment for acute pancreatitis due to gallstones. *Lancet* 1988; ii:979–83.

40. Berlinski LS, Dorazio RA, Winkley JH. Gallstone pancreatitis. *Mt Sinai J Med* 1979; 46: 364–6.

41. Osborne DH, Imrie CW, Carter DC. Biliary surgery in the same admission for gallstone-associated acute pancreatitis. *Br J Surg* 1981; 68:758–61.

42. Kelly TR, Wagner DS. Gallstone pancreatitis: a prospective randomised trial of timing of surgery. *Surgery* 1988; 104:600–5.

43. Ranson JHC. The timing of biliary surgery in acute pancreatitis. *Ann Surg* 1979; 189:654–62.

44. Tang E, Stain SC, Tang G, Froes E, Berne TV. Timing of laparoscopic surgery in gallstone pancreatitis. *Arch Surg* 1995; 130:496–500.

45. Paloyan D, Simonowitz D, Skinner DB. The timing of biliary tract operations in patients with pancreatitis associated with gallstones. *Surg Gynecol Obstet* 1975; 141:737–9.

46. Lerch MM, Saluja AK, Runzi M, Dawra R, Saluja M, Steer ML. Pancreatic duct obstruction triggers acute necrotising pancreatitis in the opossum. *Gastroenterology,*1993; 104: 853–61.

47. Senninger N, Moody FG, Coelho JCU, Van Buren DH. The role of biliary obstruction in the pathogenesis of acute pancreatitis in the opossum. *Surgery* 1986; 99:688–93.

48. Runkel NS, Rodrigues LF, LaRocco MT, Moody FG. Mechanisms of pancreatic infection in acute pancreatitis in opossums. *Curr Surg* 1990; 47:460–2.

49. Runkel NS, Rodrigues LF, Moody FG, LaRocco MT, Blasdel T. *Salmonella* infection of the biliary and intestinal tract of wild opossums. *Lab Anim Sci* 1991; 41:54–6.

50. Hirano T, Manabe T. A possible mechanism for gallstone pancreatitis: repeated short-term pancreaticobiliary duct obstruction with exocrine stimulation in rats. *Proc Soc Exp Biol Med* 1993; 202:246–52.

51. Runzi M, Saluja A, Lerch MM, Dawra R, Nishino H, Steer ML. Early ductal decompression prevents the progression of biliary pancreatitis: an expeimental study in the opossum. *Gastroenterology* 1993; 105:157–64.

52. Nowak A, Nowakowska-Duzawa E, Rybicka J. Urgent endoscopic sphincterotomy vs conservative treatment in acute biliary pancreatitis – a prospective, controlled trial. *Hepatogastroenterology* 1990; 37SII:A5.

53. Fan ST, Choi TK, Lai ECS, Wong J. Prediction of severity of acute pancreatitis: an alternative approach. *Gut* 1989; 30:1591–5.

54. Heath DI, Imrie CW. The Hong Kong criteria and severity prediction in acute pancreatitis. *Int J Pancreatol* 1994; 15:179–85.

55. Neoptolemos JP, London N, Bailey I *et al*. The role of clinical and biochemical criteria and endoscopic retrograde cholangiopancreatography in the urgent diagnosis of common bile duct stones in acute pancreatitis. *Surgery* 1987; 100:732–42.

56. Nowak A, Dzlurkowska-Marek E, Nowakowska-Dulawa E, Marek A, Kaczor R. Does acute biliary pancreatitis (ABP) worsen the results of urgent endoscopic treatment of acute obstructive cholangitis (AOC)? *10th World Congress of Gastroenterology* 1994; 68EC (abstract).

57. Freeman M *et al*. Complications of endoscopic sphincterotomy (ES): a prospective, multicentre, 30-day outcome study. *Gastroenterology* 1994; 106: A338.

58. de Virgilio C, Verbin C, Chang L, Linder S, Stabile BE, Klein, S. Gallstone pancreatitis: the role of preoperative endoscopic retrograde cholangiopancreatography. *Arch Surg* 1994; 129: 909–13.

59. Rijna H, Borgstein PJ, Meuwissen SGM, de Brauw LM, Wildenborg NP, Cuesta MA. Selective preoperative endoscopic retrograde cholangiopancreatography in laparoscopic biliary surgery. *Br J Surg* 1995; 82:1130–3.

60. Welbourn CRB, Beckly DE, Eyre-Brook IA. Endoscopic sphincterotomy without cholecystectomy for gallstone pancreatitis. *Gut* 1995; 37:119–20.

61. Winslet MC, Neoptolemos JP. The place of endoscopy in the management of gallstones. *Clin Gastroenterol* 1991; 5:99–129.

62. Andrew DJ, Johnson SE. Acute suppurative cholangitis, a medical and surgical emergency. *Am J Gastroenterol* 1970; 54:141–54.

63. Ong GB, Lakn KH, Lam SK, Lim TK, Wong J. Acute pancreatitis in Hong Kong. *Br J Surg* 1979; 66:398–403.

64. McMahon MJ, Mayer AD, Shearer MG *et al*. Cholangitis and acute pancreatitis. *Gut* 1985; 26:A648.

65. Neoptolemos JP, Carr-Locke DL, Leese T, James D. Acute cholangitis in association with acute pancreatitis: incidence, clinical features and outcome in relation to ERCP and endoscopic sphincterotomy. *Br J Surg* 1987; 74:1103–6.

16

Idiopathic recurrent pancreatitis

Pier Alberto Testoni & Alberto Tittobello

AETIOLOGY

An aetiological association can be identified in about 60–70% of patients with recurrent episodes of acute pancreatitis from the history, conventional diagnostic tests and computed tomography (CT) scan or ultrasonography (US) of the abdomen. No abnormalities are found in the remaining cases and these patients are conventionally classified as having 'idiopathic' recurrent pancreatitis. In these cases, endoscopic retrograde cholangiopancreatography (ERCP) can further improve the diagnostic accuracy by identifying some types of dysfunction of the sphincter of Oddi[1–3], small common bile duct stones[4,5], strictures of the main pancreatic duct, the presence of a pancreas divisum[6–8], a periampullary diverticulum or a variety of papillary abnormalities[9–12] as probable causes of the recurrent episodes of pancreatitis.

Dysfunction of the sphincter of Oddi

Dysfunction of the sphincter of Oddi appears to have been the most frequent cause of idiopathic relapsing pancreatitis in the majority of published series. Radiography findings consistent for dysfunction of the sphincter of Oddi are: slight dilatation of the common bile duct (CBD) (Figures 16.1–16.3) or of the main pancreatic duct (main PD) (Figures 16.4 and 16.5); delayed emptying of contrast material into the duodenum (Figure 16.6); and, in long-standing disease, the presence of a narrowed terminal CBD, suggestive of papillary stenosis (Figure 16.7). Dysmotility of the sphincter of Oddi and papillary stenosis could induce pancreatitis either by favouring the retrograde reflux of bile into the PD, as a consequence of the transient or persistent impedance to the flow of bile from the CBD into the duodenum (Opie's observation[13]), or by resultant functional obstruction to PD drainage. It has recently been documented by Cavallini *et al.*[14] that the latter event is associated with episodes of recurrent idiopathic pancreatitis. By ultrasonography after maximal stimulation with secretin (the US-S test), they demonstrated a significant increase over baseline and control values of the diameter of the main PD, throughout the observation period, in acute pancreatitis patients. In addition, serum enzyme levels in these subjects after secretin stimulation were persistently increased over controls. The investigators suggested that PD outlet obstruction, mainly at the sphincter of Oddi, may be an important pathogenetic factor in the course of the disease.

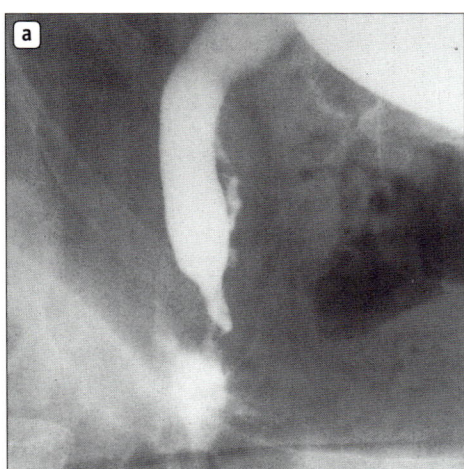
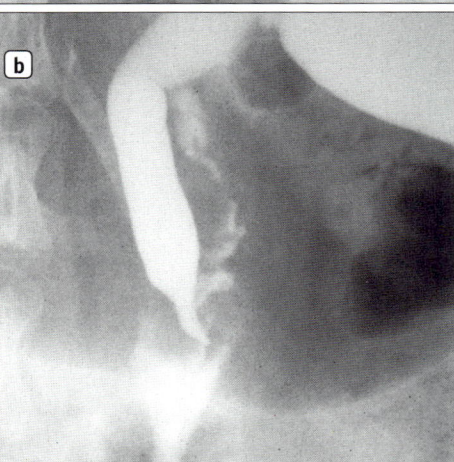

Figure 16.1 Dysfunction of the sphincter of Oddi: radiographic findings. (a) There is slight dilatation of the CBD associated with a tapering intrapapillary segment corresponding to the hypertonic sphincter. (b) Relaxation is incomplete but the contrast medium empties into the duodenum normally.

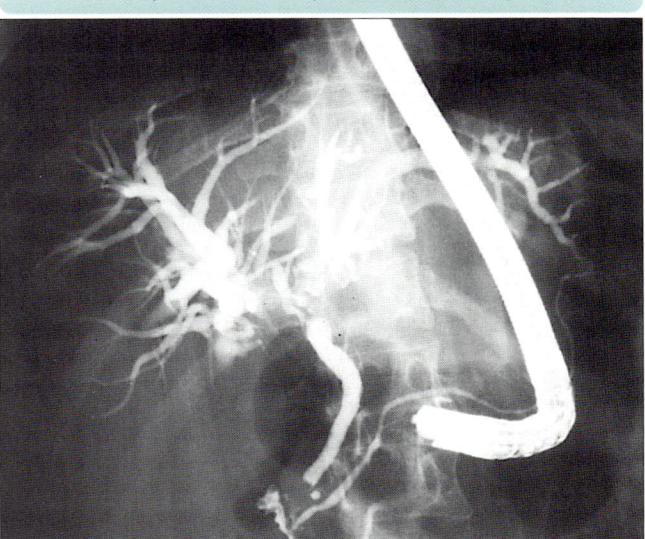

Figure 16.2 Cholangiopancreatography in a patient with recurrent pancreatitis: spasm of the CBD sphincter with slight dilatation of the biliary tree and pericholedochal cyst in the prepapillary region.

Figure 16.3 Concomitant spasm of the intrapapillary portion and of the distal part of the CBD associated with retrograde dilatation of the biliary tree.

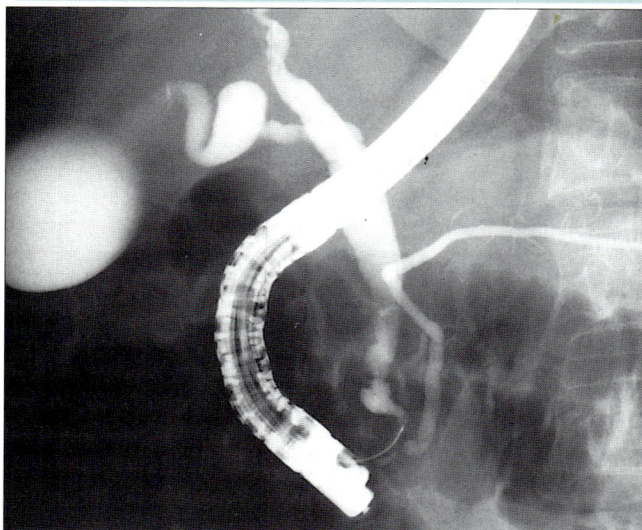

Figure 16.4 Slight dilatation of the entire main PD with delayed emptying of contrast medium into the duodenum.

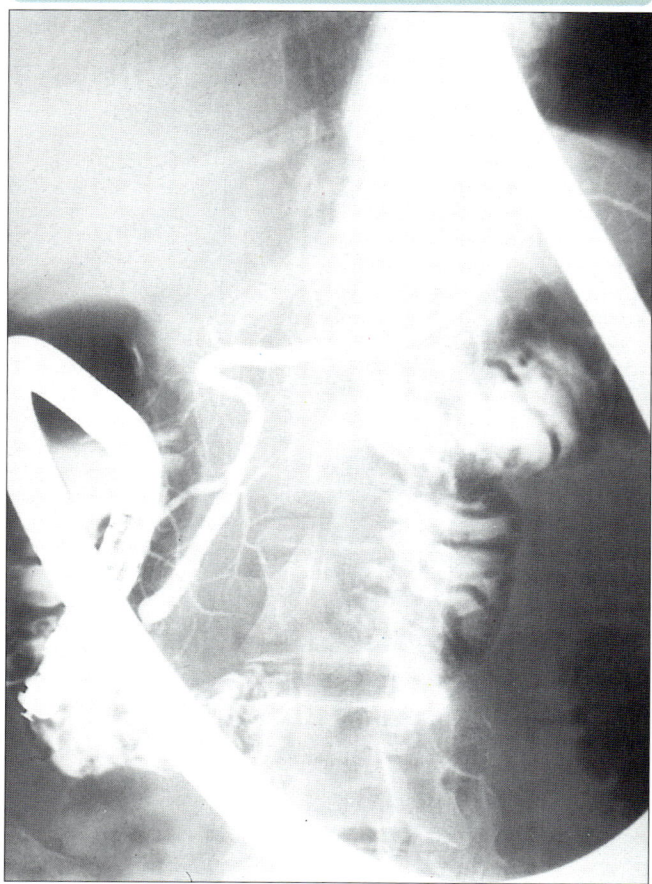

Figure 16.5 Dilatation of the entire main PD with narrowing prepapillary portion, due to hypertonia of the high pressure segment of the PD (spastic PD sphincter).

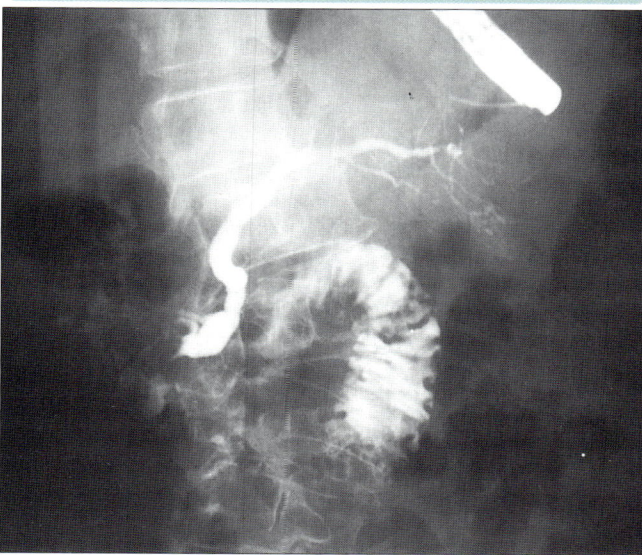

Bile duct gallstones

CBD stones are the most frequent cause of acute pancreatitis seen in community hospitals in Western Europe and in North America. The pathogenesis of biliary pancreatitis is related to the temporary impaction of migrating gallstones at the ampulla of Vater. Over a 10-year period we identified a stone disease by US and/or ERCP in 72.3% of 173 patients with a history of recurrent pancreatitis[15] (Figure 16.8). In many of these cases, long-lasting stone disease also resulted in a dysfunction of the sphincter of Oddi or in a benign papillary stenosis that might further influence the recurrence of episodes of pancreatitis. Small bile duct stones are frequently missed, even by real-time US[16,17] and can be demonstrated only at ERCP by using diluted contrast material and by a careful evaluation of the cholangiograms

(Figures 16.9 and 16.10). In a prospective series of 62 consecutive patients with idiopathic recurrent pancreatitis and no evidence of bile stones by US during the acute illness, Ros et al.[18] found ERCP diagnostic for biliary stones in 75.8% of cases.

However, in some patients thought to have idiopathic pancreatitis, small stones may not be detected even with ductal imaging techniques; in these cases microlithiasis or biliary sludges may be found only after endoscopic papillosphincterotomy (EPT) (Figure 16.11). The endoscopic procedure appears, therefore, to be at the same time both a diagnostic and a therapeutic tool. In negative cases, before performing papillosphincterotomy, microscopic examination of stimulated bile provides useful information about both the presence and the chemical composition of gallstones[19]. The finding of biliary crystal markers, either of cholesterol monohydrate or of calcium bilirubinate, could reliably diagnose microlithiasis in this situation[20,21], since it has been shown that the bile of control subjects is devoid of crystals[22,23].

In a prospective study performed by Neoptolemos et al.[24], calcium bilirubinate granules were found in 36% of patients, suggesting that small gallstones associated with pancreatitis are mostly of the non-cholesterol variety. However, another investigation showed a predominance of cholesterol microstones in these patients[18].

Figure 16.6 Concomitant dilatation of the CBD with narrowing of its distal part and of the main PD in a subject with sphincter of Oddi dysfunction.

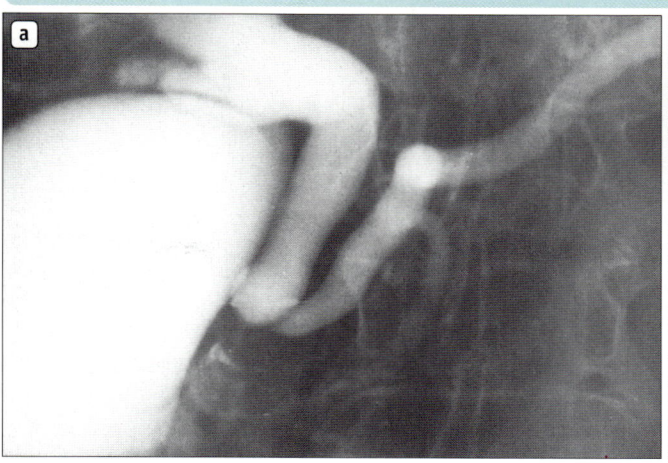

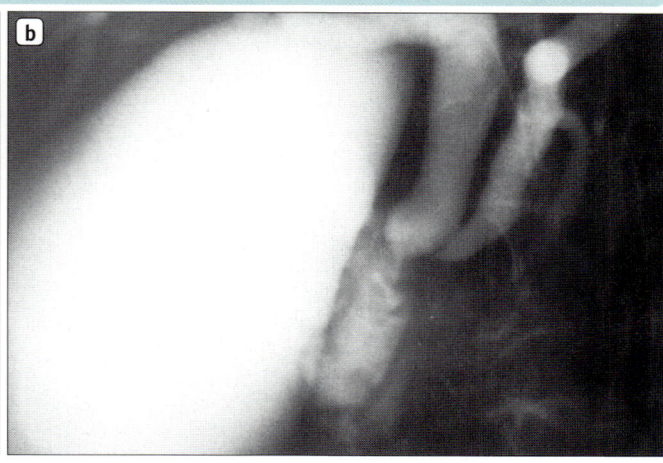

Pancreas divisum

Pancreas divisum may be associated with episodes of acute pancreatitis or upper abdominal pain, occurring either with meals or shortly after. The symptoms may be related to inadequacy of the minor papilla and its sphincter to permit outflow of the pancreatic juice. The secretion of pancreatic juice is maximal in the immediate postprandial period; in some cases, however, the symptoms occur unmpredictably at any time.

The aetiopathogenetic role of pancreas divisum in recurrent pancreatitis is still being debated, and since the first suggestion in 1977, over a hundred articles have appeared in the literature either supporting or refuting the hypothesis, with the result that the controversy continues. The overwhelming

Figure 16.7 A dilated CBD with stenosis of the intramural distal segment consistent with benign papillary stenosis.

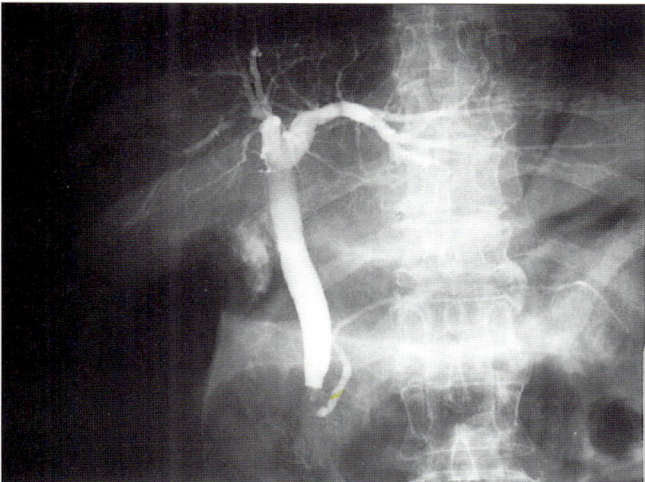

Figure 16.9 Cholangiographic finding of a small CBD stone located in the prepapillary segment; diagnosis by US of such small stones located in the intrapancreatic portion of the bile duct is still very difficult.

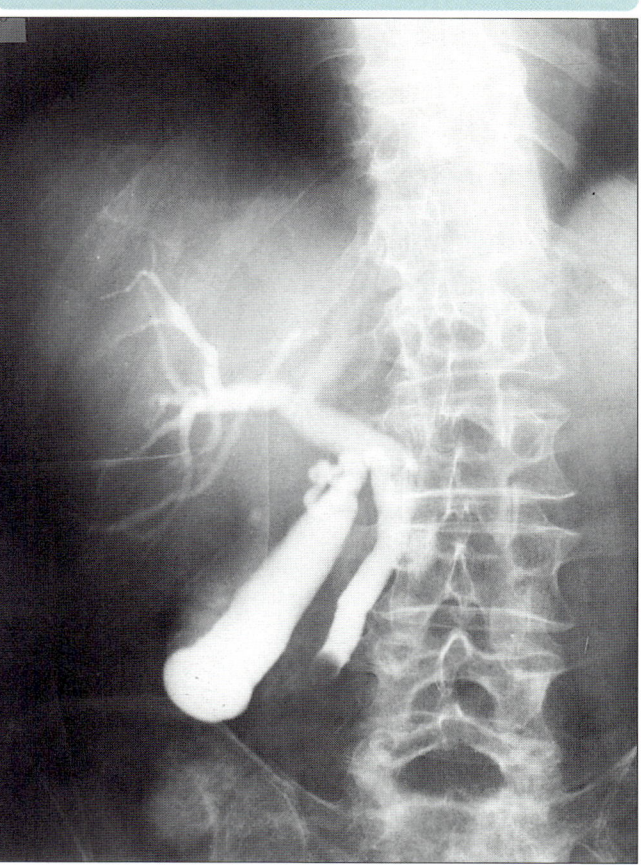

Figure 16.8 Endoscopic findings in 173 consecutive cases with recurrent episodes of acute pancreatitis. (Modified from Testoni *et al.*[15])

Diagnosis	*n*	Incidence
CBD stones		
± Papillary stenosis	125	72.3%
Benign papillary stenosis	32	18.5%
Idiopathic pancreatitis	16	9.2%
Overall cases	173	100%

Figure 16.10 Small fluctuating stone in the distal part of the CBD, associated with dysfunction of the sphincter of Oddi and dilatation of the biliary tree.

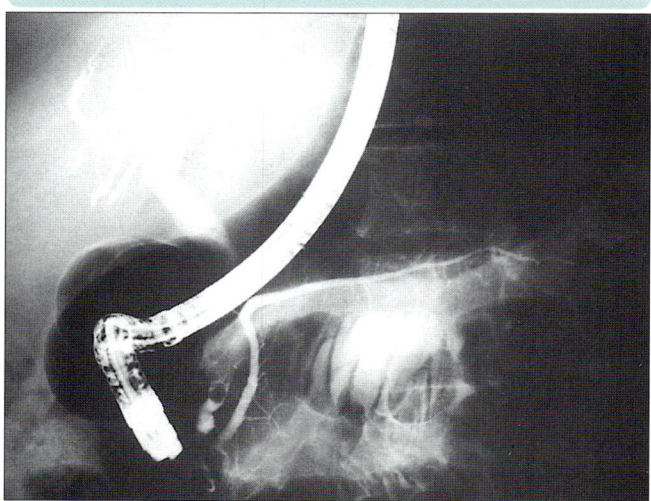

weight of opinion is more in favour of an association. Arguments for the involvement of pancreas divisum in the pathogenesis of pancreatitis and abdominal pain are based on the fact that an increased incidence of the anatomical variant has been reported in ERCP series of idiopathic relapsing pancreatitis. Clinical observation confirms the relative obstruction of outflow through the minor papilla, and that endoscopic or surgical procedures that open the minor papilla relieve the symptoms.

Arguments against the hypothesis question the evidence. There is no true association of pancreatitis with pancreas divisum; in some cases the variant is observed only by chance during ERCP. There is little direct evidence for obstruction of outflow from the dorsal duct during physiological pancreatic secretion and the response to endoscopic and surgical management is variable and unpredictable. In addition, pancreas divisum is often associated with gall bladder pathology and biliary pancreatitis, changes in the ventral PD and stenosis of the CBD sphincter (Figure 16.12)

Figure 16.11 (a) Multiple small stones extracted from the biliary tree after sphincterotomy.
(b) Microlithiasis of the CBD after sphincterotomy in a patient with benign papillary stenosis.
(c) Biliary sludge flowing out into the duodenum from the CBD after sphincterotomy.

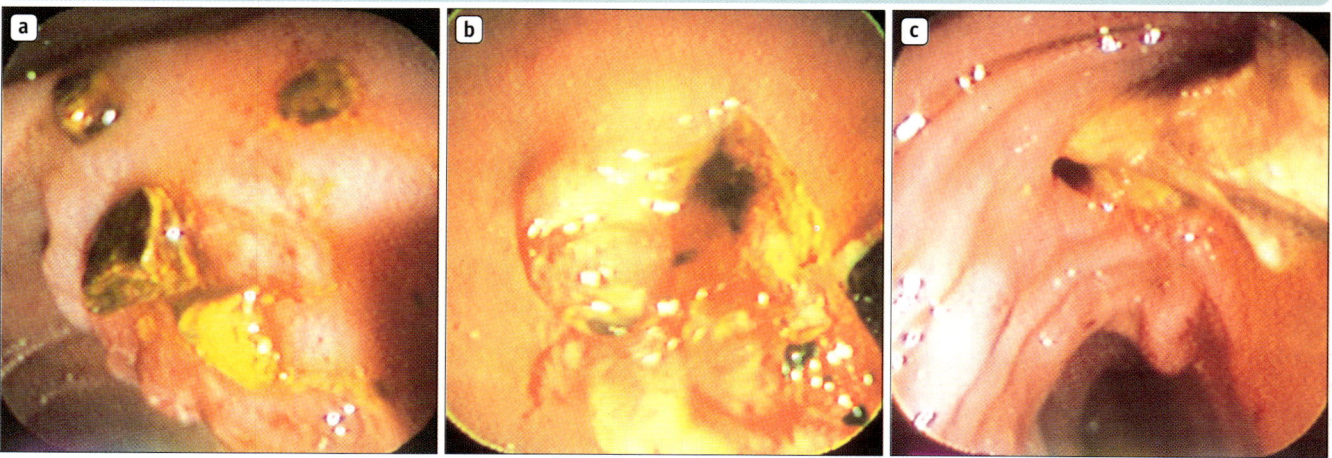

Figure 16.12 Dysfunction of the sphincter of Oddi in a patient with pancreas civisum: the opacification of the side branches, which are normally distributed, is consistent with the diagnosis of the anatomical variant.

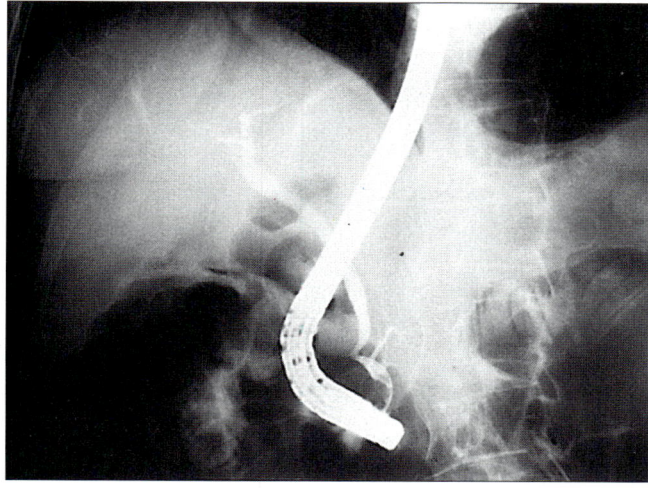

Figure 16.13 Opacification of the main PD and the duct of Santorini. There is a sigmoid configuration of the PD in the head of the gland with formation of an acute angle in correspondence with the insertion of the duct of Santorini into the main duct. The anatomical configuration is consistent with a functional pancreas divisum.

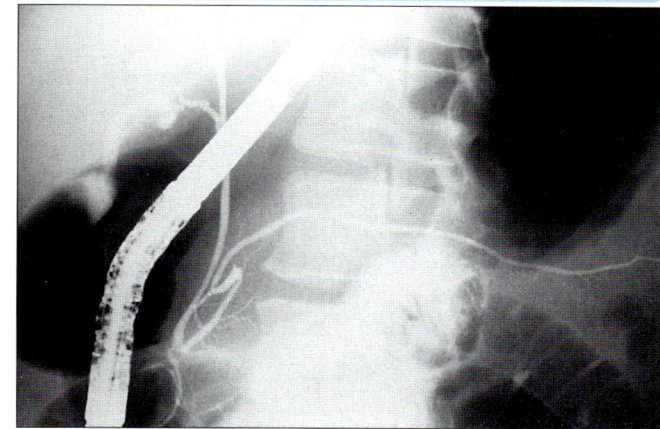

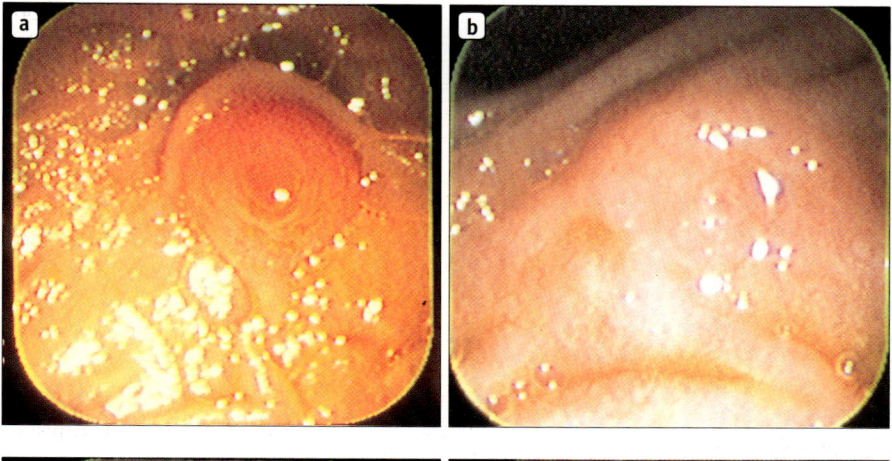

Figure 16.14 Different endoscopic appearances of a small and flat papilla of Vater, with thin orifice, which is difficult to cannulate.

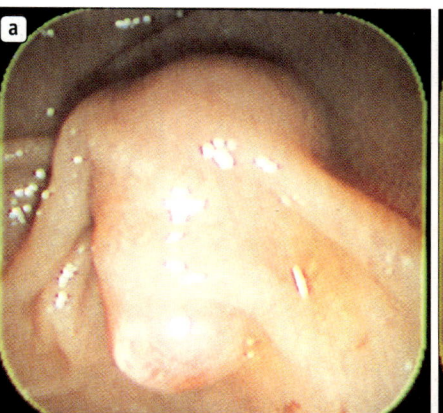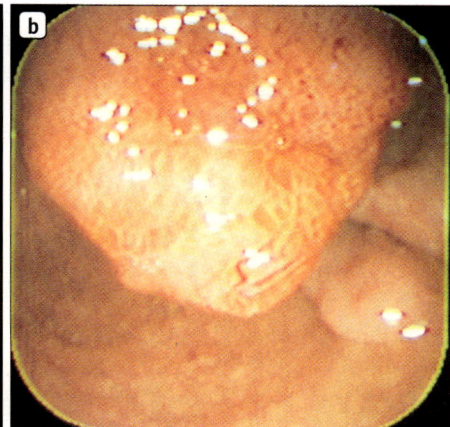

Figure 16.15 Endoscopic appearance of a prominent oedematous papilla of Vater, as a result of possible bile stone disease. (a) Image of papillo-odditis with benign stenosis, leading to a prominent, cyst-like ampulla. (b) An impacted stone is present in the ampulla, which is oedematous and projects into the duodenum. There is complete disappearance of the papillary orifice, due to compression by the stone.

and there is an unexplained association of pain with the ingestion of alcohol.

Both pancreatitis and pain can occur in the presence of a normal-appearing dorsal PD. On the other hand, subtle changes of the morphology of the duct indicate the existence of pancreatitis, even if the duct is not dilated. Since there is a predominant opinion that the pathogenesis of pain in most subjects with pancreas divisum seems to be related to the obstruction of the outlet of pancreatic flow, endoscopic drainage of the dorsal duct would be logical and effective and should always be attempted before surgery.

Variations and abnormalities of the papilla of Vater and the pancreatic excretory system

The endoscopic opacification of the PD system may reveal anatomical variations that could explain the occurrence of pancreatic pain and pancreatitis, as a consequence of impaired outflow of the pancreatic secretion into the duodenum. Variants of the course of the main PD and of fusion between the ventral and the dorsal gland (with the exception of pancreas divisum, discussed above) are the most common findings observed by pancreatography (Figure 16.13). Endoscopic examination of the descending portion of the duodenum may also document anatomical variations or abnormalities of the papilla of Vater that could induce recurrent episodes of acute pancreatitis or could be the consequences of long-standing disease. Commonly found anatomical variants in idiopathic recurrent pancreatitis are the presence of a small or flat papilla, with a small orifice, difficult to cannulate in some cases (Figure 16.14). Pathological findings of the papilla of Vater mostly suggest an unknown bile stone disease (Figures 16.15 and 16.16), whereas in rare cases there may be an ampulloma present (Figure 16.17).

The direct involvement or otherwise of periampullary diverticula in pancreatic disease is still being debated; although these diverticula are frequently found in gallstone disease and recurrent pancreatitis, it has yet to be proved that they play a role in the disease process (Figure 16.18).

After careful investigation of subjects with so-called idiopathic acute recurrent pancreatitis, the cause of the disease can be found in a large proportion of cases. Even in cases negative by ERCP or manometric recording, sphincterotomy may reveal microlithiasis or biliary sludge in the CBD, with the consequence that the term 'idiopathic' is properly justified in only very few cases.

ENDOSCOPIC TREATMENT

The majority of patients with recurrent episodes of 'idiopathic' pancreatitis in whom no organic cause can be found achieve relief of symptoms after endoscopic sphincterotomy of the CBD sphincter. A motor abnormality of the sphincter of Oddi is seen in about 50% of these subjects[5,25] with the result that, even when such an abnormality is confined to the PD segment, as in some cases[26,27], the decrease of basal pressure of the sphincter of Oddi obtained by conventional sphincterotomy is effective. Conventional sphincterotomy also results in a reduced basal PD sphincter pressure[22]. Nevertheless, persistently high PD segmental pressure may occasionally be the reason for lack of improvement after endoscopic papillosphincterotomy or surgical sphincteroplasty[28,29]. In 20% of patients with recurrent pancreatitis Raddawi *et al.*[26] found a basal pressure in the PD segment significantly greater (33.3 ± 4.2 mmHg) than that of the CBD segment (21.1 ± 2.5 mmHg) ($p < 0.05$).

Another therapeutic approach attempted for cases of hypertensive sphincter associated with episodes of recurrent pancreatitis was balloon dilatation[30]. However, the technique was not proven to be effective and was associated with a high frequency of procedure-related pancreatitis[31]. A prospective randomized trial of balloon dilatation of the sphincter of Oddi was unsuccessful in either reducing manometric pressures or improving symptoms, and carried an unacceptable rate of complications[32]. In our experience with a few cases, this therapeutic approach resulted in transient pain relief (persisting for a period of about 2 months after the procedure), followed by a process of fibrosis of the papilla of Vater and a recurrence of episodes of pancreatitis. Only endoscopic sphincterotomy provided these subjects with a stable disappearance of symptoms.

Among 173 patients with a history of previous episodes of acute pancreatitis who underwent endoscopic sphincterotomy in our centre over a 9-year period, no organic or functional alterations were found in 16 cases; these 16 patients were therefore considered to have 'idiopathic' pancreatitis. CBD stones were found in 125 subjects and a benign papillary stenosis in 32. A total of 138 subjects (79.76%) were followed for periods ranging from one to 9 years (Figure 16.19). There were further episodes of recurrent pancreatitis during the follow-up period in 2 of 16 subjects (12.5%) with previous diagnoses of idiopathic pancreatitis, suggesting that endoscopic section of the sphincter of Oddi of itself is an adequate treatment of such disease in most cases[15].

In 1983 Siegel first described[33] the results of endoscopic stenting of the main PD in 40 cases of idiopathic pancreatitis: 33 subjects obtained relief of symptoms during a mean period of follow-up of 11 months (range 3–72 months). The investigator performed pancreatic sphincterotomy with a needle-knife sphincterotome over a prosthesis previously inserted into the PD, in order to minimize the risk of perforation and bleeding that may occur more frequently during the performance of sphincterotomy of a pancreatic segment. The insertion of a pancreatic prosthesis (generally 5–7 French) decompresses the ductal system and maintains an effective opening of the high-pressure segment after the sphincterotomy has been performed. Pancreatic prostheses remain functional for a longer period of time than biliary prostheses, with duration of patency approaching an average of 6 months, in some cases up to 15 months[33]. The prosthesis may be successfully inserted into either the main PD or the duct of Santorini. Favourable

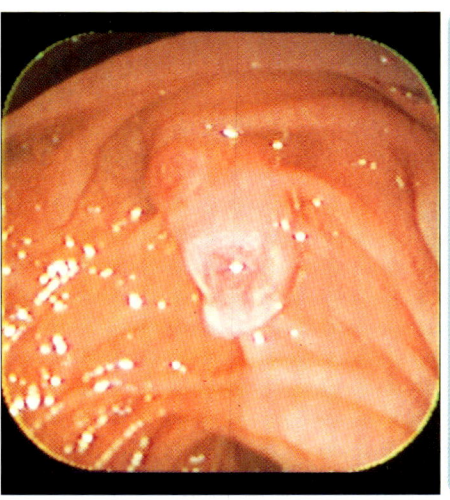

Figure 16.16 Spontaneous fistulous opening at the cephalad portion of the papilla, as the result of the recent passage of a stone into the duodenum.

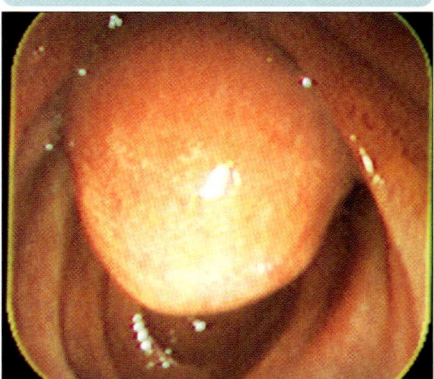

Figure 16.17 Endoscopic view of an ampullary tumour, bulging into the duodenal lumen.

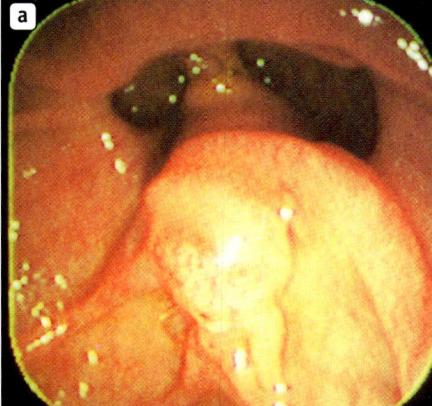

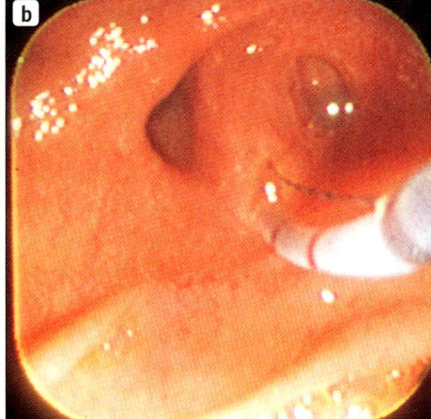

Figure 16.18 Endoscopic views of periampullary diverticula. (a) A large diverticulum completely surrounding the papilla of Vater, which is located on the inferior medial wall of the diverticulum. (b) Sphincterotomy performed between two deep diverticula.

Figure 16.19 Results of endoscopic sphincterotomy in 138 patients with recurrent pancreatitis, with follow-up periods between one and nine years. (Adapted from Testoni *et al.*[15])

Aetiology	n	Median follow-up (years)	Recurrence of pancreatitis
Bile duct stones	91	3.03	5 (5.5%)
Benign papillary stenosis	31	3.12	4 (12.9%)
'Idiopathic'	16	3.00	2 (12.5%)

Figure 16.20 Pancreatogram demonstrating a long 7-French prosthesis in place in the PD, after having traversed a narrowing segment in the prepapillary portion of the duct, in a patient with a history of recurrent idiopathic pancreatitis complicated by an attack of long-lasting acute pancreatitis and sepsis in the tail of the gland.

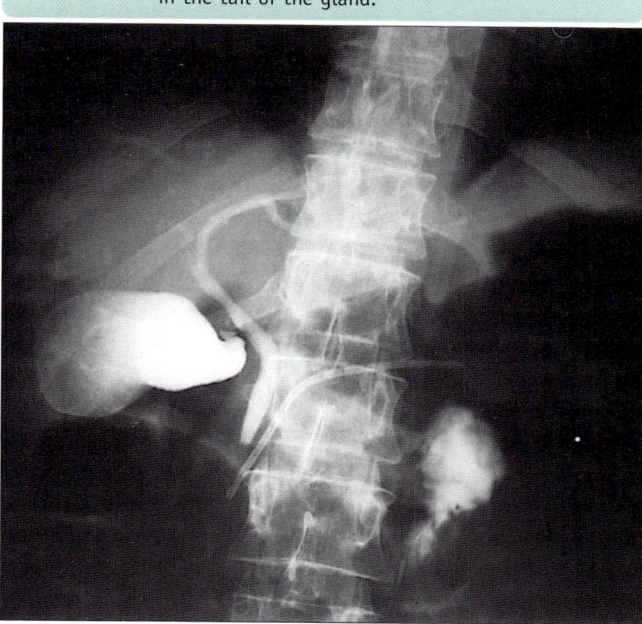

results with pancreatic stenting have also been reported by other workers[34,35].

We believe that this procedure could be performed in patients who do not benefit from standard sphincterotomy of the papilla of Vater and have positive US-S tests. It is likely that there is in these patients a stricture or a dysfunction of the high-pressure segment of the main PD, which is the cause of the recurrent episodes of pancreatitis (Figure 16.20).

Endoscopic management of pancreas divisum does not give optimal results, but the endoscopic approach should still be preferred to surgery. Stent placement across the minor papilla has been shown to be beneficial in reducing abdominal pain and episodes of pancreatitis, but the decision about endoscopic treatment is difficult to make when subjective symptoms are associated with minimal objective findings or a normal pancreatogram. Patients who present with unremitting pain and dietary restrictions and intake are the best candidates for endoscopic decompression, while it is more difficult to evaluate the stent's efficacy in relapsing pancreatitis. Stent placement has a 70% success rate, in experienced hands, and provides relief of symptoms in about 80% of patients[36]. A recent randomized controlled clinical trial in patients with acute recurrent pancreatitis documented, over a mean follow-up period of 30 months, the complete disappearance of symptoms and episodes of pancreatitis in subjects treated with endoscopic dorsal duct stenting, as compared with controls[37]. In all the studies symptoms recurred when the stent became occluded or migrated, confirming that the sphincteric dysfunction of the minor papilla is the main cause for symptoms in subjects with pancreas divisum.

Clinical results after the endoscopic therapeutic approach show that almost all cases with 'idiopathic' disease have sphincter of Oddi dysfunction, microlithiasis of the CBD, stricture of the distal segment of the main PD or anatomical variation.

COMPLICATIONS

Acute pancreatitis remains the commonest complication of diagnostic and therapeutic endoscopic procedures on the papilla of Vater. Despite efforts to reduce the known risks, by reducing chemical, mechanical and thermal trauma and avoiding acinarization or infection, it still appears to be impossible to significantly reduce the risk of post-ERCP/EPT pancreatitis. This is because the aetiology is multifactorial and the mechanisms leading to the pancreatic reaction are not yet understood in the majority of cases[38]. Patient factors that increase the risk for postprocedural complications, mainly pancreatitis, have been identified as dysfunction of the sphincter of Oddi, variant anatomy of the biliopancreatic junction, history of prior post-ERCP pancreatitis, and, probably, non-dilated CBD. Unfortunately, one or more of these factors is present in the majority of patients with idiopathic recurrent pancreatitis, with the result that the risk of complications in the endoscopic management of such disease is high. In addition, the history of recurrent idiopathic pancreatitis is of itself a risk factor for severe pancreatic reaction.

A number of investigations have found an increased risk of pancreatitis in subjects with dysfunction of the sphincter of Oddi, who have undergone diagnostic ERCP, sphincterotomy or sphincter of Oddi manometry. Leese *et al.*[39] found post-EPT complications in 16.2% of patients (33% had acute pancreatitis), in contrast with 10.3% of patients with biliary stones, and Thatcher *et al.*[40] found a complication rate of 15.6% (25% of patients had acute pancreatitis). Neoptolemos *et al.*[41] and Choudhry *et al.*[42] found pancreatitis rates of 12.3% and 31.4%, respectively, in these cases. The increased risk of pancreatitis in patients with dysfunction of the sphincter of Oddi could be the result of the presence of a hypertrophic or fibrotic sphincter that requires several attempts at

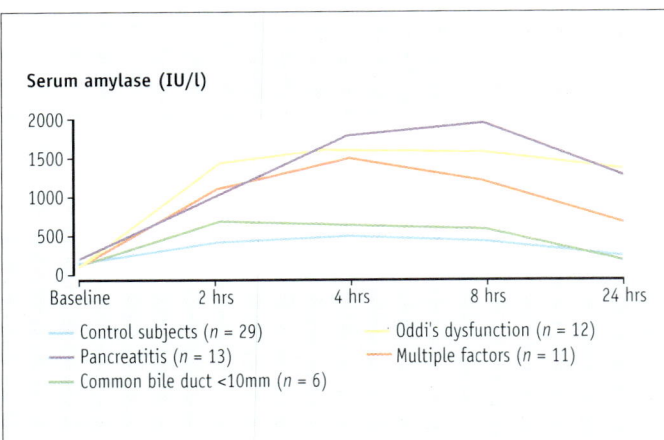

Figure 16.21 Mean serum amylase levels after ERCP/sphincterotomy in 71 consecutive patients with (42 cases) and without (29 cases) high-risk conditions for pancreatic reaction.

cannulation, repeated PD injection, an extended period of high-intensity current for sphincter ablation or the need for pre-cut sphincterotomy. In contrast, Roberts-Thomson and Tooouli[43] reported only a 4% rate of complications (bleeding and acute pancreatitis) in a series of 50 patients treated for dysfunction of the sphinter of Oddi.

A prior history of acute pancreatitis is generally believed to be a risk factor for post-ERCP/EPT pancreatic reaction or pancreatitis. In the first available multicentre trial on ERCP-related complications, Bilbao et al.[44] found that 66% of cases with post-ERCP pancreatitis had had previous pancreatitis. Similarly, Catalano et al.[45] reported that the incidence of pancreatitis after sphincter of Oddi manometry was higher in subjects with a prior history of pancreatitis. They found a pancreatitis rate of 5.3% in patients undergoing manometry, but 33% of the subgroup with idiopathic pancreatitis as the indication for the study had post-ERCP pancreatitis. In three different trials evaluating the effectiveness of somatostatin[46] and of its long-acting analogue octreotide[47,48] in prevention of pancreatic reaction after endoscopic sphincterotomy, we found that acute postprocedure pancreatitis occurred only in subjects with histories of recurrent pancreatitis and that the pancreatic reaction was more severe when there was a history of recurrent pancreatitis[48,49].

The role of the diameter of the CBD in the occurrence of postsphincteromy complications is still being debated. Generally, patients with idiopathic recurrent pancreatitis have a non-dilated biliary tree; a small-diameter (< 8mm) CBD seems, in fact, to be associated with a significantly higher rate of complications than that reported for subjects with stone disease or papillary stenosis who have dilated bile ducts. Sherman et al.[50] emphasized the association between small size of the CBD and higher incidence of complications; the complication rate was highest when dysfunction of the sphincter of Oddi was associated with a small-diameter duct, reaching 37.5%. Similar data were reported by Howerton et al.[51], who found that post-ERCP/EPT complications occurred in 14% of cases when the bile duct diameter was < 8mm compared with a 3% risk when the diameter was 8–11mm and a 5% risk when the diameter was > 11mm. In that study, the authors looked at a total of 492 patients with CBD stones and 87 patients with dysfunction of the sphincter of Oddi. On the other hand, the Duke Biliary Group found no correlation between CBD diameter and complications of sphincterotomy[52].

A recent prospective study performed by our group on 71 consecutive patients who underwent diagnostic or therapeutic ERCP was aimed at evaluating the 24-hour serum amylase response after the procedure in relation to the presence of the following risk factors: dysfunction of the sphincter of Oddi, non-dilated CBD and history of recurrent acute pancreatitis. The enzyme rise appeared to be markedly greater in subjects with one or more of such risk factors; although acute mild pancreatitis occurred in only three patients in this series, the elevated rise in serum amylase means that the patients have a more prolonged hospital stay and a more careful follow-up than subjects without risk factors (Figure 16.21).

References

1. Cooperman M, Ferrara JJ, Carey LC et al. Idiopathic acute pancreatitis: the value of endoscopic retrograde cholangio-pancreatography. *Surgery* 1981; 90:666–70.

2. Venu RP, Geenen JE, Hogan WJ et al. Idiopathic recurrent pancreatitis (IRP): diagnostic role of ERCP and sphincter of Oddi manometry. *Gastrointest Endosc* 1985; 31:153.

3. Steinberg WM. Sphincter of Oddi dysfunction: a clinical controversy. *Gastroenterology* 1988; 95: 1409–15.

4. Feller ER. Endoscopic retrograde cholangiopancreatography in the diagnosis of unexplained pancreatitis. *Arch Intern Med* 1984; 144: 797–9.

5. Venu RP, Geenen JE, Hogan WJ, Stone J, Johnson GK, Soergel K. Idiopathic recurrent pancreatitis: an approach to diagnosis and treatment. *Dig Dis Sci* 1989; 34:56–60.

6. Gregg JA. Pancreas divisum: its association with pancreatitis. *Am J Surg* 1977; 134:539.

7. Cotton PB. Congenital anomaly of pancreas divisum as a cause of obstructive pain and pancreatitis. *Gut* 1980; 21:105–14.

8. Carr-Locke DL. Pancreas divisum: the controversy goes on? *Endoscopy* 1991; 23:88–90.

9. Cotton PB, Beales JSM. Endoscopic pancreatography in management of relapsing pancreatitis. *Br Med J* 1974; 1(908):608–11.

10. Berk T, Friedman LS, Goldstein SD. Relapsing acute pancreatitis as the presenting manifestation of an ampullary neoplasm in a patient with familial polyposis. *Am J Gastroenterol* 1985; 8:627–9.

11. Willemer S, Dombrowski H, Adler G, Bussmann JF, Arnold R. Recurrent acute pancreatitis and intraluminal duodenal diverticulum. *Pancreas* 1992; 7:257–61.

12. Finnie IA, Ghosh P, Garvey C, Poston GJ, Rhodes JM. Intraluminal duodenal diverticulum causing recurrent pancreatitis: treatment by endoscopic incision. *Gut* 1994; 35:557–9.

13. Opie EL. The etiology of acute hemorrhagic pancreatitis. *Bull Johns Hopkins Hosp* 1901; 12:182

14. Cavallini G, Rigo L, Bovo P et al. Abnormal US response of main pancreatic duct after secretin stimulation in patients with acute pancreatitis of different etiology. *J Clin Gastroenterol* 1994; 18:298–303.

15. Testoni PA, Masci E, Lella F, Bagnolo F, Tittobello A. Effectiveness of endoscopic papillosphincterotomy in the treatment of acute relapsing pancreatitis. *Ital J Gastroenterol* 1991; 23:169.

16. Berk RN, Ferrucci JT, Fordtran JS, Cooperberg PL, Weissman HS. The radiological diagnosis of gallbladder disease. An imaging symposium. *Radiology* 1981; 141:49–56.

17. Venu RP, Geenen JE, Stewart EG et al. Endoscopic retrograde cholangiopancreatography: diagnosis of cholelithiasis in patients with normal gallbladder x-rays and ultrasound studies. *JAMA* 1983; 249:758–61.

18. Ros E, Navarro S, Bru C, Garcia-Pugès A, Valderrama R. Occult microlithiasis in idiopathic acute pancreatitis: prevention of relapse by cholecystectomy or ursodeoxycholic acid therapy. *Gastroenterology* 1991; 101: 701–9.

19. Juniper K, Burson EN. Biliary tract studies. II. The significance of biliary crystals. *Gastroenterology* 1957; 32:175–211.

20. Godstein F, Kucer F, Thornton J, Abramson J. Acute and relapsing pancreatitis caused by bile pigment aggregates and diagnosed by biliary drainage. *Am J Gastroenterol* 1980; 74:225–8.

21. Negro P, Flati G, Flati D, Porowska B, Tuscano D, Carboni M. Occult gallbladder microlithiasis causing acute recurrent pancreatitis. A report of three cases. *Acta Chir Scand* 1984; 150:503–6.

22. Ros E, Navarro S, Fernandez I, Reixach M, Ribò JM, Rodhès J. Utility of biliary microscopy for the prediction of the chemical composition of gallstones and the outcome of dissolution therapy with ursodeoxycholic acid. *Gastroenterology* 1986; 91:703–12.

23. Delchier JC, Benfredj P, Preaux AM, Metreau JM, Dhumeaux D. The usefulness of microscopic bile examination in patients with suspected microlithiasis: a prospective evaluation. *Hepatology* 1986; 6:118–22.

24. Neoptolemos J, Davidson BR, Winder AF, Wallance D. Role of duodenal bile crystal analysis in the investigation of "idiopathic" pancreatitis. *Br J Surg* 1988; 75:450–3.

25. Toouli J, Roberts-Thomson TC, Donts LJ. Sphincter of Oddi motility disorders in patients with idiopathic recurrent pancreatitis. *Br J Surg* 1985; 72:859–63.

26. Raddawi H, Geenen JE, Hogan WJ, Dodds WJ, Venu RP, Johnson GK. Pressure measurement from biliary and pancreatic segments of sphincter of Oddi: comparison between patients with functional abdominal pain, biliary or pancreatic disease. *Dig Dis Sci* 1991; 36:71–4.

27. Rolny P, Arleback A, Funch-Jensen P, Kruse A, Jarnerot G. Clinical significance of manometric assessment of both pancreatic duct and bile duct sphincter in the same patient. *Scand J Gastroenterol* 1989; 24:751–4.

28. Funch-Jensen P, Kruse A. Manometric activity of the pancreatic duct sphincter in patients with total bile duct sphincterotomy for sphincter of Oddi dyskinesia. *Scand J Gastroenterol* 1987; 22:1067–70.

29. Hogan WJ, Geenen JE, Kruidenier J, Wilson SD. Ineffectiveness of conventional sphincteroplasty in relieving pancreatic duct sphincter pressure in patients with idiopathic recurrent pancreatitis. *Gastroenterology* 1983; 84:1189.

30. Guelrud M, Siegel JL. Hypertensive pancreatic sphincter in a course of pancreatitis. Successful treatment with hydrostatic balloon dilatation. *Dig Dis Sci* 1984; 29:225–31.

31. Kozarek RA. Balloon dilatations of sphincter of Oddi. *Endoscopy* 1988; 20:207–10.

32. Bader M, Geenen JE, Hogan WJ. Endoscopic balloon dilatation of the sphincter of Oddi in patients with suspected biliary dyskinesia: results of a prospective randomised trial. *Gastrointest Endosc* 1986; 32:158. (Abstract.)

33. Siegel JH. Endoscopic management of pancreatic strictures: catheter dilatation and insertion of pancreatic endoprostheses. *Gastrointest Endosc* 1983; 29:174. (Abstract.)

34. McCarthy J, Geenen JE, Hogan WJ. Preliminary experience with endoscopic stent placement in benign pancreatic diseases. *Gastrointest Endosc* 1988; 34:16–18.

35. Kozarek RA, Patterson DJ, Ball TJ, Traverso LW. Endoscopic placement of pancreatic stents and drains in the management of pancreatitis. *Ann Surg* 1989; 209:261–6.

36. Siegel JH, Pullano W, Ben-Zvi JS, Cooperman AM. Effectiveness of endoscopic drainage for pancreas divisum. *Endoscopy* 1990; 20:129–32.

37. Lans JA, Geenen JE, Johanson JF, Hogan WJ. Endoscopic therapy in patients with pancreas divisum and acute pancreatitis: a prospective, randomized, controlled clinical trial. *Gastrointest Endosc* 1992; 38:430–4.

38. Sherman S, Lehman GA. ERCP- and endoscopic sphincterotomy-induced pancreatitis. *Pancreas* 1991; 6:350–67.

39. Leese T, Neoptolemos JP, Carr-Locke DL. Successes, failures, early complications and their management following endoscopic sphincterotomy: results in 394 consecutive patients from a single centre. *Br J Surg* 1985; 72:215–19.

40. Thatcher BS, Sivak MV, Tedesco FJ, Vennes JA, Hutton SW, Achkar EA. Endoscopic sphincterotomy for suspected dysfunction of the sphincter of Oddi. *Gastrointest Endosc* 1987; 33:91–5.

41. Neoptolemos JP, Bailey IS, Carr-Locke DL. Sphincter of Oddi dysfunction: results of treatment by endoscopic sphincterotomy. *Br J Surg* 1988; 75:454–9.

42. Choudhry U, Ruffolo T, Jamidar P, Hawes R, Lehman G. Sphincter of Oddi dysfunction in patients with intact gallbladder: therapeutic response to endoscopic sphincterotomy. *Gastrointest Endosc* 1993; 39:92–5.

43. Roberts-Thomson IC, Toouli J. Is endoscopic sphincterotomy for disabling biliary-type pain after cholecystectomy effective? *Gastrointest Endosc* 1985; 31:370–3.

44. Bilbao MK, Dotter CT, Lee TG, Katon RM. Complications of endoscopic retrograde cholangiopancreatography (ERCP): a study of 10.000 cases. *Gastroenterology* 1976; 70:314–20.

45. Catalano MF, Sivak MV, Falk JW. Pancreatitis after sphincter of Oddi manometry is higher in patients with prior history of pancreatitis. *Gastrointest Endosc* 1993; 39:311. (Abstract.)

46. Testoni PA, Masci E, Bagnolo F, Tittobello A. Endoscopic papillosphincterotomy: prevention of pancreatic reaction by somatostatin. *Ital J Gastroenterol* 1988; 20:70–3.

47. Testoni PA, Lella F, Bagnolo F, Buizza M, Colombo E. Controlled trial of different dosages of octreotide in the prevention of hyperamylasemia induced by endoscopic papillosphincterotomy. *Ital J Gastroenterol* 1994; 26:431–6.

48. Testoni PA, Lella F, Bagnolo F *et al*. Long-term prophylactic administration of octreotide reduces the rise in serum amylase after endoscopic procedures on Vater's papilla. *Pancreas* 1996. (In press.)

49. Testoni PA, Cicardi M, Bergamaschini L *et al*. Infusion of C1-inhibitor plasma concentrate prevents hyperamylasemia induced by endoscopic sphincterotomy. *Gastrointest Endosc* 1995; 42:301–5.

50. Sherman S, Ruffolo TA, Hawes RH, Lehman GA. Complication of endoscopic sphincterotomy. A prospective series with emphasis on the increased risk associated with sphincter of Oddi dysfunction and non-dilated bile ducts. *Gastroenterology* 1991; 101:1068–75.

51. Howerton DH, Geenen JE, Hogan WJ. Does common bile duct diameter influence the risk of post-sphincterotomy complications? *Gastrointest Endosc* 1993; 39:315. (Abstract.)

52. Edwards P, Metzler D, Troughton A. Immediate complications after endoscopic sphincterotomy: is bile duct size important? *Gastrointest Endosc* 1993; 39:313. (Abstract.)

Pancreas divisum

Jonathan Cohen & Gregory B. Haber

INTRODUCTION

The failure of fusion of the dorsal and ventral pancreatic ducts in the seventh week of embryonic development is now well recognized. The pancreatic buds, or anlages, maintain separate drainage into the duodenum through the minor or accessory papilla and the major papilla, and this has been called pancreas divisum. The description of this anatomic anomaly, present in approximately 7% of the population, has been mistakenly ascribed to Giovanni Domenico Santorini (1681–1737). However, there were several original treatises from the 17th century recognizing this variant, which pre-dated Santorini's description, referred to in the exhaustive historical review by CD Stern in 1986[1].

In most individuals with pancreas divisum, this anatomical variation has no clinical sequelae. However, there is a body of evidence supporting a causal association between pancreas divisum and pancreatic illness in a subgroup of patients[2,3,4]. The increased diagnosis of pancreas divisum with improved endoscopic techniques, coupled with increased expertise in minor papilla sphincterotomy and stenting, has fuelled the debate over whether endoscopic therapy is of value and, if so, who warrants such treatment.

In this chapter, we will review the evidence linking pancreas divisum to pancreatitis and chronic abdominal pain. We will describe the criteria for selecting those patients most likely to benefit from endoscopic therapy, with attention to the diagnostic usefulness of endoscopic assessment of the minor papilla and dorsal duct manometry, and provocative secretory studies. Therapeutic options will then be presented. Specifically, we will discuss technical considerations of minor duct papillotomy and stenting and review the experience to date with the endoscopic management of pancreas divisum. Our aims are to assess the clinical relevance of pancreas divisum and to provide an overview of how best to manage pancreatitis in this setting.

EMBRYOLOGY

Pancreas divisum is characterized by pancreatic drainage predominantly through the minor papilla via the dorsal duct (duct of Santorini), as a result of malfusion of the dorsal and ventral pancreatic anlages. The embryology of pancreas divisum was characterized by Meckel in 1812[5]. During the sixth to seventh week of gestation, the ventral pancreatic bud and bile duct rotate 180 degrees in a counterclockwise direction around the foregut and line up just inferior and adjacent to the dorsal bud. The ventral and dorsal buds and their respective ducts then fuse. The resulting main pancreatic duct is derived from the dorsal duct draining the body and tail regions and the ventral

bud draining the head and uncinate process of the pancreas. A portion of the original dorsal bud duct forms the accessory duct, which drains through the minor papilla, anterior and proximal to the papilla of Vater in the second portion of the duodenum. The accessory duct remains patent in only 30% of patients. This developmental anatomy occurs in 90% of individuals.

Pancreas divisum occurs when this fusion fails to take place, and the accessory duct alone drains the pancreatic juice from the larger dorsal pancreas. The ventral duct system is typically small, with terminal arborization. In 80% of pancreas divisum cases, non-communicating dorsal and ventral ducts are identified; in 15% the ventral duct is atretic and cannot be identified; in 5% there is 'form fruste' in which there is a partial communication between the dorsal and ventral ducts via a small filamentous duct (Figure 17.1). In view of these variations of pancreas divisum, the term 'dominant dorsal duct syndrome' has been proposed to encompass these different patterns[6].

EPIDEMIOLOGY

The overall incidence of pancreas divisum is approximately 7%. This is derived from several autopsy series, as well as endoscopic retrograde cholangiopancreatography (ERCP) series[7,8,9]. The ERCP series tend to underestimate the true prevalence of pancreas divisum because endoscopists often do not pursue a minor papilla cannulation unless trying to rule

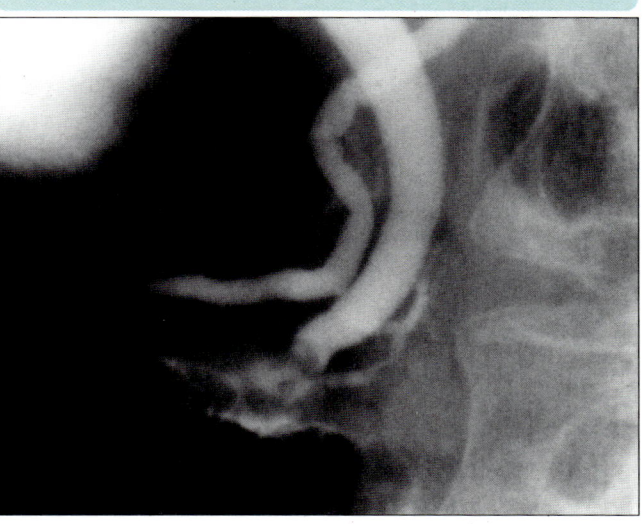

Figure 17.1 ERCP findings in a patient with a dominant dorsal duct with a filamentous communication with the ventral duct system.

out pancreatic pathology and because success at minor papilla cannulation when attempted is less than 90%. There does not seem to be any gender difference in the frequency of pancreas divisum[10]. However, there may be some geographical variation in incidence as a lower incidence of pancreas divisum has been reported in a series from Japan[11].

CLINICAL RELEVANCE OF PANCREAS DIVISUM

It has been postulated that patients with pancreas divisum are predisposed to developing pancreatitis because the minor papilla is too narrow to accommodate periods of high flow through the dorsal duct. This produces a relative outflow obstruction, resulting in acute pancreatitis or pancreatic pain. Whether this anatomical variant is an independent risk factor for pancreatitis is controversial. The arguments that would support an association have been elaborated in an excellent overview by Cotton and subsequently summarized by Carr-Locke as follows: (1) a higher prevalence of pancreas divisum in patients with idiopathic acute relapsing pancreatitis than in those with a known cause for acute relapsing pancreatitis; (2) evidence of dorsal duct outflow obstruction in patients with pancreas divisum; (3) the presence of morphological, pathological and functional changes of the dorsal pancreas in patients with pancreas divisum, when compared to the ventral pancreas; and (4) clinical resolution of symptoms in pancreas divisum patients after endoscopic or surgical drainage procedures[11,12].

The prevalence of pancreas divisum in patients with idiopathic pancreatitis

A causal relationship between pancreatitis and pancreas divisum could be supported by showing an increased prevalence of pancreas divisum among patients being investigated for an 'idiopathic' pancreatitis compared to those being investigated for other pancreaticobiliary problems. An increased incidence of pancreatitis among individuals with pancreas divisum compared to the incidence of pancreatitis among those with normal anatomy would also support this argument;

however, this is much harder to determine given the difficulty in establishing the prevalence of pancreas divisum among a truly normal population.

Tulassay and Papp[3] reported that among 2410 patients undergoing ERCP in their unit, 33 were diagnosed with pancreas divisum, of whom 14 (42%) had a history of acute pancreatitis, *versus* only 209 of 2168 (9.6%) in those with normal anatomy, suggesting an increased risk in pancreas divisum. This argument is untenable, however, without accurate data on the success of pancreatic cannulation in all ERCP patients, which was not available in this report; there is also an obvious selection bias in obtaining a pancreatogram in those with pancreatitis.

The association of pancreas divisum with pancreatitis is easier to establish from looking at the prevalence of pancreas divisum in pancreatic and non-pancreatic diseases as shown in Figure 17.2. With the exception of a subgroup (series 2) of patients reported by Burtin et al.[10], all other series are retrospective analyses and thus are subject to several pitfalls. The principal problem in these reviews is that the diagnosis of pancreas divisum is based on typical pancreatographic findings after ventral and/or dorsal ductography. Selective pancreatic cannulation is often not pursued in the absence of clinical indications. For example, in the Brussels series the success rate of pancreatography was 84.7%, and in Marseilles it was 74% in biliary indications and 92% in pancreatic indications[13,14]. In patients without pancreatic disease, a pancreatogram is often avoided to minimize the risk of post-ERCP pancreatitis. Few patients have accessory duct characterization apart from those in whom the diagnosis of pancreas divisum is being specifically investigated. This could lead to the underestimation of the incidence of pancreas divisum in patients undergoing ERCP for non-pancreatic problems. On the other hand, reluctance of some endoscopists to pursue cannulation of the accessory duct in patients being investigated for a history of pancreatitis could produce the opposite effect – an underdiagnosis of pancreas divisum in individuals with pancreatic disease.

There may be an overlap of aetiologies such as pancreas divisum and alcohol. In the Brussels series pancreas divisum is associated with alcoholic pancreatitis, occurring in 15% of

Author (ref.) PD/total ERCP	Acute pancreatitis Aetiology known	Idiopathic	Non-pancreatic disease
Cotton (4) 47/1215	9/99 (9%)	20/78 (25.6%)	6/169 (3.6%)
Richter et al. (41) 21/519	7/67 (10.4%)	8/42 (19.0%)	11/353 (3.1%)
Delhaye et al. (13) 304/5357	19/248 (6.6%)	4/60 (6.7%)	235/4257 (5.5%)
Sugawa et al. (42) 41/1529	12/521 (2.3%)	2/82 (2.4%)	27/953 (2.8%)
Bernard et al. (14) 137/1825	17/106 (16%)	28/56 (50%)	65/1087 (5.8%)
Burtin et al. (10) 62/1049	6/118 (5.1%)	3/25 (12%)	35/619 (5.7%)
Total	**70/1159 (6.0%)**	**65/343 (18.9%)**	**379/7438 (5.0%)**

Figure 17.2 Prevalence of pancreas divisum (PD) by diagnostic category.

these patients, a significantly higher proportion than that of the overall group[13]. Those centres with a high proportion of alcoholic pancreatitis may have an increased prevalence of pancreas divisum in the so-called control group, thus negating potential differences with the idiopathic group.

There has been increasing recognition of a biliary aetiology in up to 50% of patients previously classified as 'idiopathic' based on microscopic findings of cholesterol crystals and clinical follow-up after biliary intervention[15,16]. Thus, the inclusion of these cases in the idiopathic group may falsely reduce the prevalence of pancreas divisum in those with truly idiopathic pancreatitis.

A factor which augurs against an association is the age at which most patients present with pancreatitis, usually in the fourth to sixth decade, which is late for a manifestation of a congenital risk factor. Moreover, the age at presentation in this group does not differ from the age of those with a known biliary or alcoholic aetiology.

Lastly, the control population for all of these series are patients with symptoms necessitating ERCP investigation and do not represent a truly normal population. This may further confound interpretation of the data if pancreas divisum were to be associated with abdominal pain without pancreatitis, for instance. This would again falsely increase the prevalence of pancreas divisum in the control population.

Clearly there are several sources of bias in these retrospective series, which makes it difficult to draw a reliable conclusion as to the association between pancreas divisum and acute pancreatitis, but the weight of the evidence supports an association.

Outflow obstruction

Direct radiographic evidence of accessory duct outflow obstruction in patients with pancreas divisum and pancreatitis can rarely be demonstrated. Most authors have failed to find either a dilated dorsal duct or delayed emptying of the dorsal duct during ERCP[2,17,18,19]. Among 100 patients with a dominant dorsal duct and either episodic acute pancreatitis or pancreatic- type pain, Warshaw et al. found only one individual to have a dilated dorsal duct on pancreatography[6]. Although a relatively stenotic minor papilla may be able to accommodate the flow of pancreatic juice under normal circumstances, functional outflow obstruction may result when pancreatic secretion is stimulated. This may be sufficient to trigger an acute episode of pancreatitis or pain, without producing radiographic dorsal duct dilatation during periods of normal pancreatic secretion.

Ultrasonography has been used to assess delayed drainage by measuring pancreatic duct size before and after the administration of intravenous secretin. Secretin normally leads to dilatation of the pancreatic duct lasting up to 3min. A prolonged dilatation for 15–30min is considered an abnormal response. In theory, this prolonged dilatation reflects functional obstruction elicited when pancreatic secretion is stimulated by secretin.

Efforts to use secretin provocation tests to document functional dorsal duct obstruction in patients with pancreas divisum and recurrent acute pancreatitis have had mixed results[11,20,21]. Warshaw et al. have had the most successful results with this technique[6]. In their study of patients with pancreas divisum undergoing surgical sphincteroplasty, secretin–ultrasonogra-

phy correlated closely with surgical assessment of papillary stenosis, with a sensitivity of 78% and a specificity of 97%. Abnormal tests were defined as prolonged dilatation of the dorsal duct (15–30min) after administration of intravenous secretin (1IU/kg) of up to 3mm. They found prolonged dorsal duct dilatation in 39 of 72 patients with either relapsing pancreatitis or pain. More importantly, 92% of patients with abnormal secretin–ultrasonography had a beneficial clinical outcome. However, many of the patients with discrete recurrent attacks of pancreatitis benefited from surgery despite negative secretin–ultrasound tests; for patients with negative tests who presented only with chronic abdominal pain, only 21% had clinical benefit postoperatively, suggesting that the appropriate clinical history may be a better predictor of therapeutic benefit than pre-therapy evidence of outflow obstruction. In a study of 34 patients with pancreas divisum, Tulassay and Papp found a higher rate of associated pancreatitis in the group of patients with smaller baseline duct diameter (< 2mm), higher peak secretin response, and greater duration of response (> 10min), further supporting the outflow obstruction hypothesis[3].

Others have had less promising results with secretin–ultrasonography in patients with pancreas divisum and have noted a number of false-positive results in control patients[21,22]. It may be that secretin can no longer induce dilatation after the dorsal duct has become fibrotic, and that endoscopic therapy is less beneficial in patients with pancreas divisum who have chronic pancreatitis. The inherent difficulties for the radiologist in identifying the pancreatic duct and measuring millimetre differences in duct size make this test operator-dependent, and may explain the varying experience with secretin–ultrasonography[23]. Cavallini et al. found 4 of 6 patients with pancreas divisum and recurrent acute pancreatitis to have abnormally prolonged dorsal duct dilatation in response to secretin; however, they did not study control patients with asymptomatic pancreas divisum[24]. In this same study, similar abnormal secretin–ultrasound test results were observed in non-pancreas divisum patients with idiopathic recurrent acute pancreatitis as well as in a small group of patients with only one previous episode of prior pancreatitis of known aetiology. This suggests that a prior episode of pancreatitis of any aetiology may result in a positive test even in the absence of recurrent episodes of pancreatitis. A positive test may simply indicate a predisposition to develop pancreatitis when another risk factor or precipitating factor is present.

Endoscopic ultrasonography may increase the sensitivity of provocative testing in detecting evidence for outflow obstruction. One preliminary study using secretin-stimulated endoscopic ultrasound (SSEUS) tests in patients with acute relapsing pancreatitis found a correlation between an abnormal test result and a positive response to surgery, but few of the patients with normal results underwent surgery for comparison[25].

High manometric pressure recordings from the dorsal duct may be used to corroborate the existence of functional obstruction at the minor papilla. Manometry of the minor papilla is possible, but infrequently performed. The usefulness of manometry for this purpose is limited by existing technology, as the standard manometry catheter is 5 Fr or 1.5mm in diameter, which is usually too large to fit in a stenotic minor papilla (< 1mm). Staritz and Meyer zum Buschenfelde evaluated 14 patients with chronic abdominal pain, measuring intraductal pressure in the dorsal duct and ventral duct through the minor and major papilla, respectively[26]. A small probe 1.3mm in diameter was used for this study. The results from eight patients with normal anatomy were compared with those from six patients with pancreas d visum. In pancreas divisum the average dorsal duct pressure was 23.7mmHg, compared to 10.8mmHg in the ventral duct of the same patients. There was no such difference in those with normal anatomy (10.0 *versus* 10.5mmHg). These data support the outflow obstruction hypothesis.

Other results of manometry in patients with pancreas divisum have been mixed. Gregg *et al.* found elevated sphincter of Oddi pressures in some patients with pancreas divisum[27]. Lehman *et al.* performed minor papilla manometry in 19 patients with pancreas divisum and failure to benefit from prior minor papilla sphincterotomy; nine of these patients had elevated pressures, which was considered to be evidence of restenosis of the duct orifice. Minor papilla manometry was not done prior to therapy in this study, however. The value of manometry in detecting outflow obstruction and in predicting response to endoscopic therapy in pancreas divisum has not yet been prospectively evaluated and has considerable technological limitations.

Morphological and pathological changes limited to the dorsal pancreas in pancreas divisum

The occasional finding of morphological or pathological abnormalities confined to the dorsal pancreas provides compelling evidence for an association between pancreas divisum and pancreatic disease. Some ERCP series have shown that individuals with pancreas divisum and pancreatitis more often have pancreatographic changes in the dorsal duct than in the ventral duct, but this has not been a consistent finding[10,11,28] (Figure 17.3).

In one surgical series, in which careful dissection of two pancreaticoduodenal specimens allowed comparison of the ventral and dorsal portions, in both cases the changes of chronic pancreatitis were confined to the dorsal gland[29]. Subsequent work has shown histological evidence for disease, either exclusively involving the dorsal pancreas or with more severe changes in this portion of the gland[30]. However, the presence of the histopathological changes of pancreatitis in approximately 30% of needle biopsies of the ventral pancreas in patients with pancreas divisum has been used to question the importance of selective dorsal duct obstruction as a mechanism of pancreatitis in pancreas divisum[31,32]. These variable

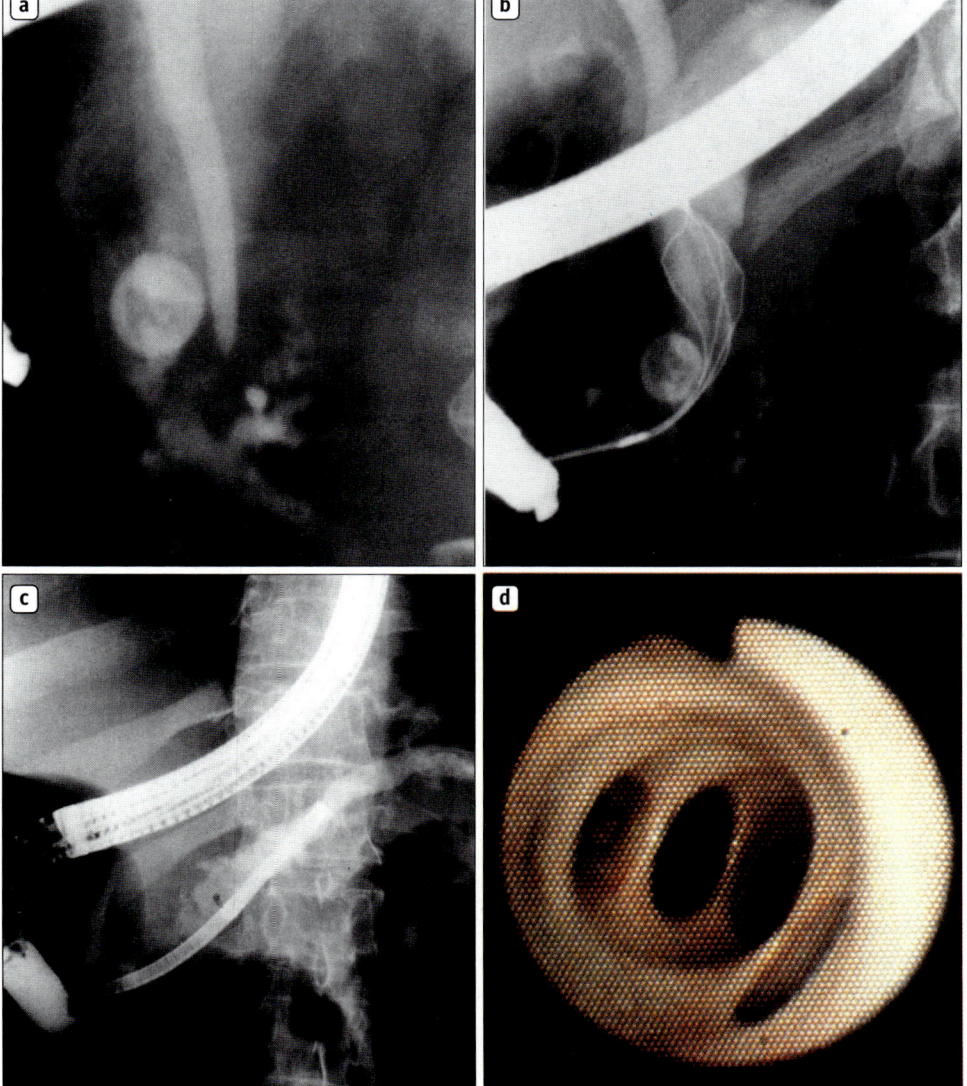

Figure 17.3
(a) ERCP in a 40-year-old man with idiopathic pancreatitis and pancreas divisum. Note the ectatic ventral duct system, the normal calibre bile duct, a large concentric calculus with a radiolucent center in the mouth of a grossly dilated dorsal duct.
(b) Unsuccessful attempt at basket entrapment of the impacted stone in the mouth of the dorsal duct.
(c) A mother-daughter scope system used for electrohydraulic lithotripsy of a pancreatic duct stone in the same patient.
(d) Pancreatoscopic views of the main pancreatic duct and side branches.

findings render tissue biopsy of the dorsal and ventral ducts of little clinical utility in deciding whether a patient's clinical presentation is attributable to pancreas divisum.

Demonstration of minor papilla stenosis, a condition that some authors consider necessary for the development of pancreatic disease in patients with pancreas divisum, also supports the association between pancreas divisum and pancreatitis. However, precise endoscopic measurement of the diameter of the orifice of the accessory duct is not possible, leaving no reliable way to determine whether the ducts is stenotic during endoscopy. The duct orifice can be evaluated during surgery by insertion of calibrated lacrimal probes. A stenotic minor papilla has been defined by some as < 1mm in diameter and by others as < 0.75mm wide. Stenosis of the minor papilla in patients with pancreas divisum, however, has been shown to be highly predictive of a successful response to surgery. In Warshaw and co-workers' series of 88 patients with pancreas divisum, 85% of patients with intraoperatively determined minor papillary stenosis benefited from surgical sphincteroplasty, as compared to 27% of patients without stenosis[6].

Results of minor papilla therapy in pancreas divisum patients

Perhaps the most compelling evidence implicating pancreas divisum as a cause of pancreatitis is the published literature on the results of therapy. Judgement must be reserved, however, as there is only a single prospective randomized trial on a small number of cases, with the remaining evidence based on less rigorous reviews. There is little doubt that some pancreas divisum patients benefit enormously from therapeutic intervention but the criteria for selection are still not well defined. Those with idiopathic acute relapsing pancreatitis have better outcomes than those with either a chronic pain presentation or an established chronic pancreatitis. There is an inherent flaw to this type of analysis in that those patients with a relapsing history often experience long periods without symptoms; whether this can be attributed to iatrogenic intervention or the natural course of this problem is not easy to differentiate without randomized prospective trials.

The Milwaukee group randomized 19 pancreas divisum patients over a 5-year period for stenting or no stenting[33]. Inclusion criteria included at least two episodes of acute pancreatitis, with amylase levels twice normal and no other identifiable cause of pancreatitis. The stent group had a 5 or 7 Fr stent replaced every 4 months for one year; the no-stent group was simply followed every 4 months, with a follow-up ERCP for pancreatitis recurrence. Ten patients received stents and nine did not, with mean follow-ups of 28.6 and 31.5 months, respectively. Six patients in the no-stent group had seven episodes of pancreatitis, compared with only one episode in the stent group (thought to be related to an occluded stent). There were two migrations into the pancreatic duct and one migration out in the stented patients but no inflammatory strictures. These results strongly support drainage therapy for pancreas divisum patients with acute pancreatitis. Perhaps the only design flaw in the study is that the follow-up was not undertaken by investigators blinded to the treatment arm.

Several other endoscopic and surgical series with a similar theme have been reported. Results of endoscopic or surgical sphincterotomy or endoscopic stenting have been most successful in those with a presentation of acute relapsing pancreatitis and of marginal benefit in those with chronic pain, without enzyme elevations. In the group with chronic pancreatitis changes the results mirror to a large extent those for treatment through the major papilla, as we have reported elsewhere in this publication. In brief, those with obstructing main duct stones or a dominant tight stricture with upstream dilatation have had good results with endoscopic and lithotripsy therapies. Early endoscopic reports focused on the technical aspects of endoscopic treatment[34,35]. Subsequently these same groups and others have reported on much larger series of patients, which will be selectively reviewed here.

Siegel et al. prospectively followed 31 pancreas divisum patients who underwent stent insertion into the dorsal pancreatic duct [36]. Five failed to respond and 26 improved, among whom 17 subsequently underwent surgical drainage procedures because of stent dependency or worsening of duct pathology. Six of these required further surgery with some form of pancreatic resection when a drainage procedure alone failed to give a sustained relief of symptoms. This publication received some heated debate in subsequent correspondence regarding some shortfalls with respect to patient data and results but the thrust of this paper was that those who did well with a stent in place did well with surgery and those who did not respond to stenting likewise did poorly with surgery.

Lehman and colleagues contributed much-needed information regarding the alternative to stenting for drainage, namely minor papilla sphincterotomy, in a large cohort of patients[37]. They reported on 52 patients treated by minor papilla sphincterotomy over a 6-year period, who presented with either pancreatic pain only and normal enzymes ($n = 24$), acute relapsing pancreatitis ($n = 17$) or chronic pancreatitis ($n = 11$), with follow-up of 1.6, 2.0, and 1.7 years, respectively. There was a marked difference in outcome depending on the mode of presentation, with minimal or no pain reported in only 26% and 27% of those presenting with either chronic pain or chronic pancreatitis, respectively. In the acute relapsing pancreatitis group, 76.5% responded to the treatment. This report also brought attention to a relatively high rate of restenosis, which was found in 10 of 18 (55.6%) patients restudied with ERCP to evaluate symptom recurrence. The true restenosis rate is unknown, as routine follow-up ERCP was not undertaken in responders.

Coleman and colleagues collected the results of the Duke experience with endoscopic treatment of pancreas divisum, and identified 46 patients over 6 years, similar to the Indianapolis experience but with follow-up in only 34 suitable patients (5 with pain only, 9 with acute relapsing pancreatitis and 20 with chronic pancreatitis)[38]. The therapy differed from the Indianapolis study in that stenting was the primary modality, with a median placement of 3 months, and only 41% of patients underwent minor papilla sphincterotomy, performed mainly to facilitate access. Effectiveness of pain relief again related to the mode of presentation, with a 40% response in pain only and 60% and 78% responses in chronic and acute relapsing pancreatitis, respectively.

The most recent large endoscopic series is the experience reported by Kozarek et al.[1] and among 39 patients treated over 5 years the results are similar to those of the prior two retrospective series, namely a 20% response in pain only

Figure 17.4 A short needle tip cannula and a wire guided catheter for minor papilla cannulation

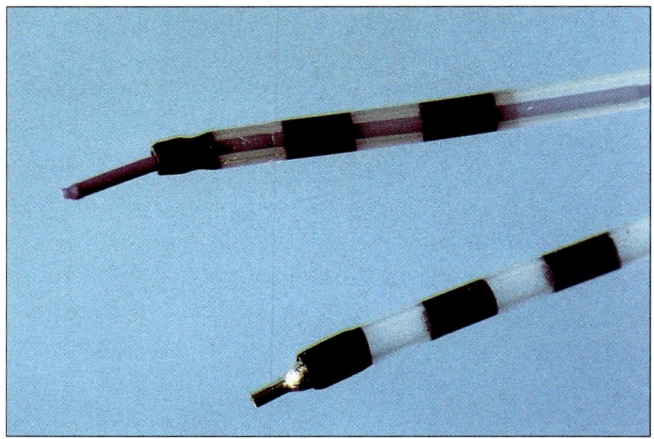

(n = 5), and 31.6% and 73.3% responses in chronic (n = 19) and acute relapsing (n = 15) pancreatitis, respectively[39].

The definitive surgical series that addresses most of the problematical issues in pancreas divisum therapy is that of Warshaw *et al*[6]. A total of 100 patients were studied over 15 years, 49 with acute relapsing pancreatitis and 51 with chronic pain; none had an alcoholic history. Minor papilla sphinctero-plasty was performed in 88 patients and among these 28 also underwent major papilla sphincteroplasty and ventral duct sep-toplasty. As in the endoscopic studies, those with acute attacks fared better than those with chronic pain, with a good out-come in 74% *versus* 38% in the pain only group. Assessment of sphincter stenosis was based on operative assessment with passage of an 0.75mm lacrimal probe or with preoperative secretin–ultrasonography. An abnormal result was loosely defined as dilatation of the pancreatic duct lasting 15–30min. There was also a system (not defined) of grading the abnor-mal results as mild, moderate, or severe. Among 62 patients who had an ultrasound–secretin study, the study was negative in 25 and 40% of these had a good outcome, but an abnor-mal result (in 37/62 patients) was highly predictive of a bene-ficial outcome, which occurred in 34 of these 37 patients (92%).

The operative assessment of stenosis using the lacrimal probe was a more reliable indicator, with a good or fair out-come in 85% of those with stenosis and in only 27% without stenosis.

There were 26 patients among 88 operated on who did poorly and the true restenosis rate in these patients is unknown, although it was proven in 7 who underwent further evaluation. Nine of the 26 underwent further pancreatic surgery. This author favoured a surgical approach over an endoscopic one, based on a high success rate and a low complication rate. However, it is not clear from the data that the restenosis rate is, in fact, lower with surgery and, based on the published data, the suc-cess rates for symptom amelioration appear comparable.

In a second surgical series, in which avoidance of sutures was considered important in order to avoid restenosis, the results of minor papilla sphincterotomy without sphinctero-plasty were reported[40]. Twenty-five patients were stratified into three groups: pain (n = 8), chronic pancreatitis (n = 3), and acute relapsing pancreatitis (n = 14). In this latter group of 13 patients

with sphincterotomy (1 minor papilla not identified), none had further attacks of pancreatitis over a 53-month follow-up. Of the eight pain-only patients, three were completely relieved of pain, and three partially relieved. In contrast to Warshaw's study, there was no correlation between the diameter of the dorsal duct orifice and the presentation with pain only or pan-creatitis. These results are some of the most successful reported (100% response in the acute pancreatitis group) and may reflect in part the stringent clinical selection process, as these 14 patients were collected over a 10-year period.

TECHNIQUES OF ENDOSCOPIC THERAPY

Cannulation

The success rate for cannulation of the minor papilla is > 80% in several recent large series. This can only be achieved with meticulous attention to both patient and equipment para-meters. Patient movement should be minimized with ample sedation; duodenal paralysis is equally important, employing the usual anticholinergics or glucagon. For this indication, a standard duodenoscope is preferred, to allow for better con-trol of the catheter during cannulation. A stable endoscope position is essential and may be achieved in either a short or long scope position, although the latter is more common.

The minor papilla can be recognized as a tiny dimple or a slightly raised mound, sometimes prominent enough to be mistaken for the major papilla. It is typically 2–4cm proximal or cephalad and 1–2cm anterior to or to the right of the major papilla. There is no tell-tale longitudinal fold but there may be an overlying transverse fold which may have to be pushed up to uncover the minor papilla. Due to the narrow calibre of the minor papillary orifice, it is necessary to use either a tapered catheter or one with a blunt needle tip 23–25 Fr in diameter and 1.5–3.0mm long (Figure 17.4). The tapered catheters go from 5 Fr down to 3 Fr and are precurved. They allow passage of a 0.018- or 0.021-inch wire. The papilla may be cannulated with the tapered catheter tip or, if very small, with the wire initially. The blunt needle-tip catheter provides a very small tip for entry and we prefer this, even though it will not accommodate a wire. The minor papilla is oriented *en face* but the direction of the catheter insertion is usually at an angle of 60–90 degrees upward, directed toward the 9–12 o'clock sector of the papilla. In the very prominent minor papillae, the dorsal duct may take off from the papillary ori-fice in a more cephalad direction, necessitating a more tan-gential angle of entry. In this circumstance a dual-channel papillotome is useful for papillotome guided wire insertion to effect the more oblique angle of entry. Selecting a site for catheter probing is of utmost importance and before prod-ding too much, which may result in a bloody field due to mucosal trauma, the papilla should be carefully inspected for evidence of a drainage point. Occasionally intravenous secretin (0.5–1.0IU/kg) may be useful to stimulate pancreatic secretions in order to find the orifice. The contrast medium injected should be of high density for better opacification of branch ducts and it is preferable that the endoscopist inject the dye him/herself so as to prevent forceful injection into a submucosal intramural plane, as well as to protect against overfilling and acinarization.

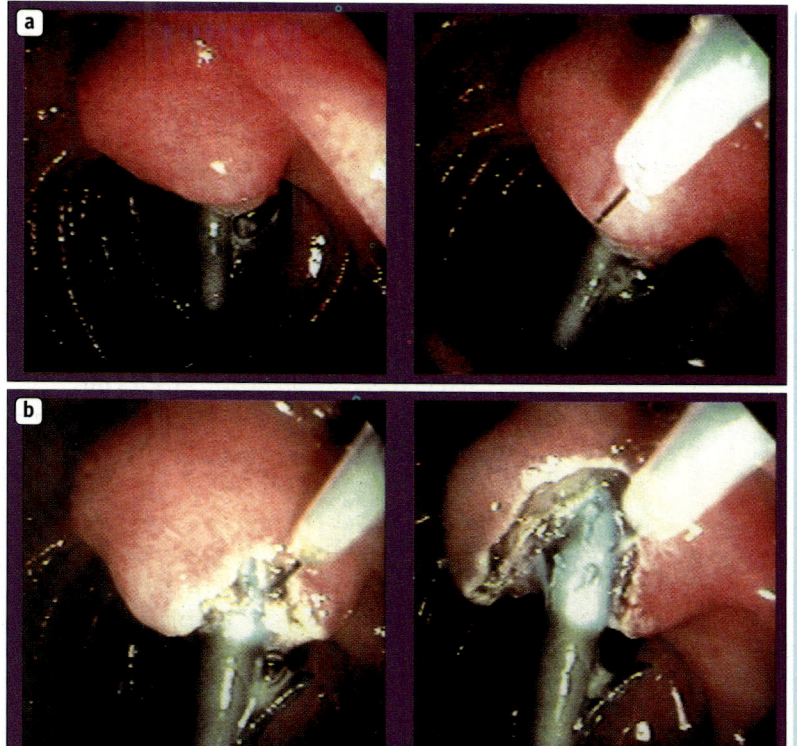

Figure 17.5
(a) A prominent minor papilla with an indwelling stent and a needle knife for sphincterotomy.
(b) Needle knife sphincterotomy over a dorsal duct stent.

Sphincterotomy

Due to the tiny orifice usually encountered, cutting the small sphincter segment is usually not possible with standard sphincterotomes. We routinely use a needle-knife wire, cutting over a previously inserted stent that serves as a guide for sphincterotomy. A short 3–4 cm stent, 5 or 7 Fr in diameter according to the calibre of the duct, is initially inserted. We routinely remove any proximal retention barbs to minimize duct trauma prior to insertion. The angle of the stent in the duodenum helps to direct the line for a needle-knife cut. The length of the cut is very difficult to define but in general it is 3–5 mm in length, unroofing the papilla to the level of the duodenal wall. The guiding stent may fall out (confirmed at follow-up X-ray) or is removed 1–2 weeks later. In the presence of an enlarged minor papilla, a dilated dorsal duct or a Santorinicoele, a 5 Fr sphincterotome, with or without a guide wire, can be used effectively (Figure 17.5).

Stent insertion

The dorsal duct often takes a sigmoid direction from the minor papilla and tends to run a straight course through the body and tail. The introduction of a guide wire is the most difficult aspect of stent insertion and is best undertaken with a small calibre (0.018–0.025-inch) hydrophilic wire, which is introduced through a tapered cannula with a 3–4 Fr tip and a 5 Fr shaft. In order to assure adequate hydration of the wire it is helpful to use a side-arm (Tuohy–Borst) valve to allow for coaxial instillation of water. In addition, it permits injection of a smaller volume of contrast medium to fill the catheter for pancreatography. Overfilling of the limited capacitance dorsal duct system may occur if the wire has to be completely withdrawn prior to contrast medium injection. The advantage of the small-calibre wire is not only its narrow diameter but also the increased flexibility of the tip, which allows for looping of

the leading edge of the wire. Given the large number of side branches, the leading loop seeks the lumen of the main duct more reliably. After the wire is advanced beyond the midbody, the tapered catheter is advanced into the duct far enough to dilate the orifice of the minor papilla. It is then withdrawn and a less tapered catheter, which will take a 0.035-inch wire, is inserted up to the midbody of the dorsal duct. The hydrophillic wire can then be exchanged for a larger wire, preferably with a stiff body (Amplatz type). The non-hydrophilic stiff wire is best suited for advancing the 5 or 7 Fr stent into the duct. A larger stent may be used if the dorsal duct is sufficiently dilated. The duration of stenting depends on the therapeutic indication. The shorter the duration, the less the risk of stent-induced ductitis and fibrosis. In a dilated dorsal duct with a dominant stricture, stent insertion is reasonable for up to 3 months, but for enlarging the minor papilla orifice it is preferable to use the stent solely as a guide for needle-knife sphincterotomy and to remove it within 2 weeks if it has not migrated out spontaneously (Figure 17.6).

Unfortunately, a stent ideal for the pancreas has not been designed but it should incorporate the features of sufficient radial force for fibrotic areas, flexibility to accommodate angulation, a mesh design to allow branch duct drainage, and a diaphragm to prevent backwash of biliary or enteric secretions. A nitinol coil or mesh would seem to have the likeliest potential to incorporate such features.

CONCLUSION

There are more unanswered than answered questions with the available information on pancreas divisum. On the basis of the available evidence, however, most of the data support an association between the anomaly of pancreas divisum and

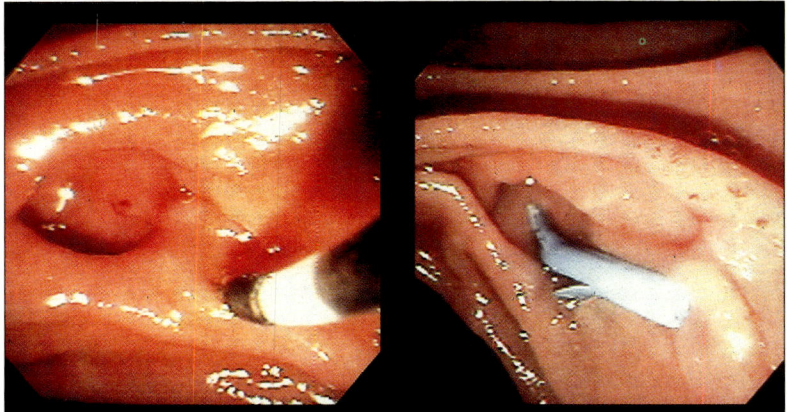

Figure 17.6 *Left.* Minor papilla orifice within a diverticulum. *Right.* Insertion of a straight stent into the dorsal duct in the 9 o'clock direction.

pancreatitis. The argument for an increased prevalence of pancreas divisum among patients with idiopathic pancreatitis is further bolstered when we consider that the number of non-pancreas divisum patients among patients with idiopathic pancreatitis is likely to be substantially fewer when the occult biliary aetiology patients are excluded, thus raising the proportion of pancreas divisum patients. The differential histopathological and morphological changes in the dorsal and ventral buds is less convincing, but most symptomatic pancreas divisum patients do not have evidence of chronic pancreatitis and it is likely that they progress to chronic disease less often, which diminishes the chance of showing structural changes. Although functional impairment assessed by provocative secretin testing is not very sensitive, some variation of this approach would appear to have the most promise of identifying those who might benefit from a drainage procedure. Whether or not surgery provides a better outcome with fewer complications is not clear. The restenosis rate after surgical sphincterotomy/-plasty is likely to be lower, but the low morbidity of endoscopic intervention tips the balance in favour of an initial endoscopic approach, with surgery reserved for those who fail endoscopic therapy or warrant resection. The final answer to this debate can only be reached through a prospective randomized comparison, which would be a daunting task given the relative scarcity of suitable patients in any single practice.

References

1. Stern CD. A historical perspective on the discovery of the accessory duct of the pancreas, the ampulla "of Vater" and pancreas divisum. *Gut* 1986; 27:203–12.
2. Gregg JA. Pancreas divisum: its association with pancreatitis. *Am J Surg* 1977; 134:539–43.
3. Tulassay Z, Papp J. New clinical aspects of pancreas divisum. *Gastrointest Endosc* 1980; 26:143–6.
4. Cotton PB. Congenital anomaly of pancreas divisum as cause of obstructive pain and pancreatitis. *Gut* 1980; 21:105–14.
5. Meckel JF. *Handbuch der pathologischen anatomie.* CH Reclaim, Leipzig; 1812.
6. Warshaw AL, Simeone JF, Schapiro RH, Flavin-Warshaw B. Evaluation and treatment of the dominant dorsal duct syndrome (pancreas divisum redefined). *Am J Surg* 1990; 159:59–66.
7. Baldwin WM. The pancreatic ducts in man, together with a study of the microscopical structure of the minor duodenal papilla. *Anat Rec* 1911; 5:197–228.
8. Dawson W, Langman J. An anatomical-radiological study on the pancreatic duct pattern in man. *Anat Rec* 1961; 139:59–68.
9. Smanio T. Proposed nomenclature and classification of the human pancreatic ducts and duodenal papillae: Study based on 200 post mortems. *Int Surg* 1969; 52:125–34.
10. Burtin P, Person B, Charneau J, Boyer J. Pancreas divisum and pancreatitis: a coincidental association? *Endoscopy* 1991; 23:55–8.
11. Cotton PB. Pancreas divisum – curiosity or culprit? *Gastroenterology* 1985; 89:1431–5.
12. Carr-Locke DL. Pancreas divisum: the controversy goes on? *Endoscopy* 1991; 23:88–9.
13. Delhaye M, Engelholm L, Cremer M. Pancreas divisum: congenital anatomic variant or anomaly? *Gastroenterology* 1985; 89:951–8.
14. Bernard JP, Sahel J, Giovannini M, Sarles H. Pancreas divisum is a probable cause of acute pancreatitis: a report of 137 cases. *Pancreas* 1990; 5:248–54.
15. Ros E, Navarro S, Bru C, Garcia-Puges A, Valderrama R. Occult microlithiasis in "idiopathic" acute pancreatitis: Prevention of relapses by cholecystectomy or ursodeoxycholic acid therapy. *Gastroenterology* 1991; 101:1701–9.
16. Lee SP, Nicholls JF, Park HZ. Biliary sludge as a cause of acute pancreatitis. *N Engl J Med* 1992; 326:589–93.
17. Warshaw AL, Richter JM, Shapiro RH. The cause and treatment of pancreatitis associated with pancreas divisum. *Ann Surg* 1983; 198:443–52.
18. Rusnak CH, Hoisie RT, Kuechler PM, McHattie JD *et al.* Pancreatitis associated with pancreas divisum: results of surgical intervention. *Am J Surg* 1988; 155:641–3.
19. Sahel J, Cros RC, Bourry J, Sarles H. Clinicopathological conditions associated with pancreas divisum. *Digestion* 1982; 23:1–8.
20. Warshaw AL, Simeone J, Schapiro RH, Hedberg SE *et al.* Objective evaluation of ampullary stenosis with ultrasonography and pancreatic stimulation. *Am J Surg* 1985; 149:65–72.
21. Lowes JR, Lees WR, Cotton PB. Pancreatic duct dilatation after secretin stimulation in patients with pancreas divisum. *Pancreas* 1989; 4:37–41.
22. Eisen GM, Coleman SD, England RE *et al.* A prospective evaluation of the secretin ultrasound test in patients undergoing endoscopic therapy for chronic pancreatitis. *Gastrointest Endosc* 1995; 41:422 (abstract).
23. Topazian M. Acute pancreatitis, pancreatic duct obstruction, and the secretin–ultrasound test (editorial). *J Clin Gastroenterol* 1994; 18:277–9.

24. Cavallini G, Rigo L, Bovo P et al. Abnormal US response of main pancreatic duct after secretin stimulation in patients with acute pancreatitis of different etiology. *J Clin Gastroenterol* 1994; 18:298–303.

25. Catalano MF, Geenen JE, Schmalz MF, Geenen DJ et al. Endoscopic ultrasound with secretin stimulation (SSEUS) in the diagnosis of obstructive chronic pancreatitis. *Gastrointest Endosc* 1995; 41:300 (abstract).

26. Staritz M, Meyer zum Buschenfelde KH. Elevated pressure in the dorsal part of pancreas divisum: the cause of chronic pancreatitis. *Pancreas* 1988; 3:108–10.

27. Gregg J, Solomon J, Clark G. Pancreas divisum and its association with choledochal sphincter stenosis: diagnosis by endoscopic retrograde cholangiopancreatography and endoscopic biliary manometry. *Am J Surg* 1984; 147:367–71.

28. Delhaye M, Engelholm L, Cremer M. Pancreas divisum: controversial clinical significance. *Dig Dis* 1988; 6:30–9.

29. Blair AJ, Russell CG, Cotton PB. Resection for pancreatitis in patients with pancreas divisum. *Ann Surg* 1984; 200:590–4.

30. Rhode J, Lowes JR, Dhillon AP, Cotton PB. Pancreas divisum pancreatitis. *J Pathol* 1986.

31. Rosch W, Koch H, Schaffner O, Demling L. The clinical significance of the pancreas divisum. *Gastrointest Endosc* 1976; 22:206–7.

32. Mitchell CJ. Pancreas divisum and pancreatitis. In *Pancreatic Disease in Clinical Practice*. Edited by CJ Mitchell, J Kelleher. Pitman Books; London:1981;404–14.

33. Lans JI, Geenen JE, Johanson JF, Hogan WJ. Endoscopic therapy in patients with pancreas divisum and acute pancreatitis: a prospective, randomized, controlled clinical trial. *Gastrointest Endosc* 1992; 38:430–4.

34. Cotton PB. Duodenoscopic papillotomy at the minor papilla for recurrent dorsal pancreatitis. *Endoscop Dig* 1978; 3:27–8.

35. Soehendra N, Kempeneers I, Nam VCh, Grimm H. Endoscopic dilatation and papillotomy of the accessory papilla and internal drainage in pancreas divisum. *Endoscopy* 1986; 18:129–32.

36. Siegel JH, Ben–Zvi JS, Pullano W, Cooperman A. Effectiveness of endoscopic drainage for pancreas divisum: endoscopic and surgical results in 31 patients. *Endoscopy* 1990; 22:129–33.

37. Lehman GA, Sherman S, Nisi R, Hawes RH. Pancreas divisum: results of minor papilla sphincterotomy. *Gastrointest Endosc* 1993; 39:1–8.

38. Coleman SD, Eisen GME, Troughton AB et al. Endoscopic treatment in pancreatic divisum. *Am J Gastroenterol* 1994; 8:1152–5.

39. Kozarek RA, Ball TJ, Patterson DJ et al. Endoscopic approaches to pancreatic divisum. *Dig Dis Sci* 1995; 40:1974–81.

40. Keith RG, Shapero TF, Saibil FG et al. Dorsal duct sphincterotomy is effective long-term treatment of acute pancreatitis associated with pancreas divisum. *Surgery* 1989; 106:660–7.

41. Richter JM, Shapiro RH, Mulley AG et al. Association of pancreas divisum pancreatitis, and its treatment by sphincteroplasty of the accessory ampulla. *Gastroenterology* 1981; 81:1104–10.

42. Sugawa C, Walt AJ, Nunez DC, et al. Pancreas divisum: Is it a normal anatomic variant? *Am J Surg* 1987; 153: 62–7.

18

Pancreatic stenting: long-term consequences *Judy Dorais & Gregory B. Haber*

INTRODUCTION

Endoscopic retrograde cholangiopancreatography (ERCP) is a widely practised technique that has been used for over 20 years[1–3]. It was not, however, until 1985 that pancreatography culminated in the endoscopic stenting of the main pancreatic duct (MPD)[4]. In the last decade, pancreatic endoprostheses have been inserted for a wide variety of pancreatic disorders. The therapeutic endpoints sought are: the prevention of pancreatitis[5]; as a guide for needle-knife pancreatic or biliary sphincterotomies[6]; to drain pseudocysts or to bypass leaks to allow fistula healing[7–16]; or to predict the response to surgery[17–20]. Long-term clinical goals are: the prolonged relief of pain; the preservation of glandular integrity; and the palliation of malignant disease.

LONG-TERM GOALS OF PANCREATIC ENDOPROSTHESES

Prolonged relief of pain

Of the three potential long-term consequences of pancreatic stenting, the prolonged relief of pain is the least controversial. The concept of duct obstruction and raised intraductal pressure as a source of pain in chronic pancreatitis was formulated in the 1950s and led to the practice of surgical decompression of the MPD[21,22]. The potential role of ductal hypertension in the pathogenesis of pain in chronic pancreatitis has evolved, from the simple demonstration of elevated distal (to the obstruction) pancreatic duct pressures[23,24], to a model approximating the chronic closed compartment syndrome[25].

Reber et al.[26] have shown that in normal cats secretory stimulation does not affect pancreatic ductal or interstitial pressures but does significantly increase pancreatic blood flow. In cats with induced chronic obstructive pancreatitis, secretory stimulation causes a significant increase in interstitial pressure and a simultaneous decrease in blood flow to the pancreas. Decompression of the MPD brings both of these parameters nearer normal values, thereby re-establishing the usual pattern of 'secretory hyperaemia'. Reber and Lo have recently presented results from the first successful, non-operative, pancreatic blood flow study in humans[27]. This procedure involves the trans-sphincteric pancreatic duct measurement of blood hydrogen, using a specially designed probe, in patients breathing 3% hydrogen in air. Computer analysis of generated signals provides a hydrogen desaturation curve which reflects pancreatic blood flow. This may prove to be a valuable tool in the future assessment of blood flow in a wide spectrum of acute and chronic pancreatic disorders. This area remains controversial despite notable advances in our understanding of the pathophysiology; this can be attributed to the inability to explain why obstructive pancreatitis is not always associated with pain, nor pain always associated with ductal obstruction. Other pain-generating mechanisms, e.g. pancreatitis-associated neuritis, have been proposed[28].

Clinically, the difficulty in assessing accurately the efficacy of stenting in long-term pancreatic pain management arises not from a paucity of available data but rather from a surplus of confounding variables. Patients comprise a heterogeneous group, both on an inter- and intra-study level, presenting with combinations of strictures, stones and other pathologies as well as diverse aetiologies of chronic pancreatitis.

The initial approach to pancreatic endotherapy was essentially derived from parallel procedures in the biliary tree. Consequently, most of the early modes of therapy were empirical in nature and highly variable. The variations included: the type of stent; duration of stenting; concomitant endoscopic biliary sphincterotomy (EBS) or endoscopic pancreatic sphincterotomy (EPS); lithotripsy technique applied; as well as any additional therapy for stones or pseudocysts.

Figure 18.1 shows the results of endoscopic therapy in patients with chronic pancreatitis, including ductal stenting and stone clearance, from 1991 to 1995[29–33]. Most of these series were retrospective reviews compiled from large therapeutic endoscopy centres, encompassing a broad range of therapeutic techniques. These pooled results are of questionable value because of their intrinsic variability.

The most uniform work to date is that of Ponchon et al.[33], who performed a prospective study with a standardized protocol including well defined inclusion/exclusion criteria and specific endpoints. In this study all patients presented with a segmental stricture in the head of the pancreas and upward homogeneous dilatation of the pancreatic duct – type IV pancreatitis according to the classification proposed by Cremer et al.[38]. Excluded from their study were patients with multiple sites of ductal stenosis, pancreatic stones, pancreas divisum and/or pseudocysts >1cm diameter. All patients were subjected to biliary and pancreatic sphincterotomies. All MPD strictures were initially dilated to 6.5Fr and then stented with a 10Fr pancreatic endoprosthesis. Subsequently, stents were exchanged every 2 months and permanently removed after a total drainage period of 6 months. Patients were evaluated for an average of 14 months after final stent removal. The results from this study are compared with less rigorous studies below.

Technical success rates are invariably high, ranging from 85% to 100%. It should be noted, however, that even in those therapeutic centres with very skilled endoscopists, technical success may require two or three attempts before a guide wire can be manipulated beyond the stricture. Tight strictures may require dilatation, using graduated catheters or dilatation balloons, before a stent can be inserted successfully.

Figure 18.1 Results of studies of pancreatic stenting between 1991 and 1995.

Author (ref)	n	Number of dominant strictures	Number with pancreas divisum	EPS/ total	Technical success	Early responders	Long-term responders		Mean duration of stenting	Mean follow-up	
							Stent in	Stent out		Stent in	Stent out
Cremer (29)	76	76	21	75/76	75/76 (99%)	71/75 (94%)	34/64	?	?	37 months	?
Duvall et al. (30)	63	58	17	27/63	100%	52/63 (83%)	46/52	= 88.5%	14 months	?	28 months
Smits et al. (31)	51	51	3	51/51	49/51 (96%)	40/49 (82%)	16/18 (38/40)	22/22 = 95%	6.3 months	18 months	28.5 months
Binmoeller et al. (32)	93	93	23	93/93	100%	69/93 (74%)	? (60/69)	49/60 =87%	15.7 months	?	3.8 years
Ponchon et al. (33)	33	33	0	33/33	28/33 (91%)	20/23 (86%)	0	12/23 (52%)	6 months	0	14 months

Clinical success rates are more variable. The primary endpoint most frequently evaluated is pain, but secondary endpoints may include the frequency of hospitalization [31,32], the change in nutritional status [29,32] and the ability to return to the work force after the stenting procedure [30]. Most authors begin by determining which proportion of the patients under study are 'immediate' or 'early' responders . As a rule, early response is evaluated in terms of response to the first stent, though the length of time this first endoprosthesis is allowed to remain in situ is quite variable from study to study. Ashby and Lo [34] removed first stents 7 days after insertion in all patients failing to show improvement. Smits et al. [31] removed stents within 3 months and Binmoeller et al. [32] within 6 months of initial ERCP in patients whose symptoms failed to improve. Early response rates were 86%, 82% and 74%, respectively, in the Ashby and Lo, Smits et al. and Binmoeller et al. studies, suggesting that the prolonged presence of a first stent in the pancreatic duct does not lead to a significantly higher proportion of 'responders'. In most recent studies the proportion of patients that are 'early' or 'immediate' responders constitute the subgroup which serves as the denominator for evaluating long-term success.

It is difficult to determine a priori which patients will, or will not, respond to pancreatic stenting. The question is crucial in determining the management strategy for patients with painful chronic pancreatitis, that is, in choosing between surgery and interventional therapy [35–37]. Cremer et al. advocate the classification of ductal changes at ERCP (pancreatitis types I–V) as the best criteria for diagnosis and selection of patients for endoscopic management [38,39]. Type IV pancreatitis, characterized by a segmental stricture in the head of the pancreas and upward homogeneous dilatation, is the best candidate for stenting. Geenen, in a study specifically designed to identify subgroups of patients who might benefit from pancreatic stent placement for pain relief, found that both pancreatic duct obstruction (due to stones or strictures <1mm) and dilatation (with MPD >6mm) were significant predictors of improvement [40]. On the other hand, in a retrospective study of 29 patients, 10 of whom had normal (nondilated) pancreatic ducts, there was no correlation between ERCP findings and clinical response to pancreatic stenting [41].

The majority of the most recent studies attempt to isolate study parameters unique among those patients responding favourably to stenting. Binmoeller et al. [32] and Smits et al. [31] found that neither demographic data (age, sex, past or current alcohol abuse, duration of disease or associated diabetes mellitus) nor ERCP findings, including the presence of strictures and/or ductal dilatation, were helpful in predicting clinical outcome.

Long-term responders constitute that subgroup of early responders who have maintained partial or complete relief from pain as a result of continuous (repeated), intermittent, or completed stenting. There are clearly major differences in defining a long-term response, with follow-up arbitrarily defined as that period subsequent to the period of stenting versus a period of follow-up commencing with the date of insertion of the initial stent. Binmoeller et al. [32] reported on the outcome of pancreatic stenting in 93 patients. Of these, 69 patients (74%) were classified as early responders and 60 of the 69 (86%) achieved sustained pain relief and were dubbed 'long-term responders' (LTRs). The mean duration of stenting in this study was 15.7 months, with a mean follow-up after stent removal of 3.8 years.

In the study of Smits et al., 49 of 51 patients with chronic pancreatitis and a dominant stricture had successful stent insertion. Pain relief with the initial stent occurred in 40 of 49 patients, giving an early response rate of 82%. In 55% of LTRs (22/40 patients) stents were removed after a mean stenting period of 6.3 months, and these patients were still doing well after a mean follow-up period of 28.5 months. The remaining 45% of LTRs (18/40) still had a stent in place for a mean of 18 months; 16 of these patients reported persisting improvement. Consequently, an impressive 96% of early responders demonstrated symptomatic improvement as a result of temporary or long-term stenting.

If one looks at the long-term success rate of these two studies on an intention-to-treat basis, that is to say the success rate for 'all comers', it then falls to 74.5% (38/51) for the study of Smits et al. and 64.5% (60/93) for the the study of Binmoeller et al. The Toronto group [30] performed a retrospective analysis of the outcome of stent therapy in a subset of patients who did not have surgical drainage procedures and compared, in follow-up, the outcomes of the early responders and the early non-responders. They reported a success rate of 88.5% (46/52 patients) 28 months after a mean stenting period of 14 months. Among the initial 11 failures, nine continued to do poorly and two patients improved spontaneously.

In contrast to the above encouraging data on the long-term consequences of endoscopic stent drainage, Ashby and Lo [34] reported a 0% success rate after a mean follow-up period of 11 months. This discrepancy may be explained, in part, by the diversity of the patient population in the Ashby and Lo study, e.g. six cases of pancreatic cancer and four of sphincter stenosis. Furthermore, only 2 of the 21 patients underwent EPS at the time of stent insertion, as opposed to 100% of the patients in the Binmoeller et al. and the Smits et al. studies.

The interesting question arises as to when to terminate pancreatic duct stenting. Binmoeller et al. report removing stents electively if follow-up pancreatography demonstrates resolution of the stricture and easy passage of a 6Fr catheter through the old stricture site. Employing these criteria, only 13 of 49 patients in whom stenting had been terminated experienced a relapse of pain; 11 of these were successfully re-treated by endoscopic drainage and subsequently became pain-free. Smits et al. use similar criteria but in addition document the rapid drainage of contrast medium from the pancreatic duct as further evidence of stricture improvement. This group reports the need to reinstitute stenting after elective discontinuation in only 13% of its LTRs. Finally, Ponchon et al. [33] found that, once stenting had been initiated, the elimination of the proximal ductal stenosis and a reduction of >2mm in the MPD diameter on follow-up ERCP were significantly associated with pain relief, whereas abstinence from alcohol and the use of pancreatic enzyme supplements were not. Ponchon's protocol did not include stent reinsertion at a later date if symptoms recurred. This could explain, in part, the lower success rate at one year (52%), compared both with the above studies and with their own success rate of 74% at completion of stent therapy. The prospective nature of Ponchon's study probably provides a more realistic assessment of outcome.

Preservation of glandular integrity

It is believed by some practitioners in the field of therapeutic endoscopy that ductal drainage might delay the development of functional impairment in patients with chronic pancreatitis. No direct evidence exits to support this claim. Animal studies [42] have shown that secretory function in cats is maintained until the diameter of the pancreatic duct is reduced by >50%; thereafter, pancreatic function deteriorates with time and with the degree of ductal stenosis.

A prospective study by Nealon and Thompson [43] of 143 patients with chronic pancreatitis, of whom 87 underwent pancreaticojejunostomy, suggested that patients with mild to moderate disease undergoing surgery had a stabilization of pancreatic function (13% progressed to severe chronic pancreatitis) compared with those patients managed without ductal decompression (78% progressed to severe disease). A small separate part of this prospective trial was randomized (17 patients): nine of these patients were operated upon and eight were not. The trend in this subgroup was similar, with

only 23% of operated patients showing progressive disease versus 75% of conservatively managed patients. Length of follow-up was impressive at 47.3 months. The authors did not use hormonal stimulation tests to evaluate pancreatic function but used less sensitive morphological tests (ERCP), exocrine function tests (bentiromide PABA and 72-hour faecal fat testing) and endocrine function tests (oral glucose tolerance test and fat meal-stimulated release of pancreatic polypeptide). Ductal decompression in patients with chronic pancreatitis cannot yet be advocated for treatment of pancreatic exocrine insufficiency or for arrest of disease progression but merits further investigation.

Palliation of malignant pancreatic disease

Virtually all that is known of the potential role of pancreatic duct stenting in malignant pancreatic disease is the result of work published by Costamagna et al. [44]. They report on 12 patients with unresectable cancer of the pancreatic head associated with upstream dilatation of the MPD and severe pancreatic 'obstructive'-like pain. Technical success was achieved in 8 of 12 cases (63%). Clinical success was observed in 7 of 8 patients, all of whom were able to discontinue narcotics. The follow-up period ranged from 26 to 575 days, with a mean of 165.5 days, wherein there was no clinical evidence of pancreatic stent clogging. As encouraging as these results may seem, it must be noted that the initial evaluation encompassed 75 patients but only 12 (16%) of the 75 were found to have the typical ERCP pattern showing MPD dilatation upstream to the neoplastic stricture – a definite minority.

More recently, Lichtenstein et al. [45] reported the results of a similar study comprising five patients. Clinical success was achieved in only those patients, three of five, that presented with pain as a meal-related symptom. The two patients with chronic, unremitting pain did not benefit from stent therapy. In the Ashby and Lo study [34] the subgroup of five patients with pancreatic cancer and upstream MPD dilatation all experienced return of their pain before death. The authors did, however, find a significantly longer (p<0.01) stent viability in the patients with pancreatic cancer – 69 days versus 25 days.

COMPLICATIONS OF PANCREATIC STENTING

The insertion of pancreatic stents may entail both short-term and long-term complications. In a review of over 500 procedures, Geenen and Rolny [46] reported that serious complications occurred in only about 3% of cases, with only four fatalities (<1%). Though complications may be of an extremely varied nature (Figure 18.2), the two most often seen are occlusion and migration.

One of the most common late complications of transpapillary pancreatic endoprostheses is clogging of the stent lumen. The occluding material is composed of calcium carbonate embedded in an organic matrix, peppered with bacterial ghosts and protein threads [47,48]. Stent viability has been found to be highly variable, ranging from days to many months. Ikenberry et al. [49] reported on a study comparing the patency of 5Fr, 6Fr and 7Fr polyethylene stents and found an almost linear progression, with time, of the number of occluded stents. By 6 weeks after insertion, 50% of the stents were clogged, and by

Figure 18.2 Immediate and delayed complications of pancreatic stenting.

Complication	Cremer et al. (29)	Duvall et al. (30)	Smits et al. (31)	Binmoeller et al. (32)	Ponchon et al. (33)	Total (%)
Immediate	n = 75	n = 63	n = 51	n = 93	n = 33	n = 316
Pancreatitis			2	4	9	15 (4.7%)
Cholangitis	3		3			6 (1.8%)
Bleeding	1		2			3 (0.9%)
Ductal trauma			1			1 (0.3%)
Infected pseudocyst				1		1 (0.3%)
Occlusion					2	2 (0.6%)
Death	0	0	0	0	0	0%
Delayed	n = 71	n = 52	n = 40	n = 69	n = 20	n = 252
Occlusion	NR	26	19	2*	3	50 (20%)
Migration	3	8	9	0*	2	22 (9%)
Pancreatitis		6				6 (2.3%)
Ductitis	NR	13	0	0	5	18 (7.1%)
De novo stones	NR	14	NR	2	NR	16 (6.3%)
Infection of pancreatic secretions	6					6 (2.3%)
Infected pseudocyst or abscess				1	2	3 (1.2%)
Death	1					1 (0.4%)

NR = not reported
* = occlusion and migration not considered as complications by the authors if situation resolved after an uneventful stent exchange

9 weeks 100% were occluded. Efforts to prolong the half-life of stents using antibiotic coatings have not met with success [50]. A recent abstract provides very preliminary evidence suggesting improved patency using a new nylon and teflon stent [51].

An equally important question concerns the frequency with which the stents require changing [52]. Some patients remain symptom-free for periods of time greatly exceeding lumen patency, possibly due to a wick-like function of the stent. Routine stent exchanges, in anticipation of occlusion, would need to be performed on a regular 6–8-week basis, entailing multiple procedures in patients slated for long-term treatment. For this reason, most endoscopists leave stents in place for 3 months once maximum stent diameter has been achieved . 'Emergent' stent exchanges expose patients to risks of recurrent pancreatitis and pancreatic infection, but these sequelae occur infrequently.

Stent migration is another important complication. Johansen et al. [53] retrospectively analysed the incidence of, and risk factors for, pancreatic stent migration. They found that sphincter of Oddi dysfunction and longer stents were associated with proximal pancreatic stent migration. No significant risk factors for distal (duodenal) migration were identified. In a later study [54], these same authors modified 51 pancreatic stents by removing the proximal (intrapancreatic) barbs and found a statistically significantly lower proximal migration rate with the altered stents, with no increase in the incidence of distal migration. This same group recently reported their experience with 178 modified stents; contrary to their initial findings, the outward migration rate was significantly greater for short, small-diameter stents. Inward migration, a much more serious complication, remained low after this modification [55].

Evidence that pancreatic ductal lesions could be induced by the stents themselves was first proposed by Kozarek in 1990 [56]. He reported an incidence of 36% for lesions related to stent occlusion (pseudocysts, diffuse duct enlargement) and direct stent trauma or side branch occlusion (irregular stenoses, side branch ectasia). Though the former type of lesion was found to resolve upon stent retrieval or exchange, the long-term consequences of the latter remained to be determined. Sherman et al. [57] published the results of an animal study which involved the stenting of normal pancreatic ducts in dogs, suggesting that the type of lesion attributed to stent trauma is probably related to stent occlusion and may be permanent.

Eisen et al. [58] reported the results of a clinical study designed to evaluate the persistence of ductal changes after stenting. The mean duration of stenting was 69 days. A remote pancreatogram performed at a mean of 189 days later in eight patients showed: complete resolution of changes in five cases (63%); no change or partial resolution of abnormalities in two cases; and worsening in one patient.

CONCLUSION

A number of optimistic conclusions have been reached concerning the efficacy of pancreatic stents without any prospective, randomized, controlled clinical trials to substantiate these claims. The only exception is the work by Lans et al. [59] which showed that, in the short term, dorsal pancreatic duct stent placement across the minor papilla in patients with pancreas divisum and acute recurrent pancreatitis resulted in significant objective clinical improvement compared with controls. No such study has evaluated the long-term consequences of pancreatic stenting. The closest approximation is the study by Ponchon et al.[33] with a 52% clinical response rate at 12 months; the results of a lengthier follow-up period for this particular patient population are eagerly awaited.

Two important points become evident as a result of the recently published studies described above. First, the exact role of EPS is unclear but as an adjunctive procedure at the time of stenting, it may contribute to long-term clinical success. Secondly, although there are no validated criteria for predicting long-term responders to pancreatic stenting, the morphological features of a very tight dominant stricture with upstream dilatation would appear to constitute the best indicator of a positive response in non-divisum patients. Finally, the potential risks of pancreatic endoprostheses have been well documented[60]. The least well understood factors, in terms of long-term consequences, are the ductal changes reminiscent of chronic pancreatitis, and these are the most worrisome. The clinical consequences of acute and/or persisting ductitis seen on the pancreatogram and the relationship, if any, to functional impairment, remain to be determined[61].

References

1. Kasugai T, Kuno N, Kizu M. Endoscopic pancreatocholangiography. *Gastroenterology* 1972; 63:217–34.
2. Classen M, Sarfany L. Endoscopic papillotomy and removal of gallstones. *Br Med J* 1975; 4:371–4.
3. Cremer M. (personal communication, 1977).
4. Siegel, JH. Evaluation and treatment of acquired and congenital pancreatic disorders: endoscopic dilation and insertion of endoprostheses. *Am J Gastroenterol* 1983; 78:696. (abstract)
5. Smithline A, Silverman W, Rogers D. Effect of prophylactic main pancreatic duct stenting on the incidence of biliary endoscopic sphincterotomy-induced pancreatitis in high-risk patients. *Gastrointest Endosc* 1993; 39:652–7.
6. Kozarek R, Ball T, Patterson D. Endoscopic pancreatic duct sphincterotomy: indications, technique, and analysis of results. *Gastrointest Endosc* 1994; 40:592–8.
7. Kozarek R, Ball T, Patterson D. Endoscopic transpapillary therapy for disrupted pancreatic duct and peripancreatic fluid collections. *Gastroenterology* 1991; 100:1362–70.
8. Kozarek R, Christie D, Barclay G. Endoscopic therapy of pancreatitis in the pediatric population. *Gastrointest Endosc* 1993; 39:665–9.
9. Kozarek R, Jiranek G, Traverso W. Endoscopic treatment of pancreatic ascites. *Am J Surg* 1994; 168:223–6.
10. Smits M, Rauw E, Tytgat G. The efficacy of endoscopic treatment of pancreatic pseudocysts. *Gastrointest Endosc* 1995; 42:202–7.
11. Deviere J, Bueso H, Baize M. Complete disruption of the main pancreatic duct: endoscopic management. *Gastrointest Endosc* 1995; 42:445–51.
12. Binmoeller K, Seifert H, Walter A. Transpapillary and transmural drainage of pancreatic pseudocysts. *Gastrointest Endosc* 1995; 42:219–24.
13. Catalano M, Geenen J, Schmalz M. Treatment of pancreatic pseudocysts with ductal communication by transpapillary pancreatic duct endoprosthesis. *Gastrointest Endosc* 1995; 42:214–18.
14. Barthet M, Sahel J, Bodiou-Bertei C. Endoscopic transpapillary drainage of pancreatic pseudocysts. *Gastrointest Endosc* 1995; 42:208–13.
15. Lichtenstein DR, Roston A, Slivka A. Pancreatic stent therapy for pancreatic fistulae. *Gastrointest Endosc* 1995; 41:426. (abstract)
16. Kozarek R, Ball T, Patterson D. Endoscopic treatment of pancreaticocutaneous fistula. *Gastrointest Endosc* 1996; A907:3626.
17. Grimm H, Meyer WH, Nam V Ch. New modalities for treating chronic pancreatitis. *Endoscopy* 1989; 21:70–4.
18. Siegel JH, Cooperman AM, Pullano W. Pancreas divisum: observation, endoscopic drainage, and surgical treatment results in 65 patients. *Surg Laparosc Endosc* 1993; 3:281–5.
19. McHenry L, Gore D, DeMaria E. Endoscopic treatment of dilated-duct chronic pancreatitis with pancreatic stents: preliminary results of a sham-controlled, blinded, crossover trial to predict surgical outcome. *Am J Gastroenterol* 1993; 88:1536. (abstract)
20. DuVall GA, Haber GB, Kortan P. Is the outcome of endoscopic therapy of chronic pancreatitis predictive of surgical success? *Gastrointest Endosc* 1996; 43:404 (A457).
21. Zollinger RM, Keith LM, Ellison EH. Pancreatitis. *New Engl J Med* 1954; 251:497.
22. Partington PF, Rochelle REL. Modified Peustow procedure for retrograde drainage of the pancreatic duct. *Ann Surg* 1960; 152:1037.
23. Madsen P, Winkler K. The intraductal pancreatic pressure in chronic obstructive pancreatitis. *Scand J Gastroenterol* 1982; 17:553–4.
24. Okazaki K, Yamamoto Y, Kagiyama S. Pressure of papillary sphincter zone and pancreatic main duct in patients with chronic pancreatitis in the early stage. *Scand J Gastroenterol* 1988; 23:501–7.
25. Widdison AL, Alvarez C, Karanjia ND. Experimental evidence of beneficial effects of ductal decompression in chronic pancreatitis. *Endoscopy* 1991; 23:151–4.
26. Karanjia ND, Widdison AL, Leung F, et al. Compartment syndrome in experimental chronic obstructive pancreatitis: effect of decompressing the main pancreatic duct. *Br J Surg* 1994; 81:259–64.
27. Lo SK, Lewis MPN, Reber HA. In-vivo endoscopic trans-sphincteric measurement of pancreatic blood flow (PBF) in humans. *Gastrointest Endosc* 1996; 43:409 (A476).
28. Bockman DE, Buchler M, Malfertheiner P. Analysis of nerves in chronic pancreatitis. *Gastroenterology* 1988; 94:1459–69.
29. Cremer M, Deviere J, Delhaye M. Stenting in severe chronic pancreatitis: results of medium-term follow-up in seventy-six patients. *Endoscopy* 1991; 23:171–6.
30. DuVall GA, Haber GB, Kortan P. Is the initial success of endoscopic therapy (ET) of chronic pancreatitis (CP) sustained in long-term follow-up? *Gastrointest Endosc* 1996; 43:404(A456).
31. Smits ME, Badiga SM, Rauws EA. Long-term results of pancreatic stents in chronic pancreatitis. *Gastrointest Endosc* 1995; 42:461–7.
32. Binmoeller KF, Jue P, Seifert H. Endoscopic pancreatic stent drainage in chronic pancreatitis and a dominant stricture: long-term results. *Endoscopy* 1995; 27:638–44.
33. Ponchon T, Bory RM, Hedelius F. Endoscopic stenting for pain relief in chronic pancreatitis: results of a standardized protocol. *Gastrointest Endosc* 1995; 42:452–6.
34. Ashby K, Lo SK. The role of pancreatic stenting in obstructive ductal disorders other than pancreas divisum. *Gastrointest Endosc* 1995; 42:306–11.
35. Ammann RW. A critical appraisal of interventional therapy in chronic pancreatitis. *Endoscopy* 1991; 23:191–3.
36. Burdick JS, Hogan WJ. Chronic pancreatitis: selection of patients for endoscopic therapy. *Endoscopy* 1991; 23:155–60.
37. Malfertheiner P, Buchler M. Indications for endoscopic or surgical therapy in chronic pancreatitis. *Endoscopy* 1991; 23:185–90.
38. Cremer M, Deviere J, Delhaye M. Non–surgical management of severe chronic pancreatitis. *Scand J Gastroenterol* 1990; 25(S175):77–84.

39. Cremer M, Deviere J, Delhaye M. Endoscopic management of chronic pancreatitis. *Acta Gastroenterol Belg* 1993; 56:192–200.

40. Burdick JS, Geenen JE, Hogan W. Pancreatic stent therapy in chronic pancreatitis: which patients benefit? *Gastrointest Endosc* 1993; 39:309. (abstract)

41. Gulliver DJ, Baker ME, Paine S. Stent placement for benign pancreatic diseases: correlation between ERCP findings and clinical response. *Am J Radiol* 1992; 159:751–5.

42. Austin JL, Pick AL, Wipfler J. Effect of chronic partial pancreatic obstruction on pancreatic duct secretory pressure and permeability in cats. *J Surg Res* 1988; 44:772.

43. Nealon WH, Thompson JC. Progressive loss of pancreatic function in chronic pancreatitis is delayed by main pancreatic duct decompression. *Ann Surg* 1993; 217:458–68.

44. Costamagna G, Gabbrielli A, Mutignani M. Treatment of "obstructive" pain by endoscopic drainage in patients with pancreatic head carcinoma. *Gastrointest Endosc* 1993; 39:774–7.

45. Lichtenstein DR, Slivka A, Banks PA. Pancreatic stent placement for palliation of "obstructive" pain in pancreatic malignancy. *Gastrointest Endosc* 1995; 41:425. (abstract)

46. Geenen J, Rolny P. Endoscopic therapy of acute and chronic pancreatitis. *Gastrointest Endosc* 1991; 37:377–82.

47. Provensal-Cheylan M, Bernard JP, Mariani A. Occluded pancreatic endoprostheses – analysis of the clogging material. *Endoscopy* 1989; 21:63–9.

48. Gopinath N, van Marle J, Smits ME. Pancreatic polyethylene stents are blocked by a proteinaceous matrix. *Gastrointest Endosc* 1995; 41:422. (abstract)

49. Ikenberry S, Sherman S, Hawes R. The occlusion rate of pancreatic stents. *Gastrointest Endosc* 1994; 40:611–13.

50. Browne S, Schmalz M, Geenen J. A comparison of biliary and pancreatic stent occlusion in antibiotic-coated vs. conventional stents. *Gastrointest Endosc* 1990; 36:A87. (abstract)

51. Jacob L, Geenen J, Henderson JD. The new nylon and teflon pancreatic stents compared to polyethylene for patency and stent induced changes in dog pancreas. *Gastrointest Endosc* 1996; 43: 408 (A469).

52. Binmoeller K, Jue P, Seifert H. Pancreatic duct stents (PDS): how often do they need to be exchanged in patients with chronic pancreatitis (CP)? *Gastrointest Endosc* 1994; 40:100. (abstract)

53. Johansen JF, Schmalz MJ, Geenen JE. Incidence and risk factors for biliary and pancreatic stent migration. *Gastrointest Endosc* 1992; 38:341–6.

54. Johanson JF, Schmalz MJ, Geenen JE. Simple modification of a pancreatic duct stent to prevent proximal migration. *Gastrointest Endosc* 1993; 39:62–4.

55. Dahman B, Geenen J, Hogan WJ. Pancreatic stents: are two barbs better than four? *Gastrointest Endosc* 1996; 43:404 (A454).

56. Kozarek RA. Pancreatic stents can induce ductal changes consistent with chronic pancreatitis. *Gastrointest Endosc* 1990; 36:93–5.

57. Sherman S, Alvarez C, Robert M. Polyethylene pancreatic duct stent-induced changes in the normal dog pancreas. *Gastrointest Endosc* 1993; 39:658–64.

58. Eisen G, Coleman S, Cotton PB. Morphological changes in the pancreatic duct after stent placement for benign pancreatic disease. *Gastrointest Endosc* 1994; 40:107. (abstract)

59. Lans JI, Geenen J, Johansen J. Endoscopic therapy in patients with pancreas divisum and acute pancreatitis: a prospective, randomized, controlled clinical trial. *Gastrointest Endosc* 1992; 38:430–4.

60. Siegel J, Veerappan A. Endoscopic management of pancreatic disorders: potential risks of pancreatic prostheses. *Endoscopy* 1991; 23:177–80.

61. Fosmark CE, Toskes PP. What does an abnormal pancreatogram mean? *Gastrointest Endosc Clin N Am* 1995; 5:105–23.

Palliative management of pancreatic cancer

Guido Costamagna

INTRODUCTION

Management of pancreatic cancer remains a major clinical issue despite the considerable progress that has been achieved in the last few years on diagnosis, staging and therapeutic options. Pancreatic cancer is the least likely malignancy to be circumscribed to its organ of origin at the time of symptomatic onset or diagnosis. Because of early spread of the disease, < 20% of patients are candidates for surgical resection at diagnosis [1, 2]: the main causes of unresectability are local vascular invasion and metastatic disease. As a consequence, most patients with pancreatic malignancies will die quite rapidly, usually within one year of diagnosis. Nevertheless, palliation of the most common complications, i.e. obstructive jaundice resulting from neoplastic compression or invasion of the common bile duct (CBD), intestinal obstruction and pain, is very often required to improve the quality of residual life in these patients [3].

Palliation of pancreatic cancer has traditionally been mostly surgical. In the 1970s percutaneous transhepatic access to the biliary ducts was developed by interventional radiologists, providing the first example of a non-surgical approach to obstructive jaundice [4]. In turn, endoscopists began to deal with these problems in the early 1980s shortly after the description by Soehendra and Reynders-Frederix [5] of a new method of stent insertion into the biliary ducts by duodenoscopy. Endoscopic techniques of biliary drainage have rapidly gained wide acceptance thanks to the development of large-channel duodenoscopes and of a huge number of dedicated accessories along with the growth of clinical experience all over the world. Today endoscopic biliary drainage is considered the first-line treatment in the clinical setting of malignant obstructive jaundice in most instances.

In more recent years techniques of endoscopic drainage of the pancreatic ducts have also been developed; they were primarily conceived for the management of chronic pancreatitis [6], but many of them were soon also applied to some specific situations in the setting of pancreatic cancer (i.e. treatment of obstructive pain, endoluminal radiotherapy). Finally, gastric outlet obstruction from duodenal invasion by pancreatic cancer, which until now has been treated by surgical gastroenterostomy, has also recently been approached by endoscopic methods thanks to the development of self-expanding metallic stents [7].

ENDOSCOPIC MANAGEMENT OF OBSTRUCTIVE JAUNDICE

Between 50 and 80% of patients with pancreatic cancer will develop obstructive jaundice in the course of the disease [1]. Itching secondary to biochemical cholestasis and/or painless progressive jaundice may often represent the first symptoms that lead the patient to clinical observation. Prolonged cholestasis induces malabsorption and anorexia with progressive malnutrition, coagulopathy, itching, hepatocellular failure, renal dysfunction and sometimes bouts of cholangitis. All these symptoms may be, at least temporarily, abolished or mitigated by biliary decompression. Prior to endoscopic retrograde cholangiopancreatography (ERCP) and stent placement it is extremely important to ascertain whether cholestatis and/or jaundice are the result of biliary obstruction or are due to multiple intrahepatic metastases, since the choice and the impact of treatment will obviously be very different.

This differential diagnosis may usually be established easily by liver ultrasonography (US) and computed tomography (CT). Magnetic resonance imaging (MRI) has recently acquired more and more importance in the setting of obstructive jaundice thanks to the improvements in magnetic resonance cholangiopancreatography (MRCP): this completely non-invasive technique not only provides information on liver and pancreatic parenchyma, but may also produce high-quality images of the biliary and pancreatic ducts, especially when dilated, without using contrast media. MRCP could replace other imaging studies in the near future.

Patients in the preterminal stage of their disease should also be excluded from aggressive treatment, which would probably be ineffective in providing substantial benefit. These patients, however, constitute a small minority: for > 90% of all unresectable cancers an aggressive palliative approach will appear worthwhile.

It is important to remember that ERCP is not an isolated technical activity but must be regarded as an integral aspect of clinical problem solving in biliopancreatic disease. Before starting an ERCP procedure the endoscopist should thus carefully review the patient's history and proceed to a complete evaluation, including indications and individual risk factors.

Technique of endobiliary stenting

The technique was first described by Soehendra and Reynders-Frederix in 1979 [5]: they used a 20cm single pigtail 7Fr angiographic catheter inserted through the neoplastic stricture over a guide wire by means of a coaxial pushing catheter. Two major problems were encountered: (a) friction between the pigtail catheter and the guide wire, and (b) a high incidence of cholangitis due to the small calibre of the stent. Both problems were solved step by step in the following years thanks to the work of some pioneer European groups, in particular by Huibregtse *et al.* in Amsterdam and Cremer *et al.* in Brussels. The Amsterdam group first developed a large-channel duodenoscope, which became commercially available in 1981, by which large-bore stents (up to 10Fr) could be inserted [8]. The design of the endoprosthesis was also modified by straightening both ends and creating two side flaps at each extremity to avoid upward or downward displacement. Further modifications in endoprosthesis shape have been suggested by Cremer, on the one hand to avoid impact of the straight end of the stent on the duodenal mucosa and on the other hand to improve the fit of the stent to the left and right hepatic ducts in hilar bile duct strictures [9].

To date, even though duodenoscopes with 4.2mm and 4.5mm operative channels fitting a 12Fr stent are available, 10 Fr. stents are the most widely used and their calibre is considered adequate [10]. Smaller calibres show a significantly lower immediate and late efficacy and therefore they should not be used except in some specific situations.

The procedure starts with a diagnostic ERCP: to date, thanks to their increased manoeuvrability, large-channel duodenoscopes are routinely employed from the beginning of the procedure. Compared to percutaneous transhepatic cholangiography (PTC), ERCP gives a better definition of bile duct strictures because opacification occurs in a caudocranial direction, from the papilla towards the intrahepatic ducts. Moreover, ERCP has the advantage of giving precise information about the infiltration of the duodenal mucosa and the papillary area (differential diagnosis of periampullary tumours and of impacted stones), and can provide opacification of the pancreatic ducts (for differential diagnosis of pancreatic carcinoma and carcinoma of the intrapancreatic CBD). Upon completion of the diagnostic ERCP, a limited sphincterotomy is performed to facilitate the introduction of catheter, guide wire and endoprosthesis. A wider sphincterotomy should be done if two or more large-bore endoprostheses are to be inserted. Endoscopic sphincterotomy (ES) is not strictly required in every case of stent insertion: it can be avoided when the papillary orifice is easily passable in order to lower the risk of bleeding, especially if coagulation defects have not been previously corrected. Bile duct cannulation is then performed with 5 or 7Fr Teflon catheters with a metal tip fitting a 0.035-inch guide wire. The guide wire has a flexible atraumatic tip, now available in different shapes (straight, J, sigmoid, cobra) to manage difficult strictures. Hydrophilic polymer-coated guide wires are nowadays routinely used as a first choice because of their extremely high efficacy. Generally, the catheter cannot be pushed through the stricture; forceful pushing is to be avoided because of the risk of creating false routes. It is best to manipulate the guide wire through the stricture and then to advance the catheter over the guide wire. If the guide wire cannot pass the stricture, or when the bile ducts above the stricture have not been opacified, a balloon catheter inflated in the CBD always allows definition of the stricture and of the overlying dilated bile ducts. The balloon catheter may also facilitate manipulation of the guide wire through asymmetrical or angular strictures. If the stricture is very tight, it is worthwhile to dilate it with bougies of increasing calibre (up to 10–11Fr) or with 'high pressure' banana balloons to be sure that the first attempt at endoprosthesis insertion will be successful. If the stricture is too firm to be dilated at the first attempt, a nasobiliary catheter (6.5Fr) is inserted and left in situ for at least 48 hours. It is generally possible to place larger stents (10Fr) after this interval during a second duodenoscopy. Dilatation manoeuvres are best performed over a stiff Teflonated guide wire. After dilatation, a 5 or 6Fr catheter is reinserted over the guide wire and the endoprosthesis can be positioned by a coaxial pushing catheter of the same calibre (10Fr) (Figure 19.1). One-step stent introduction devices are commercially available; these devices are simpler to use and allow the insertion of an endoprosthesis, avoiding time-consuming manoeuvres. However, they should probably be employed only in easy cases, after careful evaluation of the stricture's tightness.

Figure 19.1 (a) Complete obstruction of the MPD and high-grade irregular stricture of the intrahepatic CBD. This radiological finding (classically known as the 'double duct sign') is consistent with carcinoma of the head of the pancreas invading the bile duct. A metal-tipped catheter is inserted deep into the CBD. (b) The biliary tree has been opacified using a catheter–guide wire system, confirming a high-grade obstruction and dilatation of the proximal ducts. The guide wire has been left in situ and a sphincterotome has been inserted over it. (c) A straight (Amsterdam type) 10Fr stent and a coaxial 6Fr nasobiliary catheter have been inserted through the neoplastic stricture. The check cholangiography performed through the nasobiliary catheter at the end of the procedure shows good contrast medium flow via the endoprosthesis into the duodenal lumen and intrahepatic pneumobilia.

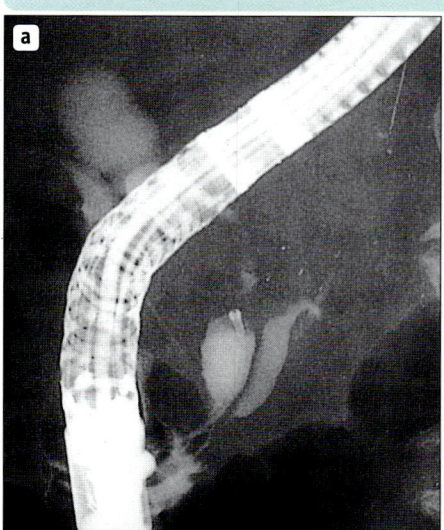
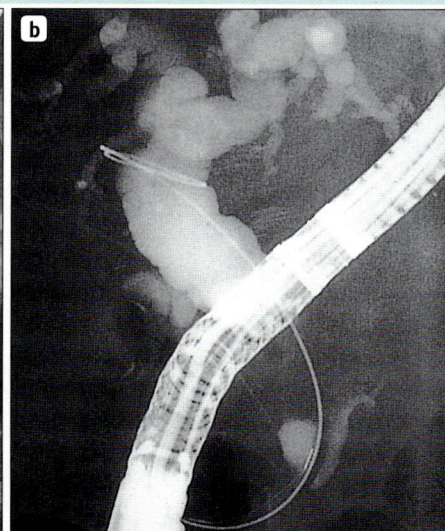
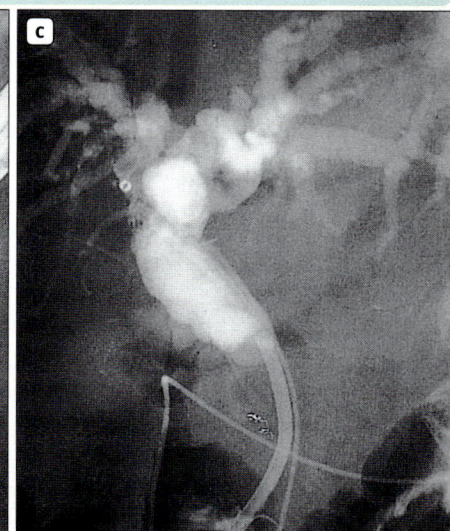

Stent insertion is mostly a 'radiological' manoeuvre: fluoroscopic control must be continuous to maintain the best and most efficacious pushing axis. In tight strictures progression of the stent is obtained by the combination of pushing the stent and pulling and/or twisting the tip of the duodenoscope. To reduce the distance between the tip of the duodenoscope and the duodenal wall and thus to avoid losing force in the duodenal lumen, it may sometimes be useful to put the patient in the supine position; the endoscopist must then turn his/her back to the radiological table and rotate the operating section of the duodenoscope clockwise 90–180 degrees in order to keep a stable position within the duodenal lumen.

We generally attempt to place along the stent and above the stricture a nasobiliary catheter (5 or 6Fr) to flush the dilated ducts and the endoprosthesis with saline solution for 24–48 hours (1000ml/24h): this catheter is also used, before removal, to perform a cholangiography and check the correct position and effectiveness of the stent (Figure 19.1c).

The percutaneous–endoscopic technique ('rendezvous' technique) may be used in cases of unsuccessful endoscopic procedure [11, 12]. Catheterization of the dilated bile ducts is performed transhepatically and a guide wire is manipulated through the stricture; an external–internal 6 or 7Fr catheter (Ring catheter) is then advanced over the guide wire until the distal tip reaches the duodenal lumen. This catheter is left *in*

situ for 48 hours. In a second stage a 350–400 cm long guide wire is introduced into the percutaneous catheter and advanced into the duodenal lumen. The guide wire is then grasped endoscopically with biopsy forceps or a polipectomy snare and withdrawn into the operative channel of the duodenoscope. The stent can then always be positioned endoscopically. This method allows the insertion of a large-bore stent avoiding major trauma to the hepatic parenchyma (Figure 19.2).

Results of plastic stenting

To date, several thousand patients around the world have been treated with endoscopic stents. The overall reported success rate of inserting a stent varies in the literature between 75% and 90% [13]. Neoplastic strictures located in the lower third of the CBD show the highest success rate (85–95%). The success rate is lower when the stricture is located in the middle third of the CBD (80–90%). The most difficult technical problems arise with strictures located in the upper third of the CBD and at the main hepatic confluence; insertion of at least one stent is successful in 75–85% of cases.

Early complications

These may be related to the limited ES (bleeding, pancreatitis, retroduodenal perforation), in less than 2% of the patients, or to stent insertion itself. Acute cholangitis is the most important complication both in frequency and severity. It is usually caused by bad drainage (Figure 19.3) resulting either from dysfunction or early clogging of the stent or from the impossibility of draining the whole biliary tree adequately when the stricture involves the hepatic hilum. Sufficient drainage of the biliary segmental branches is an essential preventive measure and can be pursued by associating endoscopic stenting and transhepatic drainage when multiple stents cannot be inserted endoscopically. The use of sterile equipment prevents nosocomial infections by multiresistant microorganisms (e.g. *Pseudomonas aeruginosa*)

Figure 19.2 Modified 'rendezvous' technique. (a) A percutaneous external–internal drainage is in place. (b) and (c) It is often possible to cannulate the CBD alongside the percutaneous catheter, which can then be removed to leave room for endoscopic stenting.

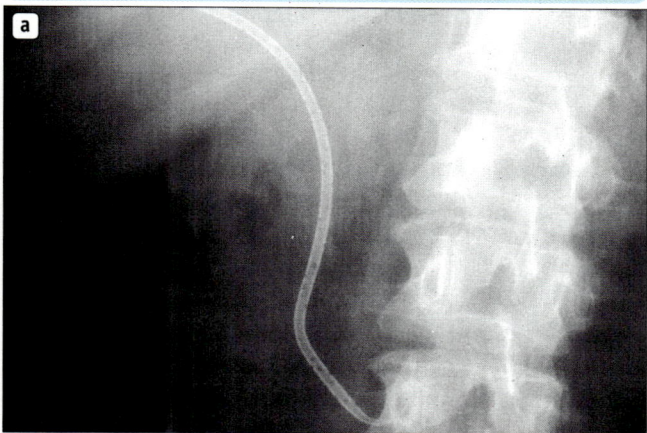

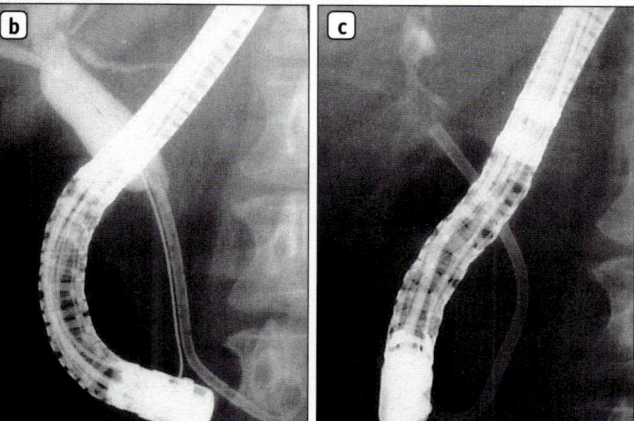

Figure 19.3 When the CBD is medially bent by the neoplastic stricture (a), the preshaped curved stent (Cremer type) is preferred (b) to fit the distorted anatomy and to avoid impaction into the bile duct wall of the proximal end of the endoprosthesis.

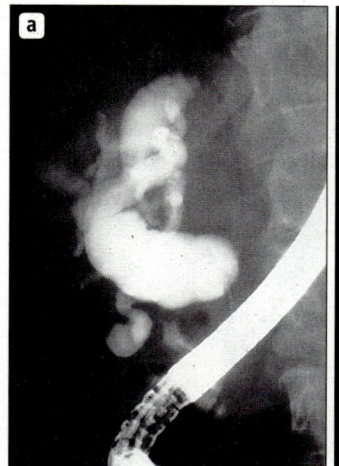

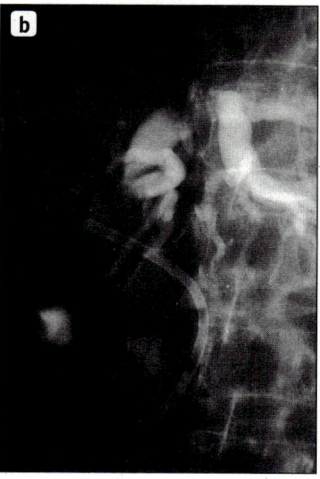

and the patient is only contaminated by his own commensal flora. It is also important to keep the number of technical acts to a strict minimum. A lower incidence of early cholangitis was observed in patients in whom implantation of the stent was done in the same session as the diagnostic examination [8, 14]. By keeping the nasobiliary perfusion catheter in position for 48 hours after implantation one can prevent the early clogging of the stent by mucous debris that is dragged upwards as the catheter is pushed through the stricture or by leucocytic aggregates which are caused by iatrogenic cholangitis. It also reduces bile viscosity by dilution.

Antibiotic prophylaxis is now recommended in each case of marked cholestasis [14]. Acute cholecystitis may also occur after stent placement, especially in patients in very poor general condition and when the cystic duct is infiltrated or compressed by a tumour.

Late complications of endobiliary stenting

The most common late complication is clogging of the stent: this occurs in at least a quarter of the patients at a mean interval of 3–5 months[13]. Acute cholangitis resulting from a clogged stent may be avoided if early symptoms of endoprosthesis dysfunction are diagnosed rapidly; ultrasonography is very helpful in assessing recurrence of biliary obstruction[15]. Clogging seems to be a bacterial related complication with deposition of a proteinaceous layer (biofilm) on the inner surface of the stent and subsequent obstruction of the lumen with calculous debris and thickened bile (sludge)[16]. Various attempts at reducing biofilm and sludge formation have been performed with different drugs (aspirin, aspirin + doxycycline, mucolytic and choleretic agents, gallstone dissolution agents); as a rule, even after *in vitro* studies suggesting possible effects, no clinical advantages could be demonstrated by any of these studies[17, 18]. Many stent-related variables that may affect occlusion have also been thoroughly investigated: length, shape, size, material and presence or absence of lateral holes have all been taken into account looking for amelioration of stent effectiveness. Some *in vitro* studies[19] and one prospective but not randomized study[20] (Christmas tree stent) have shown that the occlusion rate of plastic stents may be influenced by modifications of these variables, but prospective randomized clinical trials have not been able to substantiate these theoretical benefits [21].

Replacement of the stent is usually an easy procedure, which requires a short readmission to the hospital or may be performed on an outpatient basis (Figures 19.4–19.6). The most profitable time interval for prophylactic stent exchange has not yet been established. In clinical practice most authors

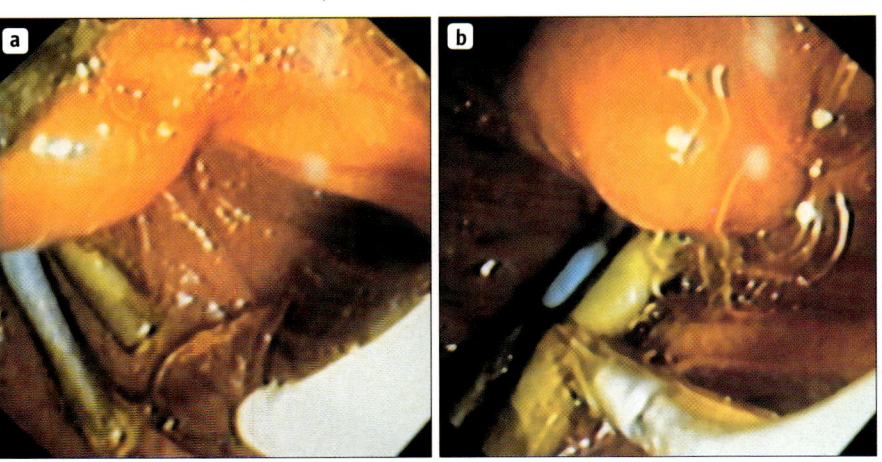

Figure 19.4 Technique of stent exchange. An asymmetrical polipectomy snare (crescent type) is the most effective device for capturing the duodenal extremity and removing multiple stents.

Figure 19.5 Technique of stent exchange. When a single short (5–7cm) stent must be removed, foreign body forceps (a) may be used to extract the stent into the duodenal lumen (b), thus avoiding withdrawal and reinsertion of the duodenoscope (c).

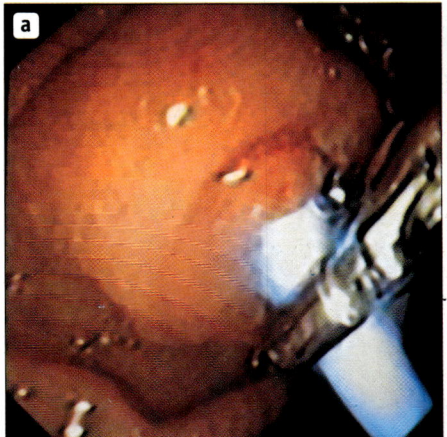
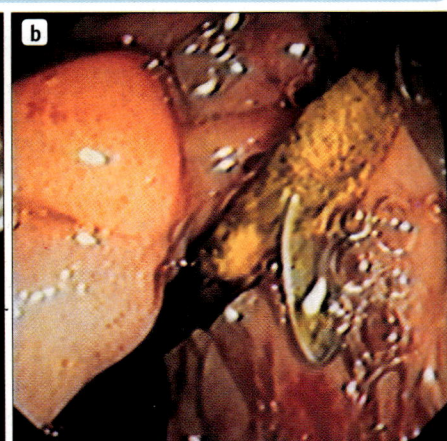
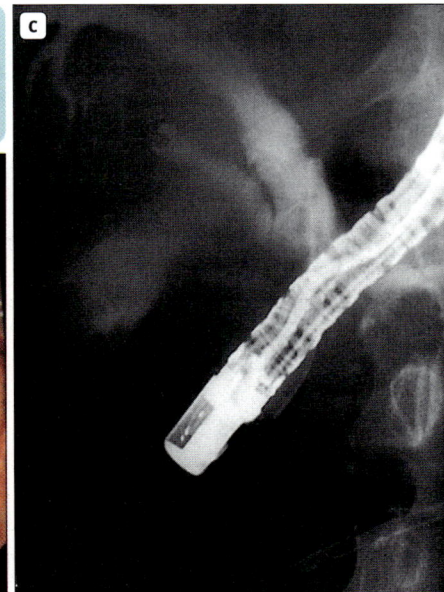

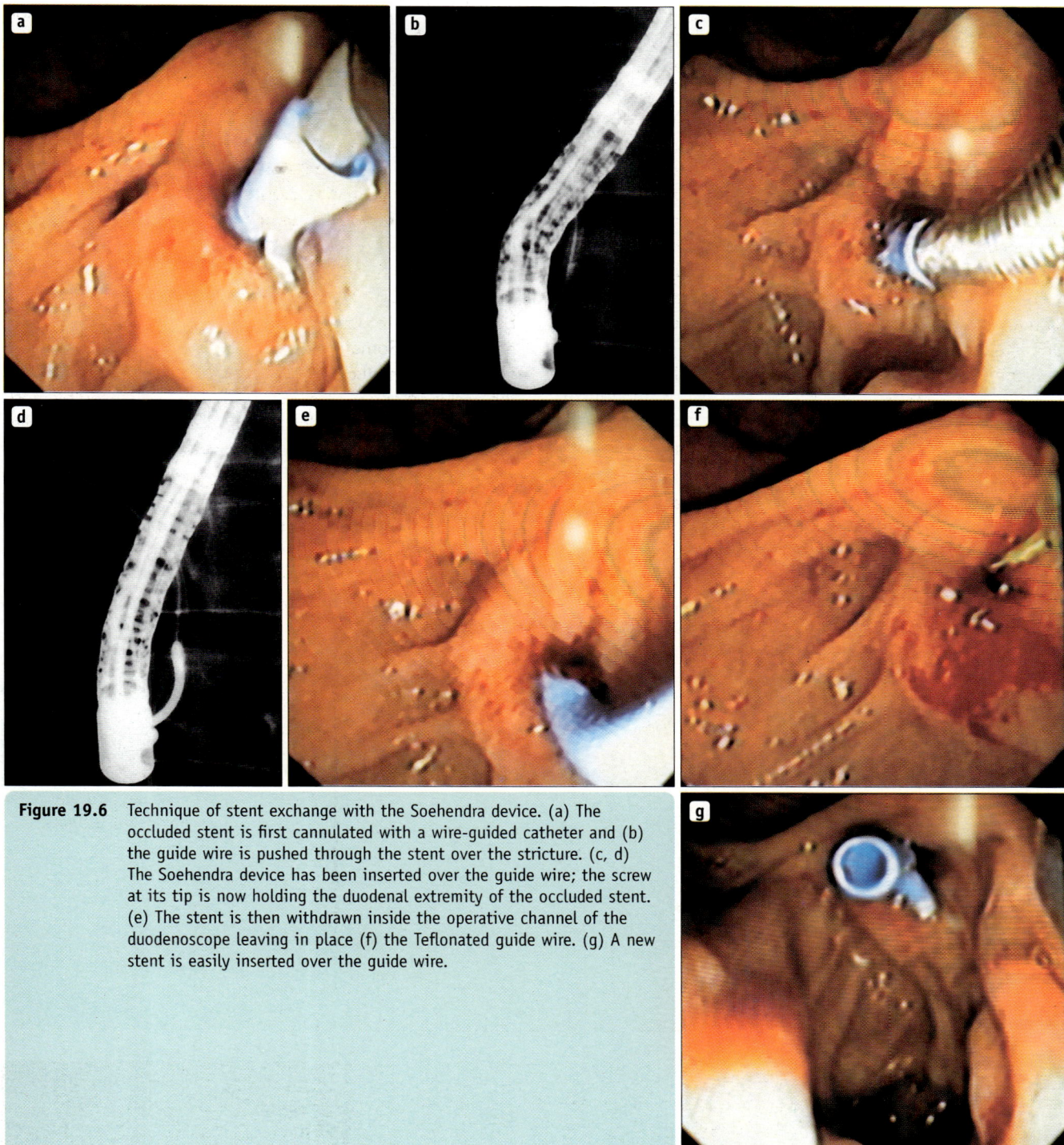

Figure 19.6 Technique of stent exchange with the Soehendra device. (a) The occluded stent is first cannulated with a wire-guided catheter and (b) the guide wire is pushed through the stent over the stricture. (c, d) The Soehendra device has been inserted over the guide wire; the screw at its tip is now holding the duodenal extremity of the occluded stent. (e) The stent is then withdrawn inside the operative channel of the duodenoscope leaving in place (f) the Teflonated guide wire. (g) A new stent is easily inserted over the guide wire.

recommend stent replacement at scheduled 3–6-month intervals. A 6-month interval has recently been proposed by Frakes *et al.*[22] in order to minimize patient discomfort and costs, avoiding useless premature procedures. Taking into account that the mean life of a stent is 3 months or more, and that the mean survival of patients with non-operable pancreatic malignancies is in most cases 6 months or less, one stent replacement is sufficient for the great majority of these patients.

Dislocation (Figure 19.7) and rupture (Figure 19.8) of the stent, acute cholecystitis and duodenal perforation have also been reported as a late complications, but their incidence is very low.

RESULTS OF ENDOSCOPIC PALLIATIVE PLASTIC STENTING IN PANCREATIC CARCINOMA

The immediate and long-term results of palliative biliary stenting in pancreatic cancer are well known (Figure 19.9). The success rate of stent insertion approximates 90% in all experiences: most of the failures are due to duodenal stricture which impairs the access to the papilla. These patients are better served by surgical biliodigestive anastomosis and concomitant gastrojejunostomy. After stent placement, jaundice and itching will resolve in the overwhelming majority of patients in a few days; an endoscopic approach is also

Figure 19.7 Plain X-ray abdominal film showing intrabiliary migration of a plastic stent

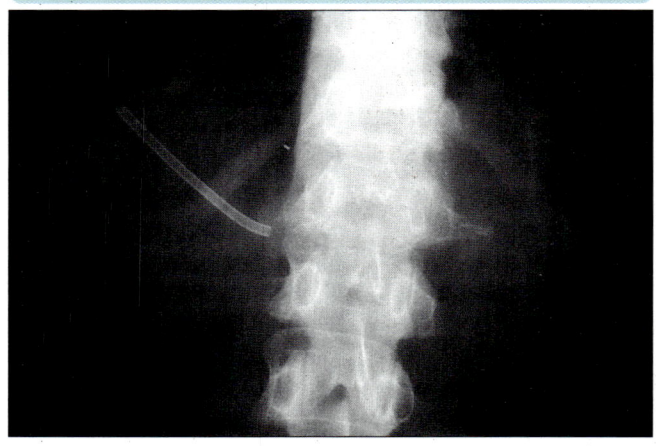

Figure 19.8 Stent rupture is a reported complication; this stent ruptured at the site of the lateral hole during extraction with the Soehendra device.

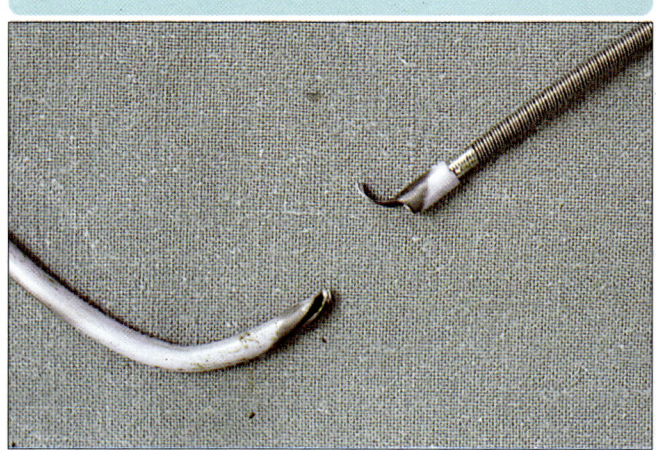

preferable to percutaneous transhepatic biliary drainage because it is less invasive and safer in terms of morbidity and 30-day mortality[23].

Palliation by endoscopic stenting has also been compared to surgical bypass in patients with non-resectable disease who are fit for surgery[24, 25]. The results of these studies favour the endoscopic approach in terms of lower morbidity and 30-day mortality. A shorter initial hospital stay is counterbalanced by the need for repeated admissions for stent exchange in case of clogging. Both successful drainage and mean survival were comparable in the two groups (Figure 19.10).

Surgical versus non-operative management has also been compared on a cost-analysis basis: in a retrospective study,

no significant difference between the two groups in survival, total hospitalization, morbidity or mortality could be verified, although patients in the non-operative group were frailer and 6 years older on average. In turn, cost analysis revealed significant savings with non-operative management[26].

To date, surgery must remain the first-line treatment whenever a hope of resection is perceived because it is the only potential curative treatment. For patients unfit for surgery or with manifestly unresectable disease, endoscopic palliation is at least as effective as surgery and can be considered as the only palliative treatment, in the absence of manifest or impending duodenal stenosis, because it carries less morbidity and mortality and requires a shorter hospital stay.

Figure 19.9 Results of endoscopic biliary plastic stenting for pancreatic carcinoma.

	Amsterdam Huibregtse et al., (8)	London Speer, Cotton, (44)	New York Siegel, Suady, (45)	Rome (personal experience 1988/89)
n	221	99	331	224
Mean age (years)	71	76	73	67
Overall technical success	90%	88%	89%	86%
Mortality of procedure	2%	—	0%	1.5%
Mortality (30 days)	9.5%	9%	18%	11%
Mean survival (weeks)	26	25	18	29
Late duodenal stenosis	7.5%	6%	0%	5%
Stent occlusion	21%	29.5%	30%	32%

Figure 19.10 Results of randomized studies comparing endoscopic and surgical biliary drainage in periampullary tumours.

	Sheperd et al. (24)		Dowsett et al. (46)	
	Endoscopy	Surgery	Endoscopy	Surgery
Patients	23	25	101	103
Technical success	91%	92%	94%	91%
Morbidity	33%	56%	10%[a]	28%[a]
Mortality (30 days)	9%	20%	7%[a]	17%[a]
Hospital stay (days)	5[a]	13[a]	9[a]	13[a]
Hospital readmissions	43%[a]	12%[a]	18%[a]	5%[a]
Late dudenal stenosis	9%[a]	4%[a]	6%[a]	1%[a]
Survival[b]	22	18	21	26

[a] $p < 0.05$

[b] weeks

METALLIC STENTS

To overcome the problem of recurrent cholestasis due to late obstruction of plastic stents by clogging, large-diameter expandable metallic stents have been developed over recent years. Two types of metallic stent have been produced: balloon-expandable and self-expandable. Little experience has been gained with balloon-expandable stents (Figure 19.11) because of their limited clinical benefit compared to plastic endoprostheses.

Self-expandable metal mesh stents have been widely used and investigated and their clinical usefulness and results are now well established and understood. Two types of self-expandable stent are currently commercially available (Figures 19.12 and 19.13), while a third type will become available in a short time (Figure 19.14). These stents are made of metal wires braided in different ways and into different shapes. They are constrained by a covering catheter during insertion and deploy to their definitive form (24–30Fr) upon removal of the insertion device. Recently a completely new metallic stent has been produced: it consists of a memory metal nitinol coiled wire which deploys to a 24Fr coil when the proximal and distal ends of the wire are freed from a fixing mechanism (Figure 19.15)[27]. Technical insertion of the Wallstent and of the Diamond stent is easier than the Gianturco–Rosch or the Instent because the insertion devices are smaller (9Fr vs 2 Fr)

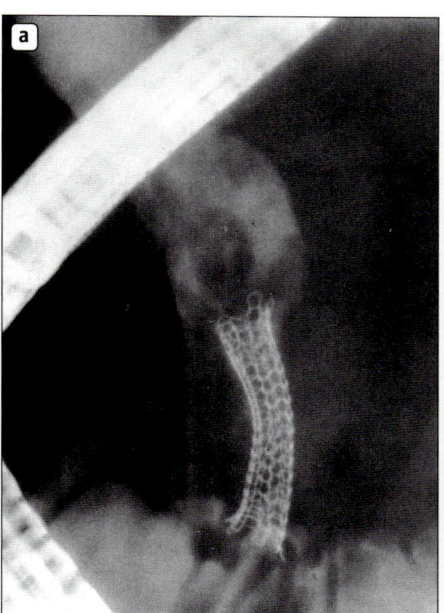
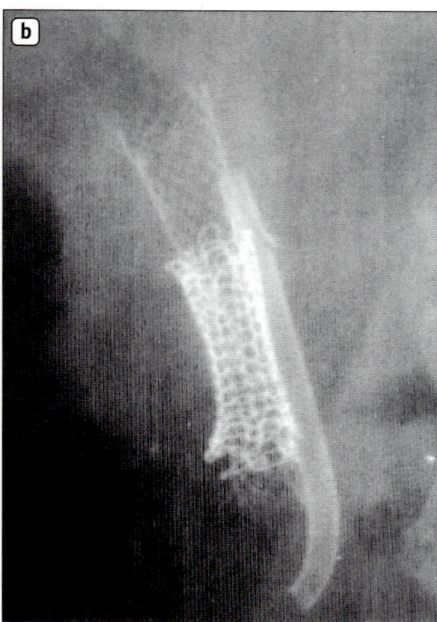

Figure 19.11 (a) Recurrent CBD stricture secondary to pancreatic head cancer with upstream dilation and intrabiliary sludge 2 months after implantation of a balloon-expandable Strecker stent. (b) Treatment consisted of the endoscopic insertion of a self-expandable Wallstent inside the Strecker stent. One 10 Fr. plastic pancreatic stent was also inserted.

Figure 19.12 (a) After removal of a clogged plastic stent, cholangiography shows high-grade dilation of the bile ducts above the stricture. (b) A self-expandable metal mesh stent (Wallstent) has been inserted through the stricture: the stent is still fully constricted in its delivery device. (c) Cholangiography via nasobiliary tube 24 hours after Wallstent deployment: the stent has already expanded, allowing good bilioduodenal flow of injected contrast medium.

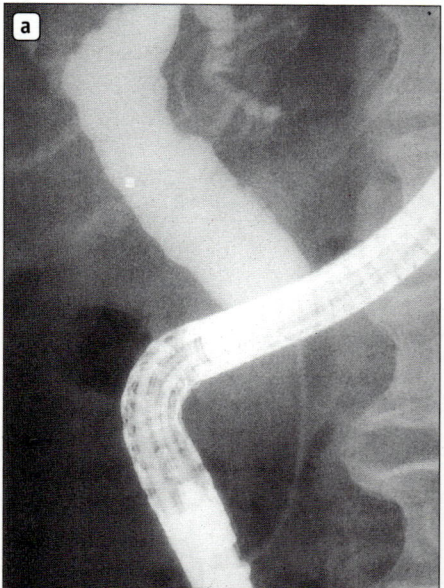
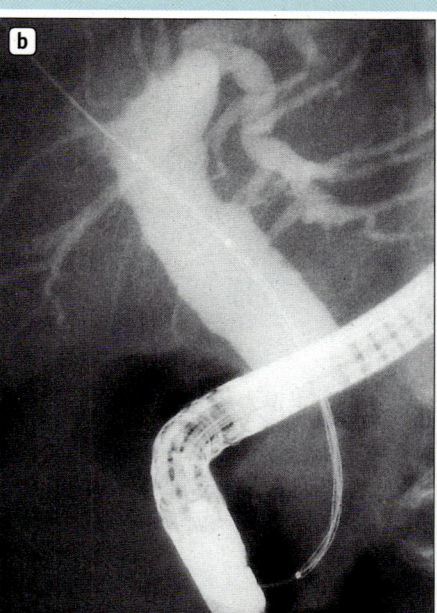
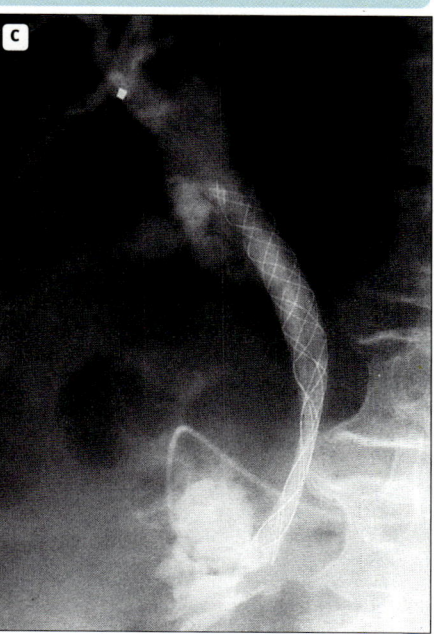

and the stents are less rigid. However, as long as only short-term results are concerned, all seem equally effective in treatment of lower bile duct obstruction. Long-term results are only well known for the Wallstent. Late complications of the use of the Wallstent leading to recurrent biliary obstruction are mainly due to tumour overgrowth (4%) and ingrowth through the wire mesh (7%)[28]. To overcome the problem of tumour ingrowth, a Wallstent with a partial plastic sheath is currently under clinical investigation.

The Wallstent has been compared to plastic stents in two prospective randomized trials (Figure 19.16) and showed longer patency and cost effectiveness [29, 30]. According to these studies the use of self-expandable metal stents may be proposed for palliative treatment of biliary obstruction in patients who will probably survive more than 3 months.

PANCREATIC STENTING

The technique of endoscopic pancreatic stenting was introduced in 1985 to resolve outflow obstruction in the pancreatic duct of patients with chronic pancreatitis who presented with continuous or recurrent pain [6]. Since that time many reports have been published; nevertheless the world experience is still limited to specialized centres particularly devoted to the management of pancreatic diseases.

In the setting of pancreatic cancer, endoscopic pancreatic stenting may be applied to palliate 'obstructive' pain or when access to the pancreatic duct is required for intraluminal brachytherapy with iridium 192.

Technique of pancreatic drainage

The technique of pancreatic drainage does not substantially differ from that applied to the biliary aspect. A biliary sphincterotomy is generally first performed to allow proper visualization of the pancreatic orifice; then a pancreatic sphincterotomy is done under visual control to get easier access to the pancreatic duct. In pancreatic cancer patients, pancreatic sphincterotomy is seldom strictly necessary. Minor papilla sphincterotomy may be needed in cases of pancreas divisum (7–10% of the population) or of 'dominant Santorini duct' anatomy (i.e. patients with a normally fused pancreas but with a distorted connection between the ventral and the dorsal duct, making the access to the main pancreatic duct easier through

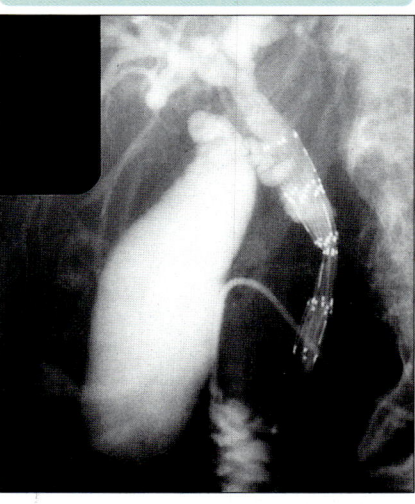

Figure 19.13 Check cholangiography via nasobiliary catheter 24 hours after endoscopic insertion of two superposed Gianturco Z-stents.

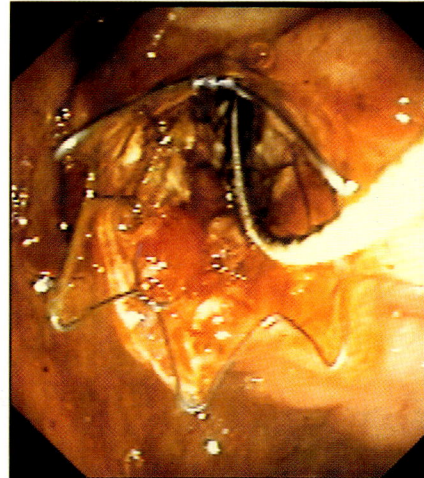

Figure 19.14 Endoscopic view of fully deployed transpapillary Diamond stent: this newly designed self-expandable metal stent is currently undergoing clinical evaluation.

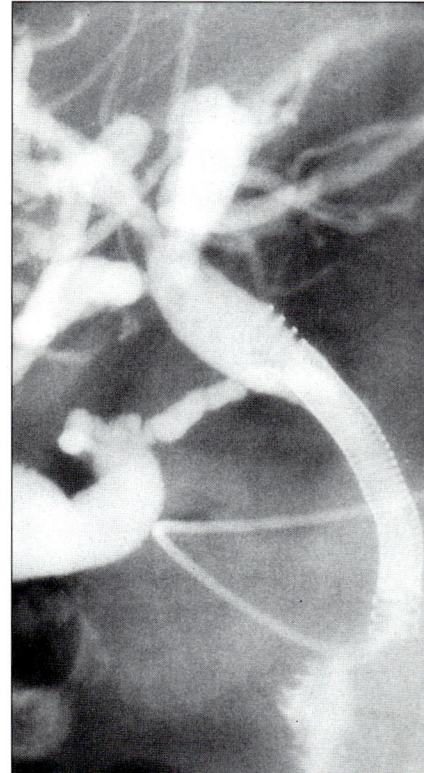

Figure 19.15 Self-expandable coiled nitinol wire stent (Instent): check cholangiography via nasobiliary tube 48 hours after positioning for pancreatic cancer. The stent is fully deployed and the bilioduodenal flow is adequate.

Figure 19.16 Results of randomized studies comparing Wallstent and plastic stents in patients with distal CBD strictures.

	Davids *et al.* (29)		Carr-Locke *et al.* (30) (Multicentre)	
	Metal	*Plastic*	*Metal*	*Plastic*
n	49	56	94	88
Technical success	96%	95%	98%	95%
Stent obstruction	33%	54%	13%	13%
Median stent patency (days)	273	126	111	62

the duct of Santorini). Deep cannulation of the MPD is then performed with a Teflon catheter and a hydrophilic guide wire (0.035 inches), which is manipulated through the stricture and advanced to the tail of the pancreas. We very often use J-tipped guide wires which have the advantage of not projecting into the secondary ducts beyond the stricture. The Teflon catheter is then advanced over the guide wire and mechanical dilatation with coaxial 9.5Fr sleeve is always performed before any attempt to place a large-bore 10Fr stent. In case of a tight stricture, Soehendra dilating catheters of increasing diameter (6–10Fr) may also be useful. Pneumatic dilatation is seldom utilized in the pancreatic duct in our experience. Large-bore 10Fr polyethylene stents that are straight (Huibregtse biliary stent) or anatomically preshaped (Cremer pancreatic stent) are used preferentially. If large-bore stents are implanted, multiple side flaps to prevent dislocation are not necessary.

We do not recommend the use of 5Fr stents because they tend to occlude in a short time. Stents of 7Fr may be used if mechanical dilatation up to 10Fr cannot be achieved. In these more difficult cases we prefer to insert a nasopancreatic drain (5–7Fr) which is left in place for 48–72 hours to dilate the stricture. After that period, insertion of a larger stent is usually easier. The length of the stent is chosen according to the location of the stricture and may vary between 4cm and 12cm. If the stricture is located in the pancreatic head, as occurs in most patients, additional side holes to prevent blockage of secondary ducts, as proposed by some authors, are not necessary. Large-bore pancreatic stents are almost always rapidly effective in decompressing the ducts immediately after their release: it is often possible to record a significant shrinkage of the ducts at the end of the procedure (Figure 19.17).

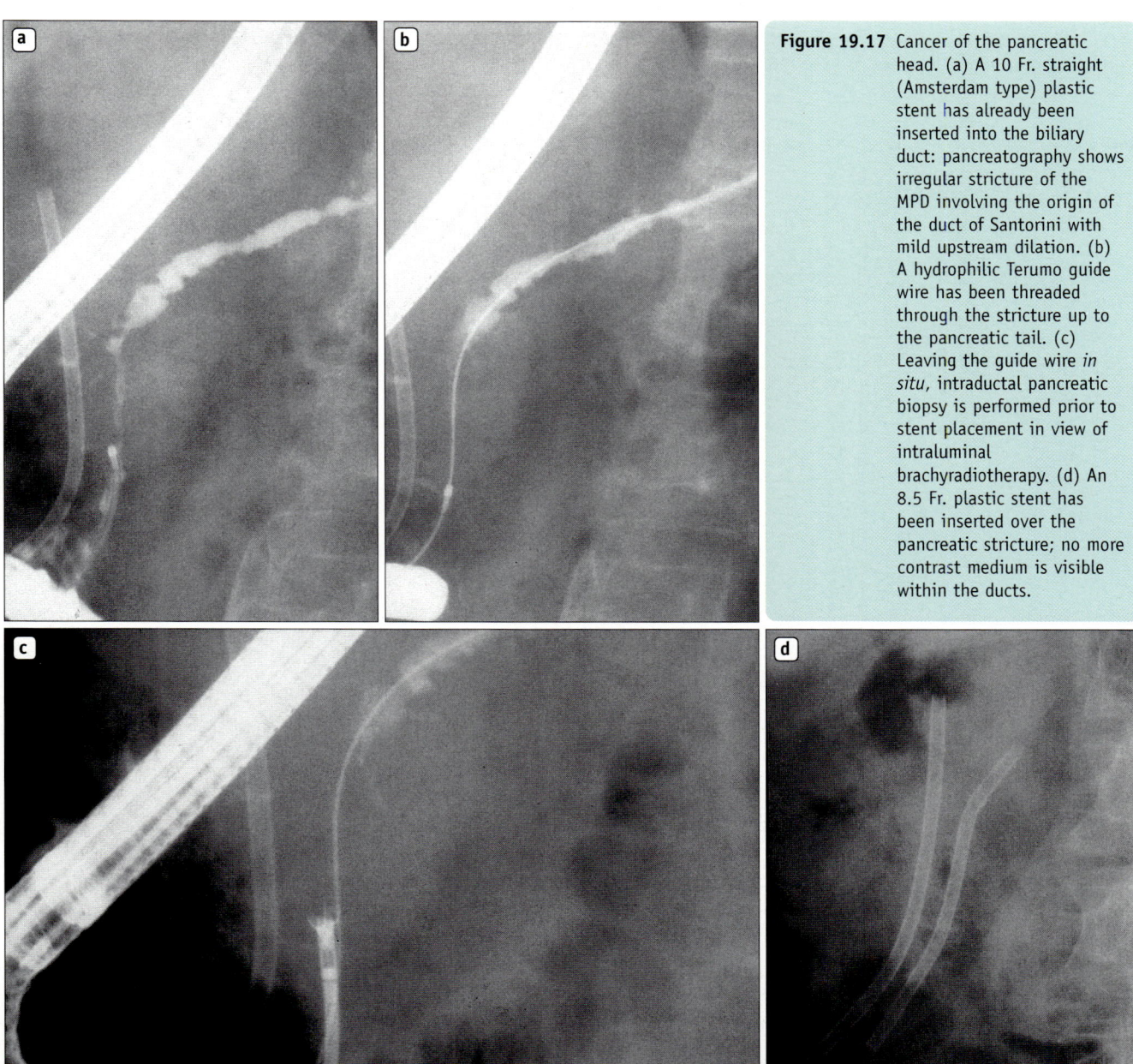

Figure 19.17 Cancer of the pancreatic head. (a) A 10 Fr. straight (Amsterdam type) plastic stent has already been inserted into the biliary duct: pancreatography shows irregular stricture of the MPD involving the origin of the duct of Santorini with mild upstream dilation. (b) A hydrophilic Terumo guide wire has been threaded through the stricture up to the pancreatic tail. (c) Leaving the guide wire *in situ*, intraductal pancreatic biopsy is performed prior to stent placement in view of intraluminal brachyradiotherapy. (d) An 8.5 Fr. plastic stent has been inserted over the pancreatic stricture; no more contrast medium is visible within the ducts.

Palliation of 'obstructive' pain

Pain occurs in 80–85% of patents with advanced stage disease[31], often being the most incapacitating and distressing symptom. Aetiology of the pain is probably multifactorial in most cases: proposed factors producing pain include neoplastic infiltration of nerve ends and pancreatic and peripancreatic tissue, obstruction of the MPD with upstream dilatation and increased parenchymal pressure secondary to ductal hypertension, superimposed pancreatic inflammation and stricture of the distal CBD[32]. The clinical characteristics of 'obstructive' pain are its correlation with meals and radiation to the back; true relapsing attacks of acute pancreatitis may also intervene, especially in the early course of the disease. Pancreatography usually shows homogeneous dilatation of the main and secondary pancreatic ducts above the malignant stricture.

As with chronic pancreatitis, ductal decompression by endoscopic stenting may dramatically improve pain symptoms in a subset of cancer patients. A single case report suggesting the usefulness of pancreatic drainage for pain control in patients with pancreatic cancer was reported by Harrison and Hamilton in 1989[33]. In turn, we reported a series of eight patients in whom a pancreatic stent was successfully inserted with impressive alleviation of pain, lasting until death in 6 out of 8[34]. Similar results have been reported in five patients by Lichtenstein and Carr-Locke in Boston[7]. Endoscopic pancreatic drainage is a safe and effective method in selected cases and should be considered as a part of the therapeutic armamentarium for pain control in pancreatic cancer patients.

Pseudocysts may be a rare cause of pain in patients with previous acute pancreatitis resulting from neoplastic obstruction of the pancreatic duct. Infrequently pancreatic fluid collections in the setting of pancreatic cancer may also impair intestinal transit by compression of the gastric and/or duodenal lumen. Non-operative drainage of pseudocysts may now be safely accomplished by endoscopic techniques. Cystogastrostomy and cystoduodenostomy by diathermic puncture of the collection through the intestinal wall can be performed when the following features are present: endoscopically visible bulging of the cyst into the intestinal lumen; fluid content; and thickness of <10mm between the intestinal lumen and the cystic cavity[35] (Figure 19.18).

Figure 19.18 Cancer of the pancreatic head. (a) A 10 Fr. preshaped plastic stent has already been inserted into the biliary duct: pancreatography shows irregular stricture of the MPD with upstream dilation and multiple cysts in the pancreatic head area consistent with carcinoma and obstructive pancreatitis. (b) A larger pseudocyst building into the duodenal cap has been opacified after transmural diathermic puncture. (c) Cremer's 8.5 Fr. cystoenterostome entering the cystic cavity over a guide wire. (d) A 10 Fr. plastic stent has been inserted to bridge the cystoduodenostomy hole: the cystic cavity is now filled with air and will collapse in the following days.

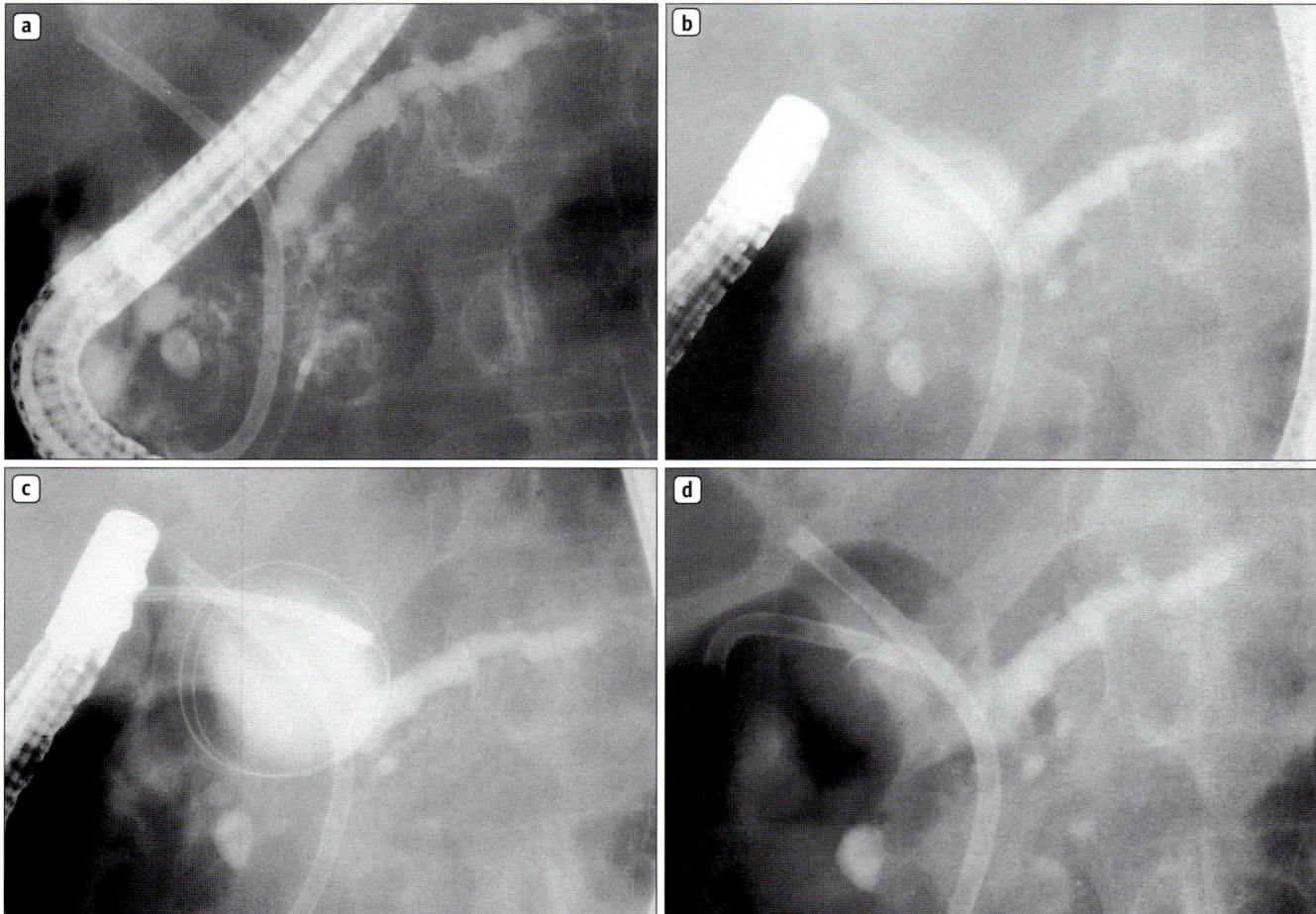

Intraluminal brachytherapy

Intraluminal brachytherapy involves placement of radioactive sources in biliary ducts and/or pancreatic ducts of patients with unresectable disease[36]. Although intraluminal brachytherapy has been used alone, in recent studies it has often been combined with external-beam radiation therapy[37, 38]. To be eligible for treatment patients must have biopsy-proven unresectable cancer, no distant metastases and a tumour development concentric to the MBD or MPD, allowing the administration of biologically effective doses of radiation. Intraluminal brachyradiotherapy may be performed either by transhepatic percutaneous drains or endoscopically[39]. Endoscopic techniques also allow the insertion of the radioactive source into the pancreatic duct, with consequent better 'geographical' positioning and advantages in terms of homogeneity of dose and sparing of the surrounding normal tissues[38, 40].

The radioactive source (iridium 192 wire) is inserted into a nasobiliary or nasopancreatic drain (8–9Fr) previously positioned across the stricture. Radiation doses (afterloading low dose rate technique) depend on the linear activity of the source, its length, the time of irradiation and the association with external beam radiotherapy. Technical details of our experience are shown in Figure 19.19.

In cancer of the pancreatic head the most appropriate duct (biliary or pancreatic), according to tumour volume, is selected for irradiation (Figures 19.20 – 19.22). In our initial experience with 13 patients, the source was positioned in the MPD in six and in the biliary duct in another six, while the remaining patient underwent treatment with two sources, one in the pancreatic duct and the other in the biliary duct. Local control of the disease may be achieved in about 60% of the patients. In our experience, patients with pancreatic cancer who underwent combined modality treatment (external beam radiotherapy with 4-day 5-fluorouracil continuous infusion chemotherapy followed by intraluminal brachytherapy) had a

Figure 19.19 Intraluminal brachytherapy with iridium 192: technical details.

Parameter	Range	Median
Dose (Gy)	20–50	47.5
Application time (h)	70–260	104.0
Linear activity (mCi/cm)	1.02–5.75	2.70
Source length (cm)	1–15	4.5

Figure 19.20 Intraluminal brachyradiotherapy with iridium 192 wire inserted into a nasobiliary tube across a biliary Wallstent.

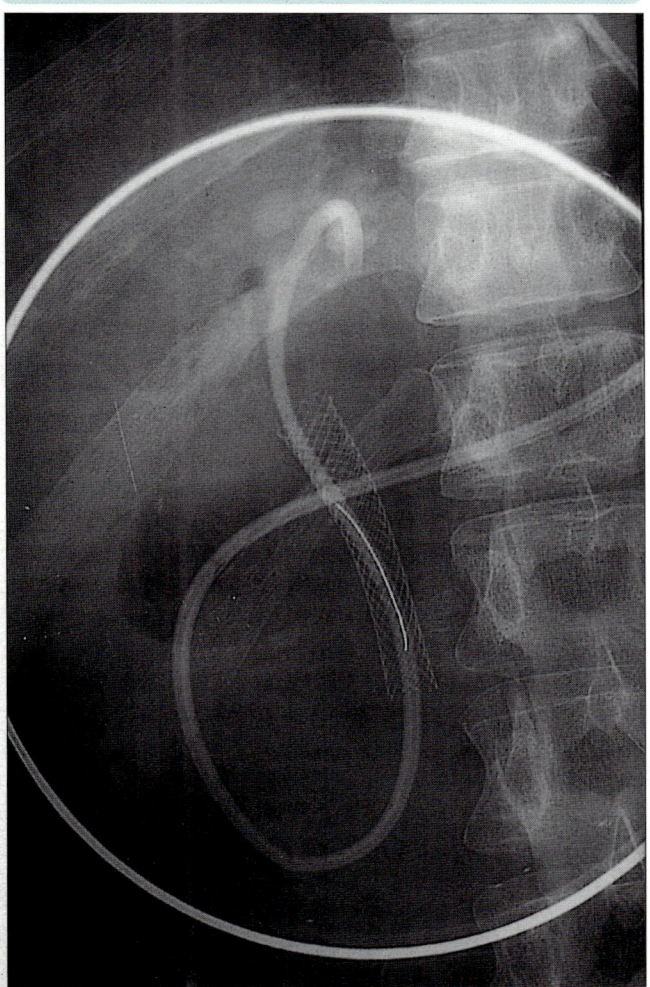

Figure 19.21 Intraluminal brachyradiotherapy for pancreatic head cancer with iridium 192 wire inserted into a nasopancreatic tube; plastic biliary and pancreatic stents are *in situ*.

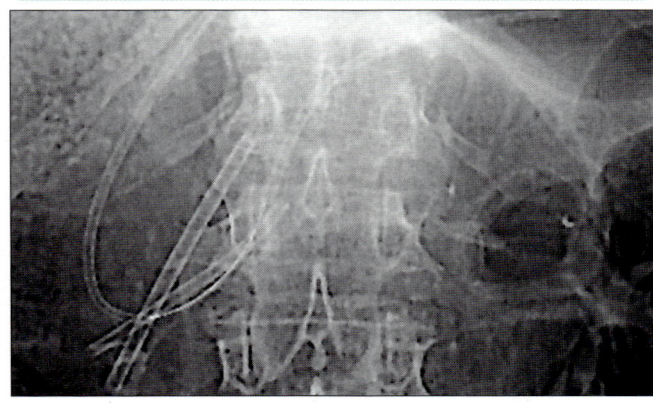

Figure 19.22 Intraluminal brachyradiotherapy for carcinoma of the pancreatic body with iridium 192 wire inserted into a nasopancreatic catheter.

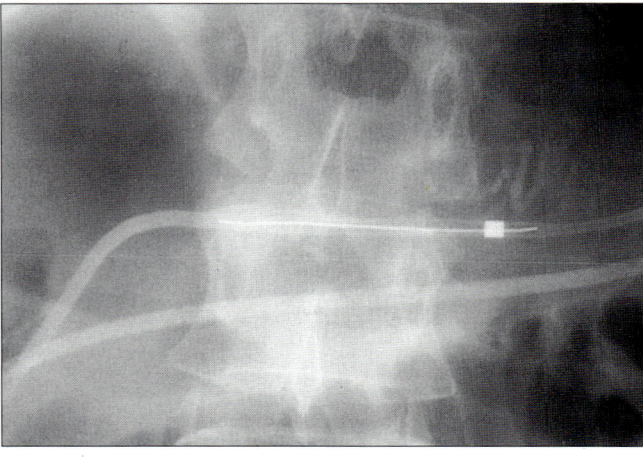

median survival of 21 months and a one-year survival rate of 83%, while patients who underwent only intraluminal brachytherapy had a median survival of 14 months and a one-year survival rate of 57% [40]. These palliative treatment modalities can thus be useful in the treatment of unresectable pancreatic cancer, allowing not only a satisfactory level of palliation but also a possible survival benefit. A larger number of patients and possibly a randomized trial would help to clarify this issue.

ENDOSCOPIC MANAGEMENT OF GASTRIC OUTLET OBSTRUCTION

Gastric outlet obstruction is an uncommon presenting complaint in patients with pancreatic cancer, but up to 13% of patients with unresectable cancer will require gastrojejunostomy for symptom palliation during the natural course of the disease[41]. Until recently, duodenal stricture secondary to pancreatic cancer was treated exclusively by surgical bypass, with complication rates as high as 20–30% reported. Recent developments in metallic stent insertion devices have prompted some authors to investigate alternative non-operative methods in gastric outlet obstruction due to direct invasion by pancreatic cancer or to recurrent cancer at the site of previous gastroenterostomy[7].

Few data are available at the moment, but the technique of self-expandable metal mesh stent insertion looks promising in this setting. Stents (mostly 16–22mm large, 6–9cm Wallstent) have been placed into the obstructed intestinal lumen either perorally, using an overtube to avoid bending of the stent shaft in the gastric cavity[42], or through a previously positioned percutaneous endoscopic gastrostomy (PEG)[43]. At the moment, this technique cannot yet be recommended as the first-line approach except for patients with formidable operative risk.

References

1. Cello JP. Carcinoma of the pancreas. In *Gastrointestinal Disease*. Edited by MH Sleisenger and JS Fordtraw. WB Saunders, Philadelphia; 1993: 1682–94.
2. Ashley SW, Reber HA. Surgical management of exocrine pancreatic cancer. In *The Pancreas: Biology, Pathobiology and Disease, 2nd Ed.* Edited by VLW Go et al. Raven Press, New York; 1993: 913–29.
3. Raijnan I, Leven B. Exocrine tumours of the pancreas. In *The Pancreas: Biology, Pathobiology and Disease, 2nd Ed.* Edited by VLW Go et al. Raven Press, New York; 1993: 899–912.
4. Molnar W, Stockum AE. Relief of obstructive jaundice through percutaneous transhepatic catheter: a new therapeutic method. *Am J Radiol* 1974: 122:346–67.
5. Soehendra N, Reynders-Frederix V. Palliative gallengangs-drainage. *Dtsch Med Wochenschr* 1979; 104:206–7.
6. Cremer M, Deviere J, Delhaye M et al. Non-surgical management of severe chronic pancreatitis. *Scand J Gastroenterol* 1990; 25(S175):7–84.
7. Lichtenstein DR, Carr-Locke DL. Endoscopic palliation for unresectable pancreatic carcinoma. *Surg Clin N Am* 1995; 75:969–88.
8. Huibregtse K, Katon RM, Coene PP, Tytgat GNJ. Endoscopic palliative treatment in pancreatic cancer. *Gastrointest Endosc* 1986; 32:334–8.
9. Deviere J, Baize M, De Toeuf J, Cremer M. Long-term follow-up of patients with hilar malignant stricture treated by endoscopic internal biliary drainage. *Gastrointest Endosc* 1988; 34:95–101.
10. Matsuda Y, Shimakma K, Akamatsu T. Factors affecting the patency of stents in malignant biliary obstructive disease: univariate and multivariate analysis. *Am J Gastroenterol* 1991; 86:843–9.
11. Kerlan RK, Ring EJ, Pogany AC, Jeffrey RB. Biliary endoprostheses insertion using a combined perioral-transhepatic method. *Radiology* 1984; 150:828–30.
12. Kerr RM, Gilliam JH III. The team approach to biliary tract intervention: current status of combined percutaneous-endoscopic techniques. *Gastrointest Endosc* 1988; 34:432–3.
13. Huibregtse K. *Endoscopic biliary and pancreatic drainage.* Thieme Verlag, Stuttgart; 1988.
14. Motte S, Deviere J, Dumonceau JM et al.. Risk factors for septicemia following endoscopic biliary stenting. *Gastroenterology* 1991; 101:1374–81.
15. Van Gansbeke D, Van Gossum A, Schils J. Sonographic monitoring of biliary endoprostheses. *Gastrointest Radiol* 1984; 9:335–9.
16. Groen AK, Out F, Huibregtse K et al. Characterization of the contents of occluded biliary endoprostheses. *Endoscopy* 1987; 19:57–61.
17. Hurwich DB, Poterucha JJ, Nixon DE et al.. Preventing biliary stent occlusion. *Gastrointest Endosc* 1992; 38:263–7.
18. Sung JY, Shaffer EA, Lam K et al. Inhibition of E.coli adhesion on biliary stents by bile salts with different hydrophobicities. *Gastrointest Endosc* 1992; 38:263–6.
19. Coene PPLO, Groen AK, Chang J et al. Clogging of biliary endoprostheses: a new perspective. *Gut* 1990; 31:913–17.
20. Seitz U, Vadeyar H, Soehendra N. Prolonged patency with a new design Teflon biliary prosthesis. *Endoscopy* 1994; 26:478–82.
21. Sung JY, Chung SCS, Tsui CP et al.. Omitting side-holes in biliary stents does not improve drainage of the obstructed biliary system: A prospective randomized trial. *Gastrointest Endosc* 1994; 40:321–4.
22. Frakes JT, Johanson JF, Stake JJ. Optimal timing for stent replacement in malignant biliary tract obstruction. *Gastrointest Endosc* 1993; 39:164–7.
23. Speer AG, Cotton PB, Russell RCG et al. Randomized trial of endoscopic versus percutaneous stent insertion in malignant obstructive jaundice. *Lancet* 1987; ii:57–62.
24. Sheperd HA, Royle G, Ross APR et al. Endoscopic biliary endoprosthesis in the palliation of malignant obstruction of the distal common bile ducts: a randomized study. *Br J Surg* 1988; 75:1166–8.
25. Smith AC, Dowsett JF, Russel RCG et al. Randomized trial of endoscopic stenting versus surgical bypass in malignant low bile duct obstruction. *Lancet* 1994; ii:1655–60.
26. Brandabur JJ, Kozarek RA, Ball TJ et al. Non-operative versus operative treatment of obstructive jaundice in pancreatic cancer: Cost and Survival analysis. *Am J Gastroenterol* 1988; 83:1132–9.
27. Goldin E, Beyar M, Safra T et al.. A new self-expandable and removable metal stent for biliary obstruction. A preliminary report. *Endoscopy* 1993; 25:59–99.
28. Huibregtse K, Carr-Locke DL, Cremer M et al. Biliary stent occlusion. A problem solved with self-expanding metal stents? *Endoscopy* 1992; 24:391–4.
29. Davids PHP, Groen AK, Rauws EAJ et al. Randomized trial of self-expanding metal stents versus polyethylene stents for distal malignant biliary obstruction. Lancet 1992; 340:1488–92.
30. Carr-Locke DL, Ball TJ, Connors PJ et al. Multicentre randomized trial of Wallstent biliary endoprosthesis versus plastic stents. *Gastrointest Endosc* 1993; 39:310–15.

31. Kiser MH, Barkin J, MacIntyre JM. Pancreatic cancer; assessment of prognosis by clinical presentation. *Cancer* 1985; 56:397–402.

32. Lebowitz AH, Lefkowitz M. Pain management of pancreatic carcinoma: a review. *Pain* 1988; 36:1–11.

33. Harrison MA, Hamilton JW. Palliation of pancreatic cancer pain by endoscopic stent placement. *Gastrointest Endosc* 1989; 35:443–5.

34. Costamagna G, Gabbrielli A, Mutignani M *et al.* Treatment of 'obstructive' pain by endoscopic drainage in patients with pancreatic head carcinoma. *Gastrointest Endosc* 1993; 39:774–7.

35. Cremer M, Deviere J, Engelholm L. Endoscopic management of cysts and pseudocysts in chronic pancreatitis: long-term follow-up after 7 years of experience. *Gastrointest Endosc* 1989; 35:1–9.

36. Zimmon DS, Barsa J, Chang J, Clemett AR. The management of hepatic duct cancer with percutaneous transhepatic biliary stent and intraluminal irradiation. *Gastroenterology* 1979; 77:49. (abstract)

37. Alden ME, Mohiuddin M. The impact of radiation dose in combined external beam and intraluminal Ir-192 brachytherapy for bile duct cancer. *Int J Radiother Oncol Biol Phys* 1994; 28:945–51.

38. Montemaggi P, Costamagna G, Dobelbower RR *et al.*. Intraluminal brachytherapy in the treatment of pancreas and bile duct carcinoma. *Int J Radiother Oncol Biol Phys* 1995; 32:437–43.

39. Classen M, Hagenmueller F. Endoprosthesis and local irradiation in the treatment of biliary malignancies. *Endoscopy* 1987; 19:25–30.

40. Montemaggi P, Morganti AG, Dobelbower RR *et al.* Role of intraluminal brachytherapy in the treatment in extrahepatic bile duct and pancreatic cancers: is it just for palliation? *Radiology* 1996; 199:861–66.

41. Sarr MG, Cameron JL . Surgical management of unresectable carcinoma of the pancreas. *Surgery* 1982; 91:123–33.

42. Feretis C, Benakis P, Dimopoulos C *et al.*. Palliation of malignant gastric outlet obstruction with self-expanding metal stents. *Endoscopy* 1996; 28:225–8.

43. Keymling M, Wagner HJ, Vakil N, Knyrim K. Relief of malignant duodenal obstruction by percutaneous insertion of metal stent. *Gastrointest Endosc* 1992; 339:439–41.

44. Speer AG, Cotton PB. Endoscopic treatment of pancreatic cancer. *Int J Pancreatol* 1988; 3:S147–S158.

45. Siegel JH, Snady H . The significance of endoscopically placed prostheses in the management of biliary obstruction due to carcinoma of the pancreas: results of non-operative decompression in 277 patients. *Am J Gastroenterol* 1986; 81:634–41.

46. Dowsett JF, Russell RGG, Hatfield ARW *et al.*. Malignant obstructive jaundice: a prospective randomized trial of surgery versus endoscopic stenting. *Gastroenterology* 1989; 96:A 128.

Complications 5

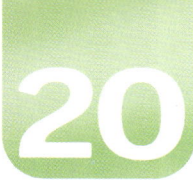

Complications of endoscopic pancreatic sphincterotomy

Stuart Sherman & Glen A. Lehman

INTRODUCTION

Since its inception and initial application in 1974, endoscopic biliary sphincterotomy has revolutionized the approach to the management of a variety of biliary tract disorders. Although endoscopic pancreatic duct sphincterotomy (EPS) has been performed since 1976[1], this technique has not been widely utilized because of concerns for prohibitive morbidity and also because of uncertainty about its indications[2]. More recently, EPS has been utilized to facilitate other endoscopic manoeuvres (e.g. placement of a pancreatic stent or drain, dilating strictures, removal of pancreatic stones, obtaining tissue from pancreatic duct strictures) and as the specific therapy for pancreatic sphincter stenosis (minor or major papilla)[3–6].

In this chapter, we will review the complications of pancreatic sphincterotomy (Figure 20.1).

Determining the incidence of pancreatitis following EPS is difficult because it is rarely performed in isolation and the other therapies (e.g. stricture dilatation, stone removal) applied simultaneously may contribute to the pancreatitis. Moreover, series reporting the use of EPS are in general small (< 50 patients) and focus on outcomes of therapy (e.g. clinical benefit of pancreatic stone removal) rather than complications. Finally, most studies are retrospective and the definitions of complications are not standardized[7]. Presumably the factors that contribute to pancreatic injury during EPS are the same factors that contribute to pancreatic injury during endoscopic retrograde cholangiopancreatography (ERCP) and biliary sphincterotomy (Figure 20.2) although this has not been studied.

MAJOR PAPILLA PANCREATIC SPHINCTEROTOMY

There are two methods of cutting the major papilla pancreatic sphincter (Figures 20.3 and 20.4)[2,8,9]. A standard pull-type sphincterotome (with or without a wire guide) is inserted into the pancreatic duct and oriented along the axis of the pancreatic duct (usually in the 1 to 2 o'clock position). Although the landmarks that determine the length of the incision are imprecise, authorities recommend cutting 5–10mm[2]. The cutting wire should not extend more than 6–7mm up the duct when applying electrocautery so as to prevent deep ductal injury. Alternatively, a needle knife can be used to perform the sphincterotomy over a previously placed pancreatic stent[2,9]. Some authorities favour performing a biliary sphincterotomy prior to the pancreatic sphincterotomy because of the high incidence of bile duct obstruction and cholangitis reported by one group if this is not done[10]. Such complications have not been found by others and have been infrequently encountered in our experience[2,9]. However, performing a biliary sphincterotomy first can expose the pancreaticobiliary septum and allow the length of the cut to be gauged more accurately.

Three recent series have focused on the complications of major papilla pancreatic sphincterotomy (Figure 20.5). Kozarek and colleagues[2] performed pancreatic sphincterotomy in 56 patients to assist in removal of pancreatic duct calculi (*n* = 26), prior to placement of a pancreatic stent for a dominant stricture (*n* = 8) or ductal leak (*n* = 12), or to treat pancreatic sphincter stenosis (*n* = 10). Fifty-four patients had chronic pancreatitis and two had acute recurrent pancreatitis but morphologically normal pancreatic parenchyma. Forty-seven patients had a pull-type pancreatic sphincterotomy (33

Figure 20.1 Complications of pancreatic sphincterotomy.

Pancreatitis
Haemorrhage
Pancreatic/Biliary sepsis
Perforation
Stent-related
    Occlusion resulting in pain and/or pancreatitis
    Migration into or out of the duct
    Duodenal erosions
    Infection
    Ductal perforation
    Stone formation
    Ductal and parenchymal changes
Late complications (> 3 months after EPS)
    Sphincterotomy restenosis
    Pancreatic duct stricture

Figure 20.2 Mechanisms of pancreatic injury in EPS-induced pancreatitis.

    Mechanical
    Chemical
    Hydrostatic
    Enzymatic
    Microbiological
    Allergic
    Thermal

Figure 20.3 Major papilla EPS using a pull-type sphincterotome. (a) Normal major papilla. (b) Pancreatic sphincterotomy performed using a pull-type sphincterotome. (c) After a pancreatic stent is placed, a biliary sphincterotomy is performed. (d) Completed pancreatic and biliary sphincterotomy.

Figure 20.4 Major papilla EPS using a needle knife. (a) Pancreatic stent in place. (b, c) Pancreatic sphincterotomy being performed with the needle knife. (d) Completed pancreatic sphincterotomy.

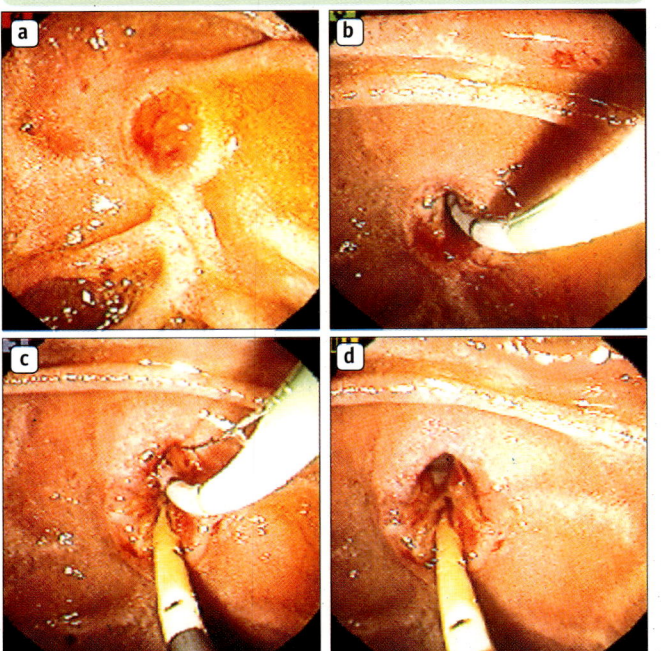

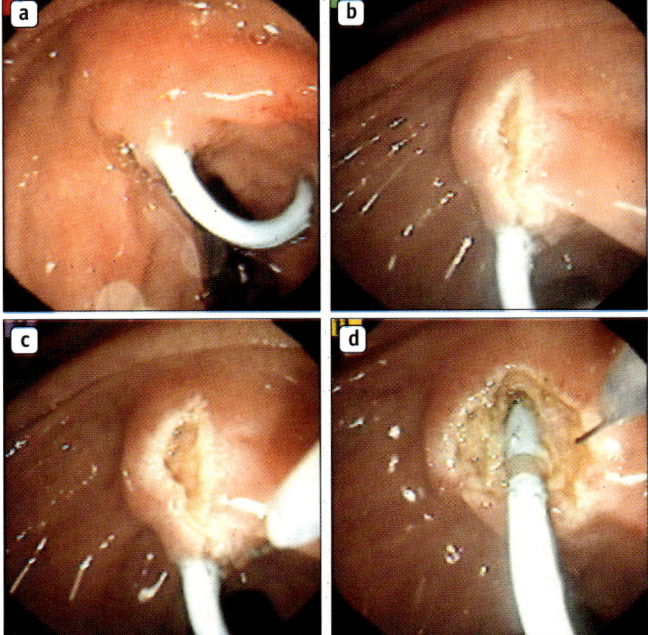

had pancreatic stents placed after the sphincterotomy) and nine had a needle-knife sphincterotomy performed over a pancreatic stent; 40W of blended current were used. The mean incision length, estimated by pullthrough of an extraction balloon or open sphincterotome, was 9mm (range 5–15mm). Mild pancreatitis occurred in four patients (7.1%), cholangitis in two (3.6%), and there were no deaths.

Esber and colleagues[9] reported complications of major papilla pancreatic sphincterotomy in 236 consecutive patients. The EPS was performed with a pull-type sphincterotome (50W blended current) in 123 patients (followed by pancreatic stent placement in 87 patients) or needle knife (40W blended current) over a pancreatic duct stent in 113

patients. A concurrent *de novo* or extended biliary sphincterotomy was performed in 90 patients (38%). The EPS was performed for treatment of pancreatic sphincter dysfunction in 174 patients (74%) and to facilitate placement of a pancreatic stent, removal of stones or stricture biopsy in 62 patients (26%). Postprocedure pancreatitis occurred in 33 patients (14%) and was graded mild in 25 (76%), moderate in 7 (21%), and severe in one (3%). All patients were managed non-operatively, and there were no deaths. Pancreatitis occurred in 15.5% (27 of 174) of patients with pancreatic sphincter dysfunction, compared to 9.7% of patients (6 of 62) with chronic pancreatitis ($p = 0.26$).

Kozarek[2] suggested that the periductular fibrosis and

Author (ref)	n	Pancreatitis	Other complications	Total complications	Mortality
Kozarek *et al.* (2)	56	4 (7.1%)	2 (3.6%)[a]	6 (10.7%)	0
Parsons *et al.* (13)	31	1 (3.2%)	0 (0.0%)	1 (3.2%)	0
Esber *et al.* (9)	236	33 (14.0%)	4 (1.7%)[b]	37 (15.7%)	0
Total	**323**	**38 (11.8%)**	**6 (1.9%)**	**44 (13.6%)**	**0 (0.0%)**

a Cholangitis in two patients
b Two mild haemorrhages and two perforations

Figure 20.5 Selected series reporting early complications of major papilla EPS.

limited amounts of nearby acinar tissue associated with chronic pancreatitis may offer protection against pancreatic injury following pancreatic sphincterotomy. This also appears to be true when patients with chronic pancreatitis undergo biliary sphincterotomy or ERCP alone. In a series of 787 patients undergoing ERCP (diagnostic with or without therapy), Chen and colleagues[11] reported that 5.5% (39 of 711) of patients with a normal pancreas developed postprocedure pancreatitis, in contrast to 0% (0 of 76; p = 0.036) of patients with chronic pancreatitis. In the Esber series[9], two patients (0.8%) developed bleeding at the time of the sphincterotomy and were managed successfully with injection of adrenaline (1:10,000) into the bleeding point. No blood transfusions were necessary. There were two (0.8%) perforations. Both patients had manometrically documented sphincter of Oddi dysfunction and underwent needle-knife pancreatic and biliary sphincterotomies (over a pancreatic stent) with extension of the biliary sphincterotomy using a wire-guided sphincterotome. Contrast extravasation was noted on follow-up ductography and a nasoduodenal tube and nasobiliary tube were placed. On observation of the major papilla, it appeared that the pancreatic sphincterotomy extended more deeply than desired and in the 9 to 11 o'clock position, i.e. off the desired axis (the duodenum was noted to be rotated in one patient). The patients were hospitalized for 3 and 9 days, respectively, and there have been no late complications after a 10-month follow-up.

Although unproven, it has been hypothesized that placement of a pancreatic stent may limit the incidence of postpancreatic sphincterotomy pancreatitis. Sherman and associates[12] prospectively compared the frequency of postprocedure pancreatitis in sphincter of Oddi dysfunction patients undergoing needle-knife sphincterotomy over a pancreatic stent (severing both the pancreatic and biliary sphincter) with those undergoing standard biliary sphincterotomy. Pancreatitis occurred in 29% of patients undergoing standard biliary sphincterotomy compared to 12% (p = 0.02) undergoing needle-knife sphincterotomy over a pancreatic duct stent. There was a trend toward less severe pancreatitis in the stented group. More data from this and other centres are necessary before this approach can be advocated for general use. The role of pancreatic stenting to reduce the incidence and severity of pancreatitis after standard pull-type pancreatic sphincterotomy awaits further investigation. Pending the results of these studies, we advocate placement of a pancreatic stent after pull-type pancreatic sphincterotomy.

Because of the stent-related complications and the need for a second endoscopy to remove the stent, Parsons and colleagues[13] evaluated the safety of performing pancreatic sphincterotomy without stenting. Thirty-one patients underwent major papilla pancreatic sphincterotomy with a pull-type sphincterotome followed by placement of a 5 Fr nasopancreatic tube. There was only one episode (3.2%) of mild pancreatitis and all drains were retrieved within 24 hours. There were no delayed episodes of pancreatitis after the drain was removed. No pancreatic sphincterotomy-induced bleeding or perforation occurred. This technique requires advancement of the guide wire and nasopancreat-

ic tube around the genu into the body of the pancreas. Variable configurations of the pancreatic duct makes this difficult in 10–20% of patients.

The study by Parsons et al.[13] partially addresses the issue of the duration of pancreatic duct stenting (or nasopancreatic tube placement) needed to protect the sphincterotomy area from oedema-induced closure of the pancreatic orifice and pancreatitis. One alternative to the nasopancreatic drain is to place an unflanged pancreatic stent (no intraductal flange) that can spontaneously dislodge. In two recent series[14,15], outward migration occurred in approximately 50% of patients at a mean time of 10 days after stent placement[15] (on abdominal X-ray evaluation performed 8–14 days after stent placement). While this technique avoids a second endoscopy in half the patients, unfortunately some stents occasionally dislodge hours after placement and even during the initial procedure. Studies are needed to define characteristics of a stent which will allow it to remain intraductal for, perhaps, 1–3 days and then spontaneously dislodge with certainty (so no follow-up endoscopy or radiographs are needed). A variety of dissolvable stents are being evaluated.

As with biliary sphincterotomy, stenosis of the pancreatic sphincterotomy may occur. In the series reported by Kozarek et al.[2], this occurred in 8 of 54 patients (14%). Patient symptoms and methods to detect the restenosis were not detailed. Adequate drainage was achieved in these patients by repeat EPS in six and surgical septotomy in two. The authors felt that this high restenosis rate was due to the relatively small incisions made at an early stage in their work (mean 6mm vs 11mm later in the series). Fuji and colleagues[16] reported one pancreatic sphincterotomy restenosis (among 10 patients) 3 months after the procedure. Other authors have not yet reported their pancreatic sphincterotomy restenosis rates.

MINOR PAPILLA PANCREATIC SPHINCTEROTOMY

Pancreas divisum, the most common congenital variant of pancreatic duct anatomy, occurs when the ductal systems of the dorsal and ventral pancreatic buds fail to fuse during the second month of gestation. With non-union of the ducts, the major portion of the pancreatic exocrine juice drains into the duodenum by way of the dorsal duct and minor papilla. As with major papilla EPS, minor papilla EPS is often done to facilitate other endoscopic manoeuvres. In addition, minor papilla EPS is being performed in a subpopulation of pancreas divisum patients in whom the minor papilla orifice appears to be critically small, resulting in pancreatic pain and/or pancreatitis[17–20]. In the latter group of patients, it is easier to determine the incidence of sphincterotomy-induced pancreatitis, as minor papilla pancreatic sphincterotomy is often performed in isolation (with or without a minor papilla stent). The technique of minor papilla EPS is similar to that of major papilla EPS except that the direction of the sphincterotomy is usually in the 10 to 12 o'clock position and the length of the sphincterotomy is limited to 4–8mm (Figures 20.6 and 20.7).

Figure 20.8 summarizes the early complication rates fol-

Figure 20.6 Minor papilla EPS using a pull-type sphincterotome. (a) Prominent minor papilla. (b) Pull-type sphincterotome passed into dorsal duct. (c) Minor papilla pancreatic sphincterotomy being performed. (d) Completed minor papilla pancreatic sphincterotomy. A dorsal pancreatic duct stent was placed after completing the sphincterotomy.

Figure 20.7 Completed minor papilla EPS performed with a needle knife over a previously placed dorsal pancreatic duct stent.

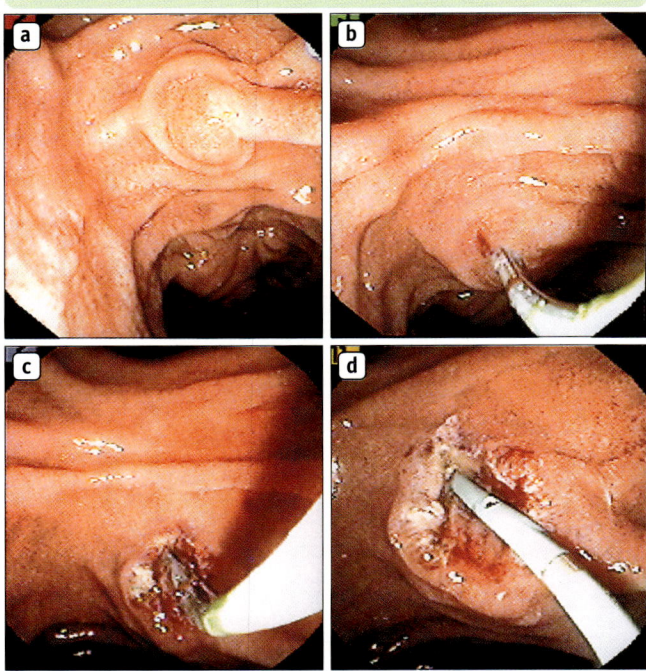

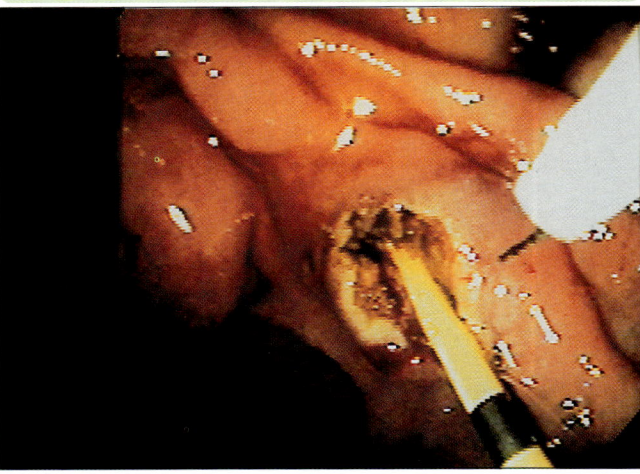

lowing minor papilla EPS in four selected series[21–24]. Pancreatitis was the most common complication, occurring in 19.6% of patients. Of the 33 episodes of postprocedure pancreatitis, 26 (79%) were graded mild, 6 (18%) moderate and one (3%) severe. One death occurred in an attempted minor papilla pancreatic sphincterotomy from complications of severe pancreatitis with abscess formation. There were only two other early complications, both haemorrhage and both managed by endoscopic therapy.

The rate of late restenosis is difficult to assess from these series. Patients are only re-evaluated for recurrent symptoms, and accurate endoscopic means to assess minor papilla patency are not well studied. Despite these limitations, however, Kozarek and colleagues[24] estimated that 3 of 26 patients (11.5%) developed restenosis of the minor papilla after EPS. This rate probably represents an underestimate of the true restenosis rate since, as noted, only patients with recurrent symptoms are re-evaluated. High-grade strictures of the terminal 10mm of the dorsal duct are estimated to occur in 2–3% of patients[17]. These strictures are particularly problematic because the narrowing extends beyond the duodenal wall and a pancreatic head resection or a ductal drainage procedure (e.g. Puestow) may be required.

Figure 20.8 Early complications of minor papilla EPS.

Author (ref)	n	Pancreatitis	Other complications	Total complications	Mortality
Lehman *et al.* (21)	52[a]	8 (13.3%)	1 (1.7%)[b]	9 (15.0%)	1 (1.7%)
Coleman *et al.* (22)	34[c,d]	18 (33.3%)	1 (1.9%)[e]	19 (35.2%)	0 (0.0%)
Sherman *et al.* (23)	16	3 (18.8%)	0 (0.0%)	3 (18.8%)	0 (0.0%)
Kozarek *et al.* (24)	39[c]	4 (10.3%)	0 (0.0%)	4 (10.3%)	0 (0.0%)
Total	**141[f]**	**33 (19.6%)**	**2 (1.2%)**	**35 (20.8%)**	**1 (0.6%)**

a 60 minor papilla sphincterotomies performed

b One haemorrhage treated with adrenaline injection and multipolar electrocoagulation

c Stent placement alone used in some patients

d 54 procedures performed

e One haemorrhage treated with adrenaline injection

f 169 procedures performed

References

1. Cremer M, Deviere J, Delhaye M, Vandermeeren A, Baize M. Non-surgical management of severe chronic pancreatitis. *Scand J Gastroenterol* 1990; 25(S175):77–84.

2. Kozarek RA, Ball TJ, Patterson DJ, Brandabur JJ, Traverso W, Raltz S. Endoscopic pancreatic duct sphincterotomy: indications, technique, and analysis of results. *Gastrointest Endosc* 1994; 40:592–8.

3. Grimm H, Meyer WH, Nam VCh, Soehendra N. New modalities for treating chronic pancreatitis. *Endoscopy* 1989; 21:70–4.

4. Watanapa P, Williamson RCN. Pancreatic sphincterotomy and sphincteroplasty. *Gut* 1992; 33:865–7.

5. Kozarek RA. Chronic pancreatitis in 1994: is there a role for endoscopic treatment? *Endoscopy* 1994; 26:625–8.

6. Kozarek RA, Traverso LW. Endotherapy of chronic pancreatitis – state of the art. *Int J Pancreatol* 1996; 19:93–102.

7. Cotton PB, Lehman GA, Vennes J *et al*. Endoscopic sphincterotomy complications and their management: an attempt at consensus. *Gastrointest Endosc* 1991; 37:383–93.

8. Fuji T, Amano H, Ohmura R, Akiyama T, Aibe T, Takemoto T. EPS – technique and evaluation. *Endoscopy* 1989; 21:27–30.

9. Esber E, Sherman S, Earle D, Pezzi J, Gottlieb K, Lehman G. Complications of major papilla pancreatic sphincterotomy: a review of 236 patients. *Gastrointest Endosc* 1995; 43:405A.

10. Delhaye M, Vandermeeren A, Baize M, Cremer M. Extracorporeal shock-wave lithotripsy of pancreatic calculi. *Gastroenterology* 1992; 102:610–20.

11. Chen YK, Walter MH, McCarter TL, Anthony M, Frankson C. Is pre-existing pancreatitis a risk factor for ERCP-induced pancreatitis? *Gastrointest Endosc* 1996; 43:404A.

12. Sherman S, Eversman D, Earle D, Bucksot L, Rusche M, Lehman G. Sphincterotomy by needle knife over pancreatic stent technique lowers the post-procedure pancreatitis frequency and severity in sphincter of Oddi dysfunction patients. *Gastrointest Endosc* 1996; 43:413A.

13. Parsons WG, Howell DA, Qasseem T, Hanson BL. Pancreatic duct sphincterotomy without stenting. *Gastrointest Endosc* 1995; 41:427A.

14. Dahman B, Geenen JE, Hogan WJ *et al*. Pancreatic stents: are two barbs better than four? *Gastrointest Endosc* 1996; 43:404A.

15. Barawi M, Olsson, M, Sherman S, Gottlieb K, Lehman G. Spontaneous dislodgement of unflanged pancreatic duct stents. *Am J Gastroenterol* 1996; 91:1928A.

16. Fuji T, Amano H, Harima K *et al*. Pancreatic sphincterotomy and pancreatic endoprosthesis. *Endoscopy* 1985; 17:69–72.

17. Lehman G, Sherman S. Pancreas divisum: diagnosis, clinical significance, and management alternatives. *Gastrointest Endosc Clin N Am* 1995; 5:145–70.

18. Gregg JA. Pancreas divisum: its association with pancreatitis. *Am J Surg* 1977; 134:539–43.

19. Bernard JP, Sahel J, Giovannini M, Sarles H. Pancreas divisum is a probable cause of acute pancreatitis: a report of 137 cases. *Pancreas* 1990; 5:248–54.

20. Cotton PB. Congenital anomaly of pancreas divisum as cause of obstructive pain and pancreatitis. *Gut* 1980; 21:105–14.

21. Lehman GA, Sherman S, Nisi R, Hawes RH. Pancreas divisum: results of minor papilla sphincterotomy. *Gastrointest Endosc* 1993; 39:1–8.

22. Coleman SD, Eisen GM, Troughton AB, Cotton PB. Endoscopic treatment in pancreas divisum. *Am J Gastroenterol* 1994; 89:1152–5.

23. Sherman S, Hawes R, Nisi R, Bucksot L, Earle D, Lehman G. Randomized controlled trial of minor papilla sphincterotomy (MiES) in pancreas divisum (PDiv) patients with pain only. *Gastrointest Endosc* 1994; 40:125A.

24. Kozarek RA, Ball TJ, Patterson DJ, Brandabur JJ, Raltz SL. Endoscopic approach to pancreas divisum. *Dig Dis Sci* 1995; 40:1974–81.

ERCP- and endoscopic biliary sphincterotomy-induced pancreatitis

Stuart Sherman & Glen A. Lehman

INTRODUCTION

Pancreatitis is the most common major complication of endoscopic retrograde cholangiopancreatography (ERCP) and endoscopic biliary sphincterotomy (EBS). Almost certainly, the aetiology of this pancreatitis is multifactorial. While most postprocedure pancreatitis is relatively mild and resolves in a few days, more serious pancreatitis may occur. Once serious pancreatitis has been provoked, secondary complications are common; resolution may require months of in-hospital care and mortality may occur. This chapter will attempt to decipher the various aetiological factors involved in ERCP- and EBS-induced pancreatitis, explore the methods to treat postprocedure pancreatitis, and look at ways to prevent this complication. When data are available, references primarily after 1985 will be cited to avoid the pre-1980 era when disinfection practices were less strict.

INCIDENCE OF POST-ERCP AND POST-EBS HYPERAMYLASAEMIA AND PANCREATITIS

Increases in serum amylase levels occur commonly after successful or unsuccessful cannulation of the papilla of Vater[1-3]. If small increases still within the normal range are included, nearly all patients undergoing pancreatography will have a rise in enzyme level. The height and frequency of hyperamylasaemia correlate with the extent of visualization of the pancreatic ductal system. In the study by Skude and colleagues[1], serum pancreatic amylase increased 1.7 times over the basal value when only the main pancreatic duct (MPD) was visualized, compared to 5.27 times when the MPD and side branches were opacified, and 7.4 times when acinarization occurred. Whereas most amylase elevations are pancreatic in origin[4], Skude et al.[1] reported a 7% incidence of increased salivary isoamylase after pancreatography. Approximately 25–40%[1,2,5] of patients will have abnormal serum amylase levels after cholangiography (without pancreatography) or failed cannulation. Amylase elevations typically peak 90 minutes to 4 hours after ERCP[6,7] and resolve within 48 hours. Increases of lipase, insulin, glucagon and cortisol, and a decrease in serum calcium levels have been reported after routine ERCP[6].

The reported incidence of pancreatitis following diagnostic ERCP has ranged from 0% to as high as 39.5% (Figure 21.1)[1,2,4,8-20]. This variable incidence is reflective of the diverse definitions of pancreatitis used in these series and the method of data collection, i.e. prospective with frequent enzyme determinations or retrospective. Mild pancreatitis probably has little significance other than the financial considerations of the short hospitalization. Although infrequent, severe pancreatitis with secondary complications of necrosis,

Author (ref)	Year	ERCP n	Pancreatitis n(%)	Surgery n(%)	Deaths n(%)	Prospective?
Nebel et al. (9)	'75	3884	51 (1.3)	0	2	No
Zimmon et al. (18)	'75	300	5 (1.7)	0	0	No
Skude et al. (1)	'76	216	2 (0.9)	0	0	Yes
Bilbao et al. (16)	'76	8681	94 (1.1)	—	0	No
Osnes et al. (8)	'77	24	0 (0.0)	0	0	Yes
Brust et al. (13)	'77	48	19 (39.5)	0	0	Yes
Montori et al. (15)	'79	8638	10 (0.1)	1	2	No
Brandes et al. (17)	'81	118	3 (2.5)	—	0	Yes
Weaver et al. (4)	'83	24	0 (0.0)	0	0	Yes
Hamilton et al. (12)	'83	1118	15 (1.3)	1	0	No
Roszler and Campbell (11)	'85	140	18 (12.9)	0	0	No
LaFerla et al. (2)	'86	71	4 (5.6)	0	0	Yes
Tyden et al. (14)	'86	47	0 (0.0)	0	0	Yes
Reiertsen et al. (10)	'87	1950	8 (0.4)	4	0	No
Sherman et al. (19)	'93	107	3 (2.8)	0	0	Yes
Johnson et al. (20)	'95	622	35 (5.6)	—	—	Yes
Total		25998	267 (1.0)	6 (0.02)	4 (0.02)	
Prospective		1277	66 (5.2)	0 (0.0)	0 (0.0)	

— *Data not reported.*

Figure 21.1 Selected series reporting the incidence of diagnostic ERCP-induced pancreatitis and the number of patients requiring surgery and/or dying. The studies are classified by the method of data collection, i.e. prospective or retrospective. (Adapted from Sherman and Lehman[44].)

Author (ref)	Year	ERCP n	Pancreatitis n(%)	Surgery n(%)	Deaths n(%)	Prospective?
Safrany (35)	'78	3618	48 (1.3)	3	9	No
Montori et al. (15)	'79	194	0 (0.0)	0	0	No
Neuhaus and Safrany (24)	'81	400	7 (1.8)	2	2	No
Cotton and Vallon (25)	'81	679	20 (2.9)	1	3	No
Viceconte et al. (26)	'81	296	0 (0.0)	0	0	No
Geenen et al. (31)	'81	1250	41 (3.3)	3	6	No
Dunham et al. (33)	'82	820	5 (0.6)	0	2	No
Arendt et al. (29)	'83	695	6 (0.9)	3	2	No
Kawai and Nakajima (34)	'83	496	3 (0.6)	0	0	No
Tedesco et al. (21)	'84	5790	122 (2.1)	5	6	No
Escourrou et al. (32)	'84	407	3 (0.7)	2	2	No
Lam (27)	'84	134	2 (1.5)	1	1	Yes
Mustard et al. (28)	'84	289	11 (3.8)	1	0	No
Roberts-Thomson (23)	'84	300	4 (1.3)	1	0	No
Leese et al. (22)	'85	394	8 (2.0)	1	1	Yes
Reiertsen et al. (10)	'87	406	0 (0.0)	0	0	Yes
Vaira et al. (30)	'89	100	9 (0.9)	0	1	No
Lambert et al. (36)	'91	602	16 (2.6)	0	2	Yes
Sherman et al. (37)	'91	423	17 (4.0)	0	0	Yes
Freeman et al. (38)	'94	1494	100 (6.7)	—	2	Yes
Total		19687	422 (2.1)	23 (0.13)	39 (0.02)	
Prospective		3453	143 (4.1)	2 (0.1)	6 (0.2)	

— Data not reported.

Figure 21.2 Selected series reporting the incidence of post-EBS pancreatitis and the number of patients requiring surgery and/or dying. The studies are classified by the method of data collection, i.e. prospective or retrospective. (Adapted from Sherman and Lehman[44].)

pseudocyst or abscess requiring prolonged hospitalization, may occur. The results in Figure 21.1 indicate that 1.0% of patients undergoing diagnostic ERCP had pancreatitis while 0.02% required surgery for a secondary complication and 0.02% died. When patients were tallied prospectively, there was a 5.2% incidence of pancreatitis, but no operations or deaths occurred.

Figure 21.2 summarizes 20 published series[10,15,21–38] of ERCP/EBS-induced pancreatitis. Pancreatitis occurred in 2.1% of patients. This complication required surgery in 0.13%, and 0.2% died. Complication rates vary according to the indication for the procedure (e.g. less frequent with biliary stones than with sphincter of Oddi dysfunction)[37,38].

The diagnosis of postprocedure pancreatitis is invariably based on the patients' signs and symptoms as well as the serum pancreatic enzyme levels. The accuracy of this approach is unknown, as histological correlation (the 'gold standard') has not been performed. Clinical assessment, using bedside examination and early Ranson criteria, has been shown to underestimate the presence and severity of post-ERCP pancreatitis (compared to computed tomography (CT) findings)[39]. Retrospective series have generally shown a lower rate of postprocedure pancreatitis (see Figures 21.1 and 21.2), suggesting that this method of analysis underestimates the true incidence of this complication.

When interpreting the data, it must be realized that the definition of pancreatitis and the grading of its severity differ among authors. Figure 21.3 presents a grading system for the severity of post-ERCP and post-EBS pancreatitis that was formulated at an international therapeutic workshop[40] in an attempt to standardize the reporting of complications. Although some authors advocate the use of Ranson's criteria[41] for grading the severity of the pancreatitis[42], several series have suggested that this classification underestimates the severity of the complication (compared to the criteria of Cotton et al.[40,43]).

Figure 21.3 A grading system for pancreatitis complicating ERCP and/or endoscopic sphincterotomy.[40] (Adapted from Cotton et al.[40].)

Grade	Description
Mild	A clinical picture of pancreatitis with an amylase level at least 3 times normal at >24 hours after the procedure, requiring unplanned admission of an outpatient or prolongation of planned admission for 2–3 days after the procedure.
Moderate	Pancreatitis requiring hospitalization of 4–10 days.
Severe	Hospitalization prolonged for >10 days or any of the following: haemorrhagic pancreatitis, phlegmon or pseudocyst, or intervention required (percutaneous drainage or surgery).

TYPES OF PANCREATIC INJURY

During ERCP and EBS the pancreas is subjected to many types of potential injury – mechanical, chemical, hydrostatic, enzymic, microbiological, allergic and thermal[44]. These factors may act independently or in concert to induce post-procedure pancreatitis.

Mechanical factors

Direct trauma from the endoscope rarely causes pancreatitis[45]. Cannulation trauma to the papilla is common and may result in sphincter of Oddi spasm[46] and/or a haemorrhagic, oedematous major papilla at the end of a difficult or prolonged case. Papillary oedema and sphincter of Oddi spasm may restrict the flow of pancreatic juice and result in pancreatitis[47]. Sphincter of Oddi or intraductal pressure studies have not been performed either before or after lengthy cannulation attempts to confirm this hypothesis.

Papillary trauma may result during cannulation attempts with the standard 5Fr cannula. Tapered-tip and needle-tip catheters, sphincterotomes and most guide wires are more pointed and/or rigid and probably increase the potential for papilla or pancreatic trauma. Good clinical judgment, based on experience, is required to help define when more vigorous cannulation techniques are likely to be productive rather than hazardous.

Repeated cannulation attempts are a major factor in papilla trauma and pancreatitis[12,48–50]. Freeman and associates[38] reported that the incidence of acute pancreatitis after EBS correlated with the difficulty of cannulation (defined by the number of attempts on the papilla). In this series, the pancreatitis rates were 3.2% (30/924), 7.1% (23/322) and 13% (19/146) for easy (≤ 5 attempts), moderate (6–15 attempts), and difficult (> 15 attempts) cannulations, respectively, ($p < 0.05$; multivariate analysis).

Deep cannulation into the pancreatic duct helps secure the catheter or guide wire position in case of patient movement or for planned catheter exchanges. However, this position increases the chances of duct or ampullary perforation with the associated intraparenchymal or submucosal injection. Submucosal contrast media injections uncommonly lead to pancreatitis. Duct perforation more commonly causes focal pancreatitis.

The incidence of hyperamylasaemia and pancreatitis is higher for pancreatography with or without cholangiography than with cholangiography alone[1,2,51,52]. In a preliminary report of 1689 patients, Johnson and associates[52] found that pancreatitis occurred in 10.9% (152 of 1391) of patients after a pancreatic duct injection compared to 1.7% of patients (5 of 298) who did not have their pancreatic duct visualized. Freeman et al.[38] reported that pancreatitis rates after EBS increased linearly with each additional pancreatic duct injection, increasing from 3.9% with no injections to 17.6% with more than 10 injections. Hamilton et al.[12] also noted that multiple pancreatic duct injections (during attempts to cannulate the bile duct), even without acinarization, were of major importance in the aetiology of acute pancreatitis following ERCP. He recommended abandoning the ERCP procedure if several attempted bile duct injections result in pancreatic opacification. Although this approach reduced the incidence of pancreatitis, the success rate of bile duct cannulation was also reduced. During difficult cannulations, the endoscopist must balance the need for specific duct visualization or deep cannulation against possible provocation of complications. Guidelines in this area remain imprecise.

Once entry into a difficult bile duct is achieved, maintenance of that position by use of a guide wire is strongly recommended if subsequent manipulation is required.

As noted, postprocedure pancreatitis may be due to sphincter of Oddi spasm and oedema. In theory, pancreatic stenting may alleviate the obstruction to pancreatic juice flow and reduce the frequency of this complication. In a randomized controlled study, 37 patients who were at high risk for development of postprocedure pancreatitis (because of traumatic manipulation of the papilla, repeated pancreatic duct injections, or difficult EBS) were treated either with placement of a nasopancreatic catheter or with conventional therapy[53]. There was a trend toward less frequent (55% for control subjects versus 37% for stented patients) and less severe postprocedure pancreatitis in the stented group.

Chemical factors

There is evidence that the contrast media used for pancreatography can provoke pancreatitis. Bub and associates[54] demonstrated morphological change in the pancreatic duct epithelium in cats within 10 minutes of contrast medium injection. Similarly, focal pancreatitis was noted microscopically but not clinically in pigs after slow contrast medium injection without acinarization[55].

Contrast media are differentially visualized from surrounding tissue because of their iodine content. The conventional agents are ionic and have high osmolality (approximately 1500mosmol/kg H_2O). The osmolality and ionic nature of these agents are believed to be the major factors responsible for many of the undesirable physiological and adverse effects that occur after intravascular administration[56].

The conventional high-osmolality contrast media are tri-iodinated compounds that dissociate into two osmotically active particles, the tri-iodinated anion (e.g. diatrizoate) and the cation (e.g. sodium or meglumine). These agents provide three iodine atoms for each pair of osmotically active particles in solution[56]. In an attempt to reduce the toxicity of the conventional contrast agents, low-osmolality agents have been developed.

There are data indicating that the new-generation contrast media cause fewer undesirable physiological effects and fewer adverse reactions after intravascular administration[56]. The low-osmolality contrast media (osmolality ranges from 350 to 700mosmol/kg H_2O) provide three iodine atoms for every osmotic particle. As a result, for an equivalent iodine concentration, the osmolality is reduced by 50% or more in comparison to the conventional agents. A 15–25-fold cost increase of the new agents has limited universal replacement of the high-osmolality agents.

It has been suggested that the potential protective effect of the non-ionic, low-osmolality contrast agents is twofold: there is reduced osmotically driven fluid transport across the acini, with an associated smaller increase in intraductal pressure; and such media may have a beneficial free radical scavenging role[57].

There are now ten prospective randomized studies comparing the incidence of pancreatic enzyme elevation and clinical pancreatitis after ERCP using the low- and high-osmolality agents[3,8,9,20–53] (Figure 21.4). Five[3,8,9,58,60,62] studies suggested that the low-osmolality media were safer,

Figure 21.4 Randomized studies comparing high- and low-osmolality contrast agents for post-ERCP pancreatitis and serum pancreatic enzyme elevation. The definition of serum pancreatic enzyme elevation and clinical pancreatitis varied in these series.

Author (ref)	Contrast media (high vs low osmolality)	n enzyme elevation/n ERCP			n clinical pancreatitis/n ERCP		
		High-osmolality	Low-osmolality	p	High-osmolality	Low-osmolality	p
O'Connor et al. (3)	diatrizoate vs iopamidol	23/25	17/25	< 0.05	0/25	0/25	ns
Cunliffe et al. (59)	diatrizoate vs oxaglate	16/48	8/46	ns	8/48	2/46	< 0.05
Hannigan et al. (61)	diatrizoate vs iopamidol	nd[a]	nd	ns	0/32	1/28	ns
Hamilton et al. (58)	diatrizoate vs metrizamide	15/33	8/17	ns	0/33	0/17	ns
Osnes et al. (8)	metrizoate vs metrizamide	nd[a]	nd	< 0.05	0/12	0/12	ns
Barkin et al. (60)	diatrizoate vs iohexol	14/15	16/22	< 0.05	3/15	0/22	ns
	diatrizoate vs ioxaglate		16/16	ns		1/16	ns
Reimer-Jensen et al. (63)	amidotrizoate vs iohexol	8/28	3/26	ns	0/28	0/26	ns
Banerjee et al. (62)	diatrizoate vs iohexol	nd	nd	ns[b]	3/25	0/24	ns
Sherman et al. (19)	diatrizoate vs iohexol	nd	nd	—	25/345	26/345	ns
Johnson et al. (20)	diatrizoate vs iopamidol	nd	nd	—	86/830	83/829	ns
Totals:		105/181 (58%)	93/180 (51.7%)		125/1393 (9.0%)	113/1390 (8.1%)	

diatrizoate = meglumine diatrizoate, nd = not determined, ns = not statistically significant (p > 0.05)
a Only the rise in serum amylase reported, b Median increments in serum amylase levels were similar, but amylase > 1000IU/l occurred in five cases in the high-osmolality group and in none in the low-osmolality group (p = 0.03).

whereas the other five[19,20,58,61,63] showed no difference between the media. In the series reported by Osnes et al.[8], O'Connor et al.[3], Barkin et al.[60] and Banerjee et al.[62], more frequent elevations in serum pancreatic enzyme levels were observed in the high-osmolality group. The occurrence of asymptomatic serum enzyme elevations probably has limited clinical significance and was not tallied in several studies. However, only the Cunliffe et al.[59] study reported a statistically significant difference in the rate of post-ERCP clinical pancreatitis. This study has been criticized[64] because of the high incidence of acinarization and pancreatitis in the high-osmolality contrast media group.

It has been suggested that the failure of these studies to show a difference in the postprocedure pancreatitis rate (when one truly exists; Type II error) may be due to an inadequate sample size[65]. However, two recently reported large, prospective, double-blind randomized trials found that the incidence and severity of postprocedure pancreatitis was similar for the high-osmolality ionic and low-osmolality non-ionic contrast agents[19,20]. Although Chong and Barkin[66] hypothesized that the ionicity rather than the osmolality played a more important role in the pathogenesis of contrast-induced pancreatitis, the two recent studies[19,20] refute this contention.

Parenchymal filling of the pancreas at ERCP provides additional information by demonstrating small parenchymal lesions[67]. However, acinarization with conventional contrast agents has been associated with a 26% incidence of pancreatitis[68]. Two non-controlled studies[67,68] used the low-osmolality agents to cause acinarization to view the pancreatic parenchyma. Four of 66 patients developed pancreatitis (6%, severity unspecified). Although this rate of pancreatitis is higher than that with standard pancreatic ductography alone, it appears to be lower than with pancreatic parenchymato-

graphy performed with the conventional agents. However, no study has been carried out comparing the incidence of pancreatitis after acinarization using the low- and high-osmolality agents.

In summary, the low-osmolality agents appear to have little effect on the incidence and severity of postprocedure pancreatitis. We currently reserve use of the newer, more expensive low-osmolality agents for patients with an allergy to iodinated contrast media.

Hydrostatic factors

Hydrostatic forces, i.e. injection pressure, during injection of contrast media or other fluid into the pancreatic duct, contribute to ductal epithelial or acinar injury. Such injury probably occurs from disruption of cellular membranes or tight junctions between cells and backflow of intraductal contents, especially into the interstitial space[69].

While it remains unclear how this rupture of the ductal system triggers pancreatitis, it appears that even seemingly innocuous substances can cause the morphological changes of pancreatitis[70]. Normal saline solution injected into the pancreatic ducts of rats at sufficient volumes and pressure to cause acinarization resulted in the histological changes of pancreatitis. Larger volumes of saline solution resulted in more severe pancreatitis. Acinarization occurs when the volume of fluid injected into the pancreatic duct exceeds the ductal capacity. Approximately 2ml is adequate to fill the MPD and secondary branches. Quantitation of the volume injected appears to be of limited clinical value, as contrast medium tends to spill into the duodenum. A rapid rate of injection and high-pressure injection contribute to the development of acinarization[70,71]. Acinarization is associated with an increased incidence of post-ERCP pancreatic

Figure 21.5 Selected series reporting the risk of pancreatitis with acinarization. The incidence shows the number of patients with acute pancreatitis from the total with or without acinarization on pancreatography. (Adapted from Sherman and Lehman[44].)

Author (ref)	Year	Contrast agent	Acinarization		No acinarization	
Roszler and Campbell (11)	'85	Meglumine/sodium diatrizoate	11/45	(24.4)	7/95	(7.4)
Cunliffe et al. (59)[a]	'87	Meglumine/sodium diatrizoate	5/12	(41.7)	3/25	(12.0)
		Meglumine/sodium ioxaglate	0/7	(0.0)	2/28	(7.1)
Hamilton et al. (12)	'83	Meglumine/sodium diatrizoate	6/54	(11.1)	9/701	(1.3)
Twomey et al. (68)	'82	Metrizamide	2/43	(4.6)	0/7	(0.0)
Lavelle et al. (67)	'85	Iopamidol	2/17	(11.8)	0/6	(0.0)
LaFerla et al. (2)	'86	Meglumine iothalamate	1/8	(12.5)	4/53	(7.5)
Total			27/186	(14.5)	25/915	(2.8)[b]

a Nineteen patients had an endoscopic sphincterotomy; the presence of acinarization in that subset was not detailed.
b $p < 0.05$ by meta analysis (odds ratio test)

enzyme level elevation and pancreatitis[2,11,12,59,67,68]. Figure 21.5 summarizes six studies since 1982 that detail this association. Freeman and associates[38] reported that acinarization was an independent risk factor for pancreatitis after EBS. Pancreatitis occurred in 29.4% of patients (10 of 34) who had acinarization compared to 5.1% (117 of 2313) who did not ($p = 0.06$; multivariate analysis).

Acinarization can be minimized by reducing the injection pressure. Kasugai et al.[71] made use of a manometer to monitor injection pressure. By opacifying the pancreatic duct at an injection pressure of 90–110mmHg (the corresponding rate of contrast injection is 0.2–0.6ml/s), the incidence of acinar filling was reduced from 22.1% to 2.6%.

Roszler and Campbell[11] showed the strong association of urographic visualization and post-ERCP pancreatitis. In this study, post-ERCP pancreatitis occurred in 4 of 85 (4.7%) patients without urographic visualization or acinarization, in 13 of 29 (45%) with urographic visualization, and in 11 of 45 (24%) with acinarization. This study adds support to the existence of a ducto-interstitial-venous pathway[72] and suggests that urographic visualization would occur if a sufficient volume of contrast were absorbed. The authors theorized that if both acinarization and urographic visualization occurred, the injection pressure and volume would be high enough to result in acinar damage and an increased occurrence of pancreatitis. Since pyelography is associated with a high risk of postprocedure pancreatitis, observation of renal opacification during ERCP is of interest.

Prevention of acinarization requires a high-resolution fluoroscopy unit that permits cessation of contrast injection once side branch filling is observed. Injection 'guns' and mechanical pumps to control injection volumes accurately are available but of uncertain value. The presence of an experienced nursing assistant who injects the contrast media or helps monitor the injection events is mandatory. Some physicians prefer to do the injection themselves.

Sphincter of Oddi manometry (SOM) may induce pancreatitis in as many as 31% of patients[73–75]. Although the aetiology of this pancreatitis appears to be multifactorial, increased pancreatic duct hydrostatic pressure resulting from prolonged perfusion of water into a closed space is believed to be the major inciting factor. In support of this theory, we and others[76] have observed a time-dependent increase in pancreatic duct pressure during prolonged manometry. To reduce the risk of this complication, we have developed a modified triple lumen 5 Fr. SOM catheter that accurately records sphincter pressure measurements while perfused fluid is aspirated[77]. As compared to the standard perfusion catheter, the aspirating manometry catheter is associated with a decreased frequency of serum pancreatic enzyme level elevation, fewer episodes of clinical pancreatitis, reduced hospital stay, and less severe pancreatitis[74]. The hydrostatic theory for post-SOM pancreatitis is further supported by the finding of a negligible incidence of pancreatitis when the bile duct is studied alone[78].

Enzymic factors

In animal models, pancreatitis can be readily provoked by retrograde pancreatic duct injection of activated trypsin, phospholipase A2, bile, and sodium taurocholate[79]. Spontaneous activation of pancreatic enzymes has been reported within acinar cells or intraductally[80]. Simultaneous secretion of protease inhibitors is thought to keep autodigestion from occurring[81]. It is unknown whether an ERCP catheter can carry a pathologically significant quantity of intestinal enzymes (particularly enterokinase) back into the pancreatic ductal system, resulting in the premature activation of zymogens to active proteolytic enzymes.

If enzyme activation at ERCP is a major causative factor in the production of pancreatitis, enzyme inhibitors might be therapeutic. Unfortunately, in two randomized studies[13,82] intravenous aprotinin (Trasylol, a protease inhibitor) prior to and after ERCP failed to reduce the incidence of pancreatic enzyme level elevation and clinical pancreatitis. On the other hand, in a randomized trial, prophylactic C-1-esterase inhibitor (one of the main circulating protease inhibitors) was shown to reduce the height of serum amylase elevation after EBS[83]. No episodes of pancreatitis occurred in the control or treated arms in this series. Additionally, gabexate meslate was shown to reduce the incidence of pancreatic enzyme elevation[84] and pancreatitis[85,86]. More studies evaluating these two protease inhibitors are awaited. Ohlsson and colleagues[87] infused recombinant human pancreatic secretory trypsin inhibitor intraductally in rats and dogs prior to or simultaneously with experimentally induced pancreatitis (with sodium taurocholate in rats and bile in dogs). This inhibitor markedly improved survival and lessened the histological damage to the pancreas, allowing the gland to return to normal after 6 weeks. The implications of the use of this protease inhibitor for the prophylaxis of ERCP- and EBS-induced pancreatitis are clear and await clinical trials.

Microbiological factors

Iatrogenic bacterial seeding (particularly with *Pseudomonas aeruginosa*) of the pancreatic or biliary tree from contaminated equipment has been well documented. Although thorough disinfection and sterilization has been emphasized, reports of this problem continue to appear in the literature[88–93]. Whether microorganisms play any part in the 'average' case of post-ERCP pancreatitis is more doubtful.

Dutta and associates[94] reported a series and summarized the results of 242 patients undergoing ERCP from the literature. Four per cent of patients were found to have positive blood cultures after ERCP and most of these were in patients with pancreatic or bile duct obstruction. Approximately one half of the organisms were *Staphylococcus epidermidis* and thought to be skin or endoscope surface contaminants. Kullman and associates[95] found that 19 of 126 (15%) diagnostic procedures and 18 of 68 (27%) therapeutic procedures were associated with bacteraemia. There was no correlation of bacteraemia with the subsequent development of pancreatitis. Gregg[96] reported that pancreatitis and pancreatic cancer patients commonly had Gram-negative organisms in their pancreatic secretions. Similar findings of Gram-negative organisms were reported in three cases of purulent pancreatitis in the setting of an obstructed pancreatic duct[97]. Chung and associates[98] described an elderly patient with intraductal candidiasis and recurrent bouts of acute pancreatitis. The authors proposed that *Candida* may contribute to symptomatic recurrent inflammation of the pancreas. Microorganisms may therefore reside in or be instilled into the ductal system. Endoscopic manipulation and contrast injection may provoke pancreatitis and/or sepsis in these settings unless drainage is successful.

Most authorities agree that patients with obstructive disease of the pancreas or biliary tree should be treated with broad-spectrum antibiotics prior to the ERCP and/or EBS[40,94,99]. With such treatment, ERCP evaluation of pancreatic pseudocysts appears safe, particularly if surgery is planned[100–102]. If obstructive disease is found during ERCP, antibiotic therapy should be started promptly after the completion of the study. Some endoscopists routinely use prophylactic intravenous antibiotics before ERCP and/or EBS with the rationale that one never knows if an obstructed duct will be identified. However, initial randomized studies of prophylactic antibiotics placed in the contrast media[103] or given systemically[17] have failed to show a lower incidence of post-ERCP pancreatic enzyme level elevation, pancreatitis or sepsis. Recently, Niederau and associates[104] showed that patients treated prophylactically with cefotaxime had less frequent pancreatobiliary sepsis than untreated patients.

Thermal factors

Both ERCP and EBS can induce pancreatic injury by all of the mechanisms discussed above; however, thermal injury is exclusive to EBS. Oedema of the surrounding tissue, produced by electrocautery, is a well recognized consequence[105]. It is thought that cautery in the vicinity of the pancreatic orifice may produce oedema of that orifice and obstruction to the flow of pancreatic juice. While the resistance to pancreatic juice flow has not been measured in this setting, this hypothesis seems reasonable. Such post-EBS oedema is probably of little consequence when the common bile duct is dilated and the greater part of the coagulation is done several millimetres away from the septum or pancreatic duct orifice. However, when pre-cutting[106–108] is used or when an EBS is performed in patients without duct dilatation, oedema is more likely to obstruct the pancreatic orifice. Two prospective randomized studies have evaluated the effect of pancreatic duct stenting on the incidence of postprocedure pancreatitis in high-risk EBS patients. Smithline and colleagues[109] placed 5–7Fr, 2–2.5cm MPD stents after performing standard biliary sphincterotomy in patients with sphincter of Oddi dysfunction and/or small-diameter common bile ducts (< 6mm). Postprocedure pancreatitis occurred in 14% of the stented patients and 18% of the controls (no stent). There was a trend toward more severe pancreatitis and longer hospitalization time for the control group. Sherman and associates[110] placed 5–7Fr, 2–2.5cm pancreatic duct stents in 93 patients undergoing pre-cut needle-knife sphincterotomy. Following the sphincterotomy, patients were randomized either for immediate stent removal or leaving the stent in place for 7–10 days. There was a significant reduction in the pancreatitis rates where the stent was left in place (21% *versus* 2%; *p* = 0.004).

Coagulation current causes more tissue injury and oedema than cutting current. Classen[111] indicated that excessive coagulation current during sphincterotomy increases the risk of pancreatitis. Two preliminary studies[112,113] evaluated the role of pure cutting current in reducing the incidence of post-EBS pancreatitis. In the study of Elta and associates[113], pancreatitis occurred in 1 of 38 patients (2.6%) undergoing EBS with pure cutting current compared to 5 of 39 (12.8%) undergoing EBS with blended current (*p* = 0.09). An increased incidence of bleeding with pure cutting current was not seen in these preliminary studies. However, more patients must be studied to determine the relative risk of haemorrhage for these two techniques.

Allergic reactions and dye absorption

Contrast media are absorbed into the circulation in sufficient quantity to produce urographic visualization in up to 50% of patients after pancreatography with acinarization and as many as 25% of patients without acinarization[11,70]. This is compatible with absorption of contrast media from the acini along the pancreatic ducto-interstitial-venous pathway[72]. Sable *et al.*[114] measured the absorption of contrast media during ERCP and showed that absorption was primarily from the pancreas, with minimal absorption from the biliary tree and small bowel mucosa. Significant amounts of contrast material were measured in the urine after pancreatic duct injection, even in the absence of urographic visualization. The concentration of absorbed dye and the rate of its appearance in the circulation are far lower than for dye entering the circulation during intentional intravenous injection, as found with studies such as intravenous pyelography and angiography.

It appears that the incidence of adverse reactions in vascular procedures is related to the rate of intravenous administration and rapid appearance in the circulation[115,116]. Moreira et al.[117] performed ERCP on 16 patients (a pancreatogram was obtained in 11) who had a history of minor reactions to contrast media. No steroid or antihistamine premedications were given and no patient had an adverse reaction during ERCP or one hour later. However, blood levels were not measured and urographic visualization was not commented on, so it is not clear whether contrast media were absorbed into the circulation[118].

ERCP contrast media reactions are believed to be rare[114,117–119], although we have observed a grand mal seizure in an allergic patient despite premedication with steroids and antihistamines. The most common allergic reaction reported is transitory exanthema[120]. The low frequency of allergic reactions is probably due to slow absorption of contrast media, as well as the relatively low total dose administered (compared to that given for pyelography or angiography).

In a retrospective study, Weiner and colleagues[121] evaluated the ability of prophylactic steroids (either 40mg prednisone orally the night before and one hour before the ERCP or 100mg hydrocortisone intravenously immediately before the ERCP) to reduce the incidence of post-ERCP pancreatitis in 824 iodine-sensitive patients. There was a significant reduction ($p < 0.05$) in the frequency of pancreatitis in the treated group (4.6%) compared to two historical control groups (7.4% and 9.1%). Sherman et al.[112] are currently performing a randomized, controlled trial evaluating the efficacy of oral prednisone in reducing the incidence and severity of postprocedure pancreatitis in patients not allergic to iodine. Pending the results of this and other studies, we feel it is probably prudent to give steroids and antihistamines to patients with a significant history of allergy to iodinated contrast media. Whether any allergic reactions are focally manifest in the pancreas, as pancreatitis, is unknown.

Patient factors

Figure 21.6 lists a variety of clinical settings that may increase the risk of post-ERCP and post-EBS pancreatitis, together with techniques attempting to minimize this complication. Since these factors are not generally correctable prior to the endoscopic study, the endoscopist should carefully weigh the risks and benefits before accepting these challenging patients.

Several investigators have found that early complications are more common when EBS is performed for sphincter of Oddi dysfunction (SOD) than for common duct stones[22,37,38,123–128]. Additionally, the mortality (two times higher for SOD) and late stenosis rate following EBS (approximately four times higher for SOD) are substantially higher in patients with SOD[126]. Freeman et al.[38] reported that SOD was an independent risk factor for post-EBS pancreatitis. Pancreatitis occurred in 19.1% of patients (52 of 272) with SOD compared to 3.6% (75 of 2075; $p < 0.001$ multivariate analysis) of patients with other indications for the EBS. Leese et al.[22] reported complications of EBS in

Factors that increase risk	Technique that may limit pancreatitis
1. Mechanical trauma to papilla	1. Limit cannulation attempts and pancreatic duct injections
2. Acinarization	2. High-resolution fluoroscopy; stop injection once side branches filled
3. Sphincter of Oddi manometry	3. Aspirating catheter; limit intraductal manometry time to <4 minutes
4. Pre-cut biliary sphincterotomy	4. Place pancreatic duct stent prior to pre-cut and leave in place for 7–10 days
5. Thermal injury	5. Cut current (?)
6. Sphincter of Oddi dysfunction or CBD small in diameter	6. See #1–5 above; limit coagulation current near pancreatic orifice during EBS
7. Recurrent or current pancreatitis of any aetiology	7. See #1–6 above; wait 1–2 weeks after pancreatitis resolves if possible
8. History of prior post-ERCP pancreatitis	8. See #7 above
9. History of contrast media reaction	9. Premedicate with steroids; give antihistamines; consider using low-osmolality non-ionic contrast media
10. Pseudocyst	10. Prophylactic antibiotic therapy; limit contrast media filling of pseudocyst; consider pseudocyst decompression within 24 hours

Figure 21.6 Patient and procedural factors that increase the risk of ERCP- and EBS-induced pancreatitis, and techniques that may avoid or limit this complication.

16.2% of patients with SOD (33% had acute pancreatitis), in contrast to 10.3% of patients with CBD stones. In a series of 423 patients undergoing EBS, Sherman and associates[37] reported an overall complication rate of 6.9%, with pancreatitis occurring in 4.0%. However, the complication rate was 10.8% when the EBS was performed for SOD, in contrast to 4.3% for all other indications. A total of 76.5% of the episodes of pancreatitis occurred in the SOD group. The risk of a complication was considerable for a small-diameter common bile duct (< 5mm), particularly when the EBS was performed for SOD (37.5%). In another series, EBS-induced pancreatitis occurred in 13.1% of patients with a normal-calibre duct in contrast to 2.2% with a dilated bile duct (> 10mm)[128]. In contrast, Wilson *et al.*[129] and Cotton *et al.*[130] reported that the complication rate following EBS for bile duct stones was higher or the same (respectively) when the bile duct was dilated.

Several theories have been advanced to explain the increased incidence of pancreatitis when sphincterotomy is performed for SOD. Gregg[76] noted that the hypertrophic or fibrotic sphincter in patients with SOD may increase the risk of pancreatitis, as extended periods of high-intensity current may be required for sphincter ablation. Mechanical factors may also be important. It has been our impression that the common bile duct is more difficult to cannulate deeply and selectively in SOD patients. This may result in repeated cannulation attempts, multiple pancreatic duct injections, and mechanical trauma to the pancreatic orifice[37,38]. Additionally, the basal pancreatic sphincter pressure may be elevated in up to 85% of patients with elevated biliary sphincter pressures[131–133]. Thus, residual pancreatic sphincter stenosis after EBS may predispose to pancreatitis. In a preliminary report, Tarnasky and colleagues[134] evaluated the role of pancreatic sphincterotomy or pancreatic duct stenting in patients with residual pancreatic sphincter hypertension after EBS. Pancreatitis occurred in 1 of 13 patients (8%) who were treated, compared to 4 of 7 patients (57%; *p* < 0.05) who were not. These data support the notion that untreated pancreatic sphincter hypertension may predispose to postprocedure pancreatitis. However, these results need to be confirmed in a larger series and by other centres. Because EBS for SOD is associated with a relatively high incidence of major complications, some authorities recommend a trial of medical management.

A prior history of acute pancreatitis is believed to be a risk factor for ERCP-, EBS- and SOM-induced pancreatitis[9,16,18,50,74,135,136]. In the series reported by Bilbao *et al.*[16], previous pancreatitis had occurred in 66% of patients with post-ERCP pancreatitis. Data from Chen and colleagues[135] suggested that patients with a prior history of pancreatitis (regardless of the cause) tended to develop less severe postprocedure pancreatitis than patients without this history. The authors hypothesized that intralobular and/or periductal fibrosis secondary to prior pancreatitis may limit the degree of ERCP-induced pancreatic acinar damage. Freeman and colleagues[38] reported that post-EBS pancreatitis occurred in 37 of 422 patients (8.8%) with a prior history of pancreatitis and in 90 of 1925 (4.7%) without this history. While these differences were statistically significant in the univariate analysis (*p* < 0.001), prior pancreatitis was

not an independent predictor in the multivariate model. Although prior ERCP-induced pancreatitis is thought to be a risk for this complication on a subsequent ERCP, data on this point are limited. Howerton and associates[136] determined the incidence of postprocedure pancreatitis among 739 patients undergoing ERCP with or without therapy and SOM. Pancreatitis occurred in 3 of 40 patients (8%) with a prior history of postprocedure pancreatitis, and 34 of 699 (5%, *p* > 0.05) without this history. In the study by Freeman and associates[38], prior ERCP-induced pancreatitis was not found to be an independent risk factor for the development of EBS-induced pancreatitis.

Ongoing acute pancreatitis is considered a relative contraindication for the performance of ERCP/EBS[137]. However, since their introduction in 1978 for patients with acute gallstone pancreatitis, ERCP and EBS have proved safe in this setting, and effective[138,139]. In a randomized prospective controlled trial of endoscopic treatment for acute biliary pancreatitis, there was no increased morbidity associated with the endoscopic intervention (despite pancreatic duct filling in 50% of severe cases and 90% of mild cases)[138]. Moreover, urgent EBS and stone removal (if stones were present in the common duct at the time of ERCP) resulted in a reduction in the major complication rate and hospital stay for those patients with severe attacks. Other series of patients undergoing ERCP during an acute pancreatitis episode also suggested that the course of the disease was not worsened by the procedure[140–142]. Moreover, additional pathology of the pancreas may be discovered and useful information in cases possibly requiring surgery (e.g. fistulization) may be provided[143,144]. Although ERCP is of value in defining the cause of acute pancreatitis, it has not been shown to predict the clinical outcome[142].

There has been concern that pancreatography in the setting of a pseudocyst could convert the cavity into a pancreatic abscess, which has a markedly higher morbidity and mortality than the pseudocyst alone[137]. However, data from O'Connor and associates[100] suggest that ERCP is relatively safe, particularly if surgery is planned. In that study there was a 4% incidence of pancreatic sepsis after ERCP. More importantly, there were no episodes of clinical sepsis in patients not operated on (0 of 5) after ERCP and only 2 cases (of 16) when surgery was delayed beyond 24 hours. In a follow-up study[101], it was found that the complication rates were not significantly different among patients having both ERCP and surgery, surgery alone, or ERCP alone. However, when pancreatography is performed in the presence of a pseudocyst, we recommend broad-spectrum prophylactic antibiotic therapy, limited pseudocyst injection, and consideration (within 24–48 hours) of pseudocyst drainage by surgical, endoscopic or percutaneous means. In the setting of necrotizing pancreatitis of suspected gallstone aetiology, we recommend not injecting the pancreatic duct unless laparotomy (and generally necrosectomy) are already planned.

A Swedish group emphasized caution when performing pancreatography in patients with homozygous alpha-1-antitrypsin deficiency[145]. This group reported two cases of haemorrhagic pancreatitis (one death) following ERCP, presumably due to the absence of circulating antiprotease. However,

Pseudomonas aeruginosa was cultured in both cases, suggesting instrument contamination. Conn and associates[146] reported that post-ERCP pancreatitis occurred in 3 of 10 patients with serum alpha-2-macroglobulin (the other key circulating pancreatic protease inhibitor) levels below 243mg/dl but in no patients with higher levels[146]. This study also suggested that low levels of circulatory alpha-2-macroglobulin may predispose to postprocedure pancreatitis.

MANAGEMENT OF POST-ERCP AND POST-EBS PANCREATITIS

A transient increase of abdominal pain with or without serum amylase level elevation is common after ERCP with or without therapy and is generally ignored, with patients permitted at least a clear liquid diet. If the pain is more severe and is associated with abdominal tenderness, distension and an amylase level elevation more than 3–5 times normal, pancreatitis is commonly diagnosed (in the absence of free air or other causes of pain) and will usually require hospital admission or prolongation of the hospital stay. If the patient appears acutely ill in the first 12–24 hours after the procedure, retroduodenal perforation must be differentiated from pancreatitis. However, this may be difficult if a small perforation is missed at post-EBS ductography and no free air is present on the plain abdominal X-ray film[33,147]. At the first suspicion of perforation, a computed tomography (CT) scan, with oral and intravenous contrast media, should be done to distinguish perforation from pancreatitis[148]. Moreover, the CT scan may provide an early diagnosis and prognosis for acute pancreatitis[149,150].

Most post-procedure pancreatitis is graded as mild (see Figure 21.3). It usually resolves within 3 days and is associated with fewer than three Ranson criteria[41]. We usually treat these patients with gut rest, intravenous fluids and liberal parenteral analgesics. Diagnostic undertakings are generally not needed other than simple screening laboratory studies.

If the symptom complex is more severe and associated with ileus, fever, and/or significant third spacing of fluid, moderate to severe pancreatitis is diagnosed. In addition to the above mentioned therapy, we usually treat these patients with broad-spectrum antibiotics as bacteria may have been introduced during the ERCP. Nasogastric suction is often necessary when nausea and vomiting are significant. Parenteral hyperalimentation should also be used if it appears that the pancreatitis is not improving after 3–5 days. Intensive care unit monitoring and placement of a Swan–Ganz catheter may be required to clarify the intravascular fluid status in patients who have a rising blood urea nitrogen level, pulmonary infiltrates and effusions. If the patient continues to have a toxic course, especially with a temperature above 39°C and a white cell count > 20,000/l, the possibility of bacterial infection is significant. Surgical consultation should be obtained. A CT scan should be performed to look for fluid collections and extraluminal gas (as a sign of abscess or perforation), and to evaluate the general amount of pancreatic oedema/necrosis.

Recent interest has centred on the identification of pancreatic and peripancreatic necrosis by CT scan using rapid bolus intravenous contrast medium[151]. Non-enhanced areas of pancreas are thought to represent parenchyma that is either necrotic or at significant risk of necrosis[152]. The quantity of necrotic tissue is directly correlated with the likelihood of bacterial infection, development of systemic complications and mortality[153,154]. Infection or pancreatic necrosis may occur in 40–70% of patients[155].

If peripancreatic fluid or inflammatory solid tissue changes are found on CT scan in patients who are acutely ill, percutaneous aspiration[156] for culture and sensitivity, as well as a Gram stain, should be strongly considered. Using ultrasonography (US) or CT scan guidance, this technique has been shown to be safe and reliably distinguishes between fluid collections that are sterile and those that are infected[157]. Gerzof *et al.*[156] showed the benefits of needle aspiration of fluid or solid areas to differentiate severe sterile pancreatitis from pancreatic infection. This series pointed out that patients appear to have equal toxicity whether bacterial infection is present or not. Because of the significant morbidity and mortality associated with pancreatic infection, aspiration is necessary to guide further therapy. Gram stains revealed an organism in 41 of 42 infected aspirates. All 42 infected aspirates were confirmed by culture. All 50 sterile aspirates were judged to be true negatives on the basis of cultures obtained either at surgery, at the time of repeated aspiration, or by resolution of the pancreatic mass without surgery. Interestingly, 20 of the 36 patients had positive aspirates within 2 weeks of the onset of pancreatitis.

Like other intra-abdominal infections, most pancreatitis-related infections are polymicrobic, with coliforms being the most frequently isolated pathogens. *Staphylococcus aureus*, anaerobes and *Candida* spp are found in 10–20% of cases[158].

Büchler and colleagues[159] analysed the human pancreatic tissue concentration of 10 different bactericidal antibiotics that cover the spectrum of bacteria commonly found in pancreatic infection. Ciprofloxacin, ofloxacin and imipenem had high tissue concentrations as well as high bactericidal activity against most of the organisms recovered. Although antibiotic therapy should be instituted or continued, pending culture results, surgical debridement followed by percutaneous drainage (of residual fluid collections) and lavage of the infected area is the mainstay of treatment[158]. Percutaneous drainage guided by US or CT scan can be performed, particularly in patients who are at a prohibitive operative risk or in patients with localized abscess with safe percutaneous access routes[160]. Because several reports have indicated a high failure rate of percutaneous therapy of infected pancreatic necrosis and pancreatic abscesses[161,162], surgical intervention has been advocated[157,163–166]. The surgical approaches are varied and depend on the extent of necrosis and/or infection, size, location of fluid collections, and operator preferences[158]. Management of such complex patients usually requires a team approach, with a radiologist, surgeon and multiple members of a medical group of gastroenterologists, pulmonologists and nephrologists participating. Patients who have culture-negative aspirates can often be managed medically, but will usually require prolonged hospitalization. Recent data have suggested that early (< 72 hours) administration of imipenem reduces the incidence of pancreatic sepsis in patients with pancreatic necrosis[167].

Patients with post-ERCP pancreatitis who have persistent pain and multiple peripancreatic fluid collections after 4–6 weeks of gut rest and hyperalimentation may have disruption of the MPD. Endoscopic stenting of the MPD and/or transpapillary catheter placement to divert juice flow may resolve such fluid collections[168]. The frequency with which such endoscopic measures totally resolve the inflammatory process is uncertain. Many patients already enduring an endoscopy-associated complication are reluctant to try endoscopic therapy.

PREVENTION OF ERCP/EBS-ASSOCIATED PANCREATITIS

Complications from ERCP and EBS are expected and are, in part, unavoidable. However, attempts must be made to limit the occurrence of these unfavourable events. Unfortunately, only a few techniques have been identified or developed to reduce the incidence of pancreatitis. Careful selection criteria may eliminate patients whose risk:benefit ratio is unfavourable. Figure 21.6 lists the technical factors that logically may reduce the incidence of pancreatitis in high- (and probably low-) risk patients, although controlled studies in humans to evaluate these techniques and confirmatory studies have not been performed in all settings. Overall, the most important techniques to reduce the risk of pancreatitis appear to be limiting the number of cannulation attempts and pancreatic duct injections, avoiding acinarization, limiting coagulation current near the pancreatic duct orifice, pancreatic duct stent placement prior to pre-cut EBS (and leaving the stent in place for 7–10 days), meticulous endoscope disinfection, use of an aspirating SOM catheter when

Figure 21.7 Methods to reduce the incidence of sphincter of Oddi manometry-induced pancreatitis.

Avoid pancreatic manometry

Limit pancreatic manometry to < 4 minutes

Decrease the rate of water perfusion

Drain the pancreatic duct after manometry

Use a microtransducer manometry catheter

Use an aspirating catheter

manometry of the pancreatic duct sphincter is being performed, and, perhaps, premedication with oral steroids and antihistamines for patients with previous contrast media reactions[40,44]. Unfortunately, in SOD patients undergoing EBS (the group at greatest risk for postprocedure pancreatitis), no method has been developed that has been definitively shown to reduce the incidence of postprocedure pancreatitis. Figure 21.7 lists other methods to reduce the incidence of postmanometry pancreatitis[75].

Clinical judgment, preferably based on extensive endoscopic experience, must be exercised especially in difficult cannulation or sphincterotomy settings. Limiting cannulation attempts or other possible hazardous manoeuvres may not be practical and may result in a high failure rate. This may, in turn, result in more percutaneous transhepatic diagnostic and therapeutic manoeuvres, exploratory surgeries, referral to specialized ERCP centres, or untreated primary disease states. Such procedural and patient management decisions continue as part of the 'art of medicine'.

References

1. Skude G, Wehlin L, Maruyama T, Ariyama J. Hyperamylasemia after duodenoscopy and retrograde cholangiopancreatography. *Gut* 1976; 17: 127–32.

2. LaFerla G, Gordon S, Archibald M, Murray WR. Hyperamylasemia and acute pancreatitis following endoscopic retrograde cholangiopancreatography. *Pancreas* 1986; 1:160–3.

3. O'Connor HJ, Ellis WR, Manning AP, Lintott DJ, McMahon MJ, Axon ATR. Iopamidol as contrast medium in endoscopic retrograde pancreatography: a prospective randomized comparison with diatrizoate. *Endoscopy* 1988; 20:244–7.

4. Weaver DW, Sugawa C, Bouwman DL, Altshuler J. Isoamylase analyses in patients undergoing ERCP. *Gastrointest Endosc* 1983; 29:175A.

5. Blackwood WD, Vennes JA, Silvis SE. Post-endoscopy pancreatitis and hyperamylasuria. *Gastrointest Endosc* 1973; 20:56–8.

6. Tulassay Z, Papp J, Koranyi L, Szathmari M, Tamas G. Hormonal and biochemical changes following endoscopic retrograde cholangiopancreatography. *Acta Gastroenterol Belg* 1981; 44:538–43.

7. Bordas JM, Toledo V, Mondelo F, Rodes J. Prevention of pancreatic reactions by bolus samatostatin administration in patients undergoing endoscopic retrograde cholangiopancreatography and endoscopic sphincterotomy. *Hormone Res* 1988; 29:106–8.

8. Osnes M, Skjennald A, Larsen S. A comparison of a new nonionic (metrizamide) and a dissociable (metrizoate) contrast medium in endoscopic retrograde pancreatography (ERP). *Scand J Gastroenterol* 1977; 12:821–5.

9. Nebel OT, Silvis SE, Rogers G, Sugawa C, Mandelstam P. Complications associated with endoscopic retrograde cholangiopancreatography: results of the 1974 ASGE survey. *Gastrointest Endosc* 1975; 22:34–6.

10. Reiertsen O, Skjoto J, Jacobsen CD, Rosseland AR. Complications of fiberoptic gastrointestinal endoscopy – five years' experience in a central hospital. *Endoscopy* 1987; 19:1–6.

11. Roszler MH, Campbell WL. Post-ERCP pancreatitis: association with urographic visualization during ERCP. *Radiology* 1985; 157:595–8.

12. Hamilton I, Lintott DJ, Rothwell J, Axon ATR. Acute pancreatitis following endoscopic retrograde cholangiopancreatography. *Clin Radiol* 1983; 34:543–6.

13. Brust R, Thomson ABR, Wensel RH, Sherbaniuk RW, Costopoulos L. Pancreatic injury following ERCP: failure of prophylactic benefit of Trasylol. *Gastrointest Endosc* 1977; 24:77–9.

14. Tyden G, Nyberg B, Sonnenfeld T, Thulin L. Effect of somatostatin on hyperamylasemia following endoscopic pancreatography. *Acta Chir Scand* 1986; 530(S):43–5.

15. Montori A, Viceconte G, Viceconte GW, Bogliolo G. ERCP and EPT: Italian experience. *Endoscopy* 1979; 11:142–5.

16. Bilbao MK, Dotter CT, Lee TG, Katon RM. Complications of endoscopic retrograde cholangiopancreatography (ERCP): a study of 10,000 cases. *Gastroenterology* 1976; 70:314–20.

17. Brandes JW, Scheffer B, Lorenz-Meyer H, Korst HA, Littmann KP. ERCP: complications and prophylaxis: a controlled study. *Endoscopy* 1981; 13:37–40.

18. Zimmon DS, Falkenstein DB, Riccobono C, Aaron B. Complications of endoscopic retrograde cholangiopancreatography. *Gastroenterology* 1975; 69:303–9.

19. Sherman S, Hawes RH, Rathgaber SW et al. Post-ERCP pancreatitis: randomized prospective study comparing a low and high osmolality contrast agent. *Gastrointest Endosc* 1994; 40:422–7.

20. Johnson GK, Geenen JE, Bedford RA et al. A comparison of nonionic versus ionic contrast media: results of a prospective multicenter study. *Gastrointest Endosc* 1995; 42:312–16.

21. Tedesco FJ, Vennes JA, Dreyer M. Endoscopic sphincterotomy: the USA experience. In *Endoscopic Surgery*. Edited by H Okabe, T Honda, F Oshiba. Elsevier Science: New York. 1984:41–6.

22. Leese T, Neoptolemos JP, Carr-Locke DL. Successes, failures, early complications and their management following endoscopic sphincterotomy: results in 394 consecutive patients from a single centre. *Br J Surg* 1985; 72:215–19.

23. Roberts-Thomson IC. Endoscopic sphincterotomy of the papilla of Vater: an analysis of 300 cases. *Aust NZ J Med* 1984; 14:611–17.

24. Neuhaus B, Safrany L. Complications of endoscopic sphincterotomy and their treatment. *Endoscopy* 1981; 13:197–9.

25. Cotton PB, Vallon AG. British experience with duodenoscopic sphincterotomy for removal of bile duct stones. *Br J Surg* 1981; 68:373–5.

26. Viceconte G, Viceconte GW, Pietropaolo V, Montori A. Endoscopic sphincterotomy: indications and results. *Br J Surg* 1981; 68:376–80.

27. Lam SK. A study of endoscopic sphincterotomy in recurrent pyogenic cholangitis. *Br J Surg* 1984; 71:262–6.

28. Mustard R, Mackenzie R, Jamieson C, Haber GB. Surgical complications of endoscopic sphincterotomy. *Can J Surg* 1984; 27:215–17.

29. Arendt R, Bosseckert H, Rogos R, Schulz JH, Schentke U, Schwenke U. Experience with endoscopic sphincterotomy in the GDR: a collective study of 6 centres. *Endoscopy* 1983; 15:173–4.

30. Vaira D, d'Anna L, Ainley C et al. Endoscopic sphincterotomy in 1000 consecutive patients. *Lancet* 1989; ii:431–3.

31. Geenen JE, Vennes JA, Silvis SE. Resumé of a seminar on endoscopic sphincterotomy (ERS). *Gastrointest Endosc* 1981; 27:31–8.

32. Escourrou J, Cordova JA, Laxorthes F, Frexinos J, Ribet A. Early and late complications after endoscopic sphincterotomy for biliary lithiasis with and without the gallbladder 'in situ'. *Gut* 1984; 25:598–602.

33. Dunham F, Bourgeois N. Gelin M, Jeanmart J, Toussaint J, Cremer M. Retroperitoneal perforations following endoscopic sphincterotomy: clinical course and management. *Endoscopy* 1982; 14:92–6.

34. Kawai K, Nakajima M. Present status and complications of EST in Japan. *Endoscopy* 1983; 15:169–72.

35. Safrany L. Endoscopic treatment of biliary-tract diseases: an international study. *Lancet* 1978; 2:983–5.

36. Lambert ME, Betts CD, Hill J et al. Endoscopic sphincterotomy: the whole truth. *Br J Surg* 1991; 78:473–6.

37. Sherman S, Ruffolo TA, Hawes RH, Lehman GA. Complications of endoscopic sphincterotomy: a prospective series with emphasis on the increased risk associated with sphincter of Oddi dysfunction and nondilated bile ducts. *Gastroenterology* 1991; 101:1068–75.

38. Freeman M, Nelson D, Sherman S et al. Complications of endoscopic biliary sphincterotomy. *N Engl J Med* 1996; 335:909–918.

39. Uzer M, Kopecky K, Wass J et al. Correlation between clinical assessment and computed tomography (CT) findings in detection of acute pancreatitis (AP) occurring after ERCP. *Am J Gastroenterol* 1993; 88:1543A.

40. Cotton PB, Lehman G, Vennes J et al. Endoscopic sphincterotomy complications and their management: an attempt at consensus. *Gastrointest Endosc* 1991; 37:383–93.

41. Ranson JHC, Rifkind KM, Roses DF, Fink SD, Eng K, Spencer FC. Prognostic signs and the role of operative management in acute pancreatitis. *Surg Gynecol Obstet* 1974; 139:69–81.

42. Rolny P, Anderberg B, Ihse I, Lindstrom E, Olaison G. Pancreatitis following endoscopic sphincter of Oddi manometry. *Gastrointest Endosc* 1992; 38:201–2.

43. Sherman S, Lehman GA. Pancreatitis after sphincter of Oddi manometry. *Gastrointest Endosc* 1991; 37:214–15.

44. Sherman S, Lehman GA. ERCP- and endoscopic sphincterotomy-induced pancreatitis. *Pancreas* 1991; 6:350–67.

45. Deschamps JP, Allemand H, Magnificat RJ, Camelot G, Gillet M, Carayon P. Acute pancreatitis following gastrointestinal endoscopy without ampullary cannulation. *Endoscopy* 1982; 14:105–6.

46. Polack EP, Fainsinger MH, Bonnano SV. A death following complications of roentgenologic nonoperative manipulation of common bile duct calculi. *Radiology* 1977; 123:585–6.

47. Saari A, Kivisaari L, Standertskjold-Nordenstam CG, Brackett K, Schroder T. Experimental pancreatography: a comparison of three contrast media. *Scand J Gastroenterol* 1988; 23:53–8.

48. Bedford RA, Johnson GK, Geenen JE et al. Does additive diagnostic or therapeutic therapy influence the incidence of post-ERCP pancreatitis. *Am J Gastroenterol* 1993; 88:1525A.

49. Cohen N, Lipshutz W, Wright S, Aronchick C. Pancreatic duct occlusion: a possible etiologic factor in pancreatitis post-ERCP and sphincter of Oddi manometry (SOM). *Gastrointest Endosc* 1989; 35:190A.

50. Podolsky I, Haber GB, Kortan P, Gray R. Risk factors for pancreatitis following ERCP: a prospective study. *Am J Gastroenterol* 1987; 82:972A.

51. Alam K, Schubert TT, Wong DK. Risk factors for the development of post-ERCP pancreatitis. *Gastrointest Endosc* 1992; 38:246A.

52. Johnson G, Cass O, Geenen J et al. Post-ERCP pancreatitis: a comparative study of patients with and without pancreatic duct injections at the time of ERCP. *Gastrointest Endosc* 1993; 39:319A.

53. Shakoor T, Hogan WJ, Geenen JE. Efficacy of nasopancreatic catheter in the prevention of post-ERCP pancreatitis: a prospective randomized controlled trial. *Gastrointest Endosc* 1992; 38:251A.

54. Bub H, Burner W, Riemann JF, Stolte M. Morphology of the pancreatic ductal epithelium after traumatization of the papilla of Vater or endoscopic retrograde pancreatography with contrast media in cats. *Scand J Gastroenterol* 1983; 18:581–92.

55. Kivisaari L, Alitalo I. The immediate effects of retrograde pancreatography on the pancreas. *Eur J Radiol* 1984; 4:58–60.

56. King BF, Hartman GW, Williamson B, LeRoy AJ, Hattery RR. Low-osmolality contrast media: a current perspective. *Mayo Clin Proc* 1989; 64:976–85.

57. Banerjee AK. Different contrast agents and development of pancreatitis after endoscopic retrograde pancreatography. *Am J Gastroenterol* 1992; 87:683–4.

58. Hamilton I, Lintott DJ, Rothwell J, Axon ATR. Metrizamide as contrast medium in endoscopic retrograde cholangiopancreatography. *Clin Radiol* 1982; 33:293–5.

59. Cunliffe WJ, Cobden I, Lavelle MI, Lendrum R, Tait NP, Venables CW. A randomized, prospective study comparing two contrast media in ERCP. *Endoscopy* 1987; 19:201–2.

60. Barkin JS, Casal GL, Reiner DK, Goldberg RI, Phillips RS, Kaplan S. A comparative study of contrast agents for endoscopic retrograde pancreatography. *Am J Gastroenterol* 1991; 86:1437–41.

61. Hannigan BF, Keeling PWN, Slavin B, Thompson RPH. Hyperamylasemia after ERCP with ionic and non-ionic contrast media. *Gastrointest Endosc* 1985; 31:109–10.

62. Banerjee AK, Grainger SL, Thompson RPH. Trial of low versus high osmolality contrast media in endoscopic retrograde cholangiopancreatography. *Br J Clin Pract* 1990; 44:445–7.

63. Reimer Jensen A, Malchow–Moller A, Matzen P *et al*. A randomized trial of iohexol versus Amidotrizoate in endoscopic retrograde pancreatography. *Scand J Gastroenterol* 1985; 20:83–6.

64. Rambow A, Staritz M, Meyer zum Buschenfelde KH. Contrast media for ERCP. *Endoscopy* 1988; 20:126–7.

65. Cotton PB, Brazer SR. Different contrast agents and development of pancreatitis after endoscopic retrograde pancreatography. *Am J Gastroenterol* 1992; 87:682.

66. Chong J, Barkin JS. Analysis of comparative studies using different contrast agents for endoscopic retrograde cholangiopancreatography. *Dig Endosc* 1992; 5:206–12.

67. Lavelle MI, Tait NP, Walsh T, Alderson D, Record CO. Demonstration of pancreatic parenchyma by digital subtraction techniques during endoscopic retrograde cholangiopancreatography. *Clin Radiol* 1985; 36:405–7.

68. Twomey B, Wilkin RA, Levi AJ. Pancreatic parenchymography using metrizamide. *Gut* 1982; 23:462A.

69. Bockman DE, Schiller WR, Anderson MC. Route of retrograde flow in the exocrine pancreas during dutal hypertension. *Arch Surg* 1971; 103:321–9.

70. Kivisaari L. Contrast absorption and pancreatic inflammation following experimental ERCP. *Invest Radiol* 1979; 14:493–7.

71. Kasugai T, Kuno N, Kizu M. Manometric endoscopic retrograde pancreatography: technique, significance and evaluation. *Am J Dig Dis* 1974; 19:485–502.

72. Waldron RL, Luse SA, Wollowick HE, Seaman WB. Demonstration of a retrograde pancreatic pathway: correlation of roentgenographic and electron microscopic studies. *Am J Roentgenol* 1971; 111:695–9.

73. Rolny P, Anderberg B, Ihse I, Lindstrom E, Olaison G, Arvill A. Pancreatitis after sphincter of Oddi manometry. *Gut* 1990; 31:821–4.

74. Sherman S, Troiano FP, Hawes RH, Lehman GA. Sphincter of Oddi manometry: decreased risk of clinical pancreatitis with use of a modified aspirating catheter. *Gastrointest Endosc* 1990; 36:462–6.

75. Hawes RH, Lehman GA. Complications of sphincter of Oddi manometry and their prevention. *Gastrointest Endosc Clin N Am* 1993; 3:107–18.

76. Gregg JA. Function and dysfunction of the sphincter of Oddi. In *ERCP: Diagnostic and Therapeutic Applications*. Edited by IM Jacobson. Elsevier Science, New York. 1989: 139–70.

77. Sherman S, Troiano FP, Hawes RH, Lehman GA. Does continuous aspiration from an end and side port in a sphincter of Oddi manometry (SOM) catheter alter recorded pressures? *Gastrointest Endosc* 1990; 36:500–3.

78. Sherman S, Hawes RH, Troiano FP, Lehman GA. Pancreatitis following bile duct sphincter of Oddi manometry: utility of the aspirating catheter. *Gastrointest Endosc* 1992; 30:347–50.

79. Steer ML. Experimental models of pancreatitis. In *Acute Pancreatitis: Experimental and Clinical Aspects of Pathogenesis and Management*. Edited by G Glazer G, JHL Ranson. Baillière Tindall, London. 1988: 207–26.

80. Leach SD, Gorelick FS, Modlin IM. New perspectives on acute pancreatitis. *Scand J Gastroenterol* 1992; 27(S192):29–38.

81. Eddeland A, Wehlin L. Secretin/cholecystokinin-stimulated secretion of trypsinogen and trypsin inhibitor in pure human pancreatic juice collected by endoscopic retrograde pancreatic catheterizations. *Hoppe Seylers Z Physiol Chem* 1978; 359:1653–8.

82. Koch H, Belohlavek D, Schaffner O, Tympner F, Rosch W, Demling L. Prospective study for the prevention of pancreatitis following endoscopic retrograde cholangiopancreatography (ERCP). *Endoscopy* 1975; 7:221–4.

83. Testoni PA, Cicardi M, Bergamachini L *et al*. Intusion of C1-inhibitor plasma concentrate prevents hyperamylasemia induced by endoscopic sphincterotomy. *Gastrointest Endosc* 1995; 42:301–5.

84. Benini L, Angelini G, Lavarini E *et al*. Effect of a new enzyme inhibitor (gabexate mesilate – FOY) on hyperenzymemic induced by ERCP. A double blind study. *Digestion* 1985; 32:165A.

85. Matsunaga E, Sata Y, Nakashima H. Prophylactic effects of FOY in post-ERCP pancreatitis. *Gendai Iryo* 1979; 11:1213–16.

86. Cavallini G, Tittobello A. Gabexate mesilate (Foy) in the prevention of pancreatic damage secondary to endoscopic maneuvers on Vater's papilla. Results of an Italian randomized double-blind multicenter study. *Gastroenterology* 1995; 108:348A.

87. Ohlsson K, Olsson R, Bjork P *et al*. Local admistration of human pancreatic secretory trypsin inhibitor prevents the development of experimental acute pancreatitis in rats and dogs. *Scand J Gastroenterol* 1989; 24:693–704.

88. Godiwala T, Andry M, Agrawal N, Ertran A. Consecutive *Serratia marcescens* infections following endoscopic retrograde cholangiopancreatography. *Gastrointest Endosc* 1988; 34:345–7.

89. Classen DC, Jacobson JA, Burke JP, Jacobson JT, Evans RS. Serious Pseudomonas infections associated with endoscopic retrograde cholangiopancreatography. *Am J Med* 1988; 84:592–6.

90. Allen JI, O'Connor Allen M, Olsen MM *et al*. Pseudomonas infection of the biliary system from use of a contaminated endoscope. *Gastroenterology* 1987; 92:759–63.

91. Doherty DE, Falko JM, Lefkovitz N, Rogers J, Fromkes J. *Pseudomonas aeruginosa* sepsis following retrograde cholangiopancreatography (ERCP). *Dig Dis Sci* 1982; 27:169–70.

92. Deviere J, Motte S, Dumonceau JM, Serruys E, Thys JP, Cremer M. Septicemia after endoscopic retrograde cholangiopancreatography. *Endoscopy* 1990; 22:72–5.

93. Struelens MJ, Rost F, Deplano A *et al*. *Pseudomonas aeruginosa* and Enterobacteriaceae bacteremia after biliary endoscopy: an outbreak investigation using DNA macrorestriction and analysis. *Am J Med* 1993; 95:489–98.

94. Dutta SK, Cox M, Williams RB, Eisenstat TE, Standiford HC. Prospective evaluation of the risk of bacteremia and the role of antibiotics in ERCP. *J Clin Gastroenterol* 1983; 5:325–9.

95. Kullman E, Borch K, Lindstrom E, Ansehn S, Ihse I, Anderberg B. Bacteremia following diagnostic and therapeutic ERCP. *Gastrointest Endosc* 1992; 38:444–9.

96. Gregg JA. Detection of bacterial infection of the pancreatic ducts in patients with pancreatitis and pancreatic cancer during endoscopic cannulation of the pancreatic duct. *Gastroenterology* 1977; 73:1005–7.

97. Ayela P, Ponchon T, Valette PJ, Chavaillon A. Sepsis following injection of obstructed pancreatic ducts. *Endoscopy* 1989; 21:242.

98. Chung RT, Schapiro RH, Warshaw AL. Intraluminal pancreatic candidiasis presenting as recurrent pancreatitis. *Gastroenterology* 1993; 104:1532–4.

99. Hershey SD, Sugawa C, Cushing R, Ledgerwood AM, Lucas CE. The value of prophylactic antibiotic therapy during endoscopic retrograde cholangiopancreatography. *Surg Gynecol Obstet* 1982; 155:801–3.

100. O'Connor M, Kolars J, Ansel H, Silvis S, Vennes J. Preoperative endoscopic retrograde cholangiopancreatography in the surgical management of pancreatic pseudocysts. *Am J Surg* 1986; 151:18–23.

101. Kolars JC, O'Connor Allen M, Ansel J, Silvis SE, Vennes JA. Pancreatic pseudocysts: clinical and endoscopic experience. *Am J Gastroenterol* 1989; 84:259–64.

102. Lehman GA. Endoscopic management of pancreatic pseudocysts continues to evolve. *Gastrointest Endosc* 1995; 42:273–5.

103. Colleen MJ, Hanan MR, Maher JA, Stubrin SE. Modification of endoscopic retrograde cholangiopancreatography (ERCP) septic complications by the addition of an antibiotic to the contrast media. *Am J Gastroenterol* 1980; 74:493–6.

104. Niederau C, Pohlmann U, Lubke H, Thomas L. Prophylactic antibiotic treatment in therapeutic or complicated diagnostic ERCP: results of a randomized controlled clinical study. *Gastrointest Endosc* 1994; 40:533–7.

105. Sivak MV Jr. Endoscopic management of bile duct stones. *Am J Surg* 1989; 158:228–40.

106. Shakoor T, Geenen JE. Pre-cut papillotomy. *Gastrointest Endosc* 1992; 38:623–7.

107. Tweedle DEF, Martin DF. Needle knife papillotomy for endoscopic sphincterotomy and cholangiography. *Gastrointest Endosc* 1991; 375:518–21.

108. Dowsett JF, Polydorou AA, Vaira D *et al*. Needle knife papillotomy: how safe and how effective? *Gut* 1990; 31:905–8.

109. Smithline A, Silverman W, Rogers D et al. Effect of prophylactic main pancreatic duct stenting on the incidence of biliary endoscopic sphincterotomy-induced pancreatitis in high-risk patients. *Gastrointest Endosc* 1993; 39:652–7.

110. Sherman S, Earle D, Bucksot L, Baute P, Gottlieb K, Lehman G. Does leaving a main pancreatic duct stent in place reduce the incidence of precut biliary sphincterotomy (ES)-induced pancreatitis? A final analysis of a randomized prospective study. *Gastrointest Endosc* 1996; 43:412A.

111. Classen M. Endoscopic papillotomy. In *Gastroenterologic Endoscopy*. Edited by M Sivak. WB Saunders, Philadelphia. 1987: 631–51.

112. Paschricha PJ, Tietjen TG, Kallos AN. Pure cutting vs blended current for endoscopic sphincterotomy: a prospective blinded controlled trial. *Gastrointest Endosc* 1994; 40:31A.

113. Elta GA, Barnett JL, Brown KA. Pure cut electrocautery current for sphincterotomy causes less post-procedure pancreatitis than blended current. *Gastrointest Endosc* 1995; 41:395A.

114. Sable RA, Rosenthal WS, Siegel J, Jankowski RH. Absorption of contrast medium during ERCP. *Dig Dis Sci* 1983; 28:801–6.

115. Shehadi WH. Adverse reactions to intravascularly administered contrast media: a comprehensive study based on a prospective survey. *Am J Roentgenol* 1975; 124:145–52.

116. Saltzman GH, Sundstrom KA. The influence of different contrast media for cholography on blood pressure and pulse rate. *Acta Radiol* 1960; 54:353–64.

117. Moreira VF, Merono E, Larraona JL et al. ERCP and allergic reactions to iodized contrast media. *Gastrointest Endosc* 1985; 31:293.

118. Ladas SD, Rokkas T, Kaskarelis J, Hatzioannou J, Raptis S. Absorption of iodized contrast media. *Gastrointest Endosc* 1986; 32:376.

119. Classen M, Phillip J. Newer endoscopic techniques for image diagnosis and management of hepatobiliary disease. *Semin Liver Dis* 1982; 2:67–74.

120. Lorenz R. Allergic reaction to contrast medium after endoscopic retrograde pancreatography. *Endoscopy* 1990; 22:196.

121. Weiner GR, Geenen JE, Hogan WJ, Catalano MF. Use of corticosteroids in the prevention of post-ERCP pancreatitis. *Gastrointest Endosc* 1995; 42:579–83.

122. Sherman S, Lehman G, Earle D et al. Does prophylactic steroid administration reduce the frequency and severity of post-ERCP pancreatitis?: randomized, prospective, multicenter study. *Gastrointest Endosc* 1996; 43:320A.

123. Siegel JH. Endoscopic papillotomy in the treatment of biliary tract disease. *Dig Dis Sci* 1981; 26:1057–64.

124. Neoptolemos JP, Bailey IS, Carr-Locke DL. Sphincter of Oddi dysfunction: results of treatment by endoscopic sphincterotomy. *Br J Surg* 1988; 75:454–9.

125. Thatcher BS, Sivak MV, Tedesco FJ, Vennes JA, Hutton SW, Achkar EA. Endoscopic sphincterotomy for suspected dysfunction of the sphincter of Oddi. *Gastrointest Endosc* 1987; 33:91–5.

126. Classen M. Endoscopic papillotomy – new indications, short- and long-term results. *Clin Gastroenterol* 1986; 15:457–69.

127. Krims PE, Cotton PB. Papillotomy and functional disorders of the sphincter of Oddi. *Endoscopy* 1988; 20:203–6.

128. Chen YK, Foliente RL, Santoro MJ, Walter MH, Collen MJ. Endoscopic sphincterotomy-induced pancreatitis: increased risk associated with nondilated bile ducts and sphincter of Oddi dysfunction. *Am J Gastroenterol* 1994; 89:327–33.

129. Wilson MS, Tweedle DEF, Martin DF. Common bile duct diameter and complications of endoscopic sphincterotomy. *Br J Surg* 1992; 79:1346–7.

130. Cotton PB, Geenen J, Sherman S et al. Sphincterotomy for stone is safer than advertised, even in young patients with small ducts. A multicenter prospective study. *Gastrointest Endosc* 1994: 40:104A.

131. Silverman WB, Ruffolo TA, Sherman S, Hawes RH, Lehman GA. Correlation of basal sphincter pressures measured from the bile duct and the pancreatic duct in patients with suspected sphincter of Oddi dysfunction. *Gastrointest Endosc* 1992; 38:440–3.

132. Raddawi HM, Geenen JE, Hogan WJ, Dodds WJ, Venu RP, Johnson GA. Pressure measurements from biliary and pancreatic segments of the sphincter of Oddi. Comparison between patients with functional abdominal pain, biliary or pancreatic disease. *Dig Dis Sci* 1991; 36:71–4.

133. Rolny P, Arleback A, Funch-Jensen P, Kruse A, Jarnevot G. Clinical significance of manometric assessment of both pancreatic duct and bile duct sphincter in the same patient. *Scand J Gastroenterol* 1989; 24:751–4.

134. Tarnasky P, Cunningham J, Cotton P, Hoffman B, Freeman J, Hawes R. Is pancreatic duct obstruction secondary to pancreatic sphincter hypertension (PSH) the cause of post-ERCP pancreatitis in patients with sphincter of Oddi dysfunction. *Gastrointest Endosc* 1995; 41:430A.

135. Chen YK, Abdulian JD, Escalante-Glorsky S, Youssef AI, Foliente RL, Collen MJ. Clinical outcome of post-ERCP pancreatitis: relationship to history of previous pancreatitis. *Am J Gastroenterol* 1995; 90:2120–3.

136. Howerton DW, Geenen JE, Hogan WJ. Post-ERCP pancreatitis: is there increased risk at repeat ERCP. *Gastrointest Endosc* 1993; 39:315A.

137. Ferguson DR, Sivak MV. Indications, contraindications and complications of ERCP. In *Gastroenterologic Endoscopy*. Edited by M Sivak. WB Saunders, Philadelphia. 1987: 581–8.

138. Neoptolemos JP, London NJ, Carr-Locke DL, Bailey IA, James D, Fossard DP. Controlled trial of urgent endoscopic retrograde cholangiopancreatography and endoscopic sphincterotomy versus conservative treatment for acute pancreatitis due to gallstones. *Lancet* 1988; ii:979–83.

139. Fan S-T, Lai ECS, Mok FPT, Lo C-M, Zheng S-S, Wong J. Early treatment of acute biliary pancreatitis by endoscopic papillotomy. *New Engl J Med* 1993; 328:228–32.

140. Scholmerich J, Gross V, Johannesson T et al. Detection of biliary origin in acute pancreatitis. Comparison of laboratory tests, ultrasonography, computed tomography, and ERCP. *Dig Dis Sci* 1989; 34:830–3.

141. Brambs HJ, Scholmerich J, Gross V et al. ERCP in acute pancreatitis. A preliminary report. *Dig Surg* 1988; 5:156–9.

142. Scholmerich J, Lausen M, Lay L et al. Value of endoscopic retrograde cholangiopancreatography in determining the cause but not the course of acute pancreatitis. *Endoscopy* 1992; 24:244–7.

143. Tonak J, Lux G, Gebhardt CH. A surgical approach to hemorrhagic necrotizing pancreatitis based on endoscopic retrograde pancreatography. *Gastrointest Endosc* 1986; 32:104–6.

144. Neoptolemos JP, London NJM, Carr-Locke DL. Assessment of main pancreatic duct integrity by endoscopic retrograde cholangiopancreatography in patients with acute pancreatitis. *Br J Surg* 1993; 80:94–9.

145. Svenberg T, Haggmark T, Strandvik B, Slezak P. Hemorrhagic pancreatitis after ERCP in patients with alpha 1-antitrypsin deficiency. *Lancet* 1988; i:772.

146. Conn M, Goldenberg A, Concepcion L, Mandeli J. The effect of ERCP on circulating pancreatic enzymes and pancreatic protease inhibitors. *Am J Gastroenterol* 1991; 86:1011–14.

147. Sarr MG, Fishman EK, Milligan FD, Siegelman SS, Cameron JL. Pancreatitis or duodenal perforation after peri-Vaterian therapeutic endoscopic procedures: diagnosis, differentiation, and management. *Surgery* 1986; 100:461–6.

148. Kulman JE, Fishman EK, Milligan FD, Siegelman SS. Complications of endoscopic sphincterotomy: computed tomographic evaluation. *Gastrointest Radiol* 1989; 14:127–32.

149. Balthazar EJ. CT diagnosis and staging of acute pancreatitis. *Radiol Clin North Am* 1989; 27:19–37.

150. Claiven PA, Hauser H, Meyer P, Rohner A. Value of contrast-enhanced computerized tomography in the early diagnosis and prognosis of acute pancreatitis: a prospective study of 202 patients. *Am J Surg* 1988; 155:457–66.

151. Freeny PC. Incremental dynamic bolus computed tomography of acute pancreatitis. *Int J Pancreatol* 1993; 13:147–58.

152. Fernandez del-Castillo C, Rattner DE, Warshaw AL. Acute pancreatitis. *Lancet* 1993; 342:475–9.

153. Beger AG. Surgery in acute pancreatitis. *Hepatogastroenterology* 1991; 38:92–6.

154. Banks PA. Modern concepts in acute pancreatitis. *Mt Sinai J Med* 1993; 60:170–4.

155. Rattner DW, Legermate DA, Lee MJ, Muller PR, Warshaw AL. Early surgical debridement of symptomatic pancreatic necrosis is beneficial irrespective of infection. *Am J Surg* 1992; 163:105–9.

156. Gerzof SG, Banks PA, Robbins AH *et al.* Early diagnosis of pancreatic infection by computed tomography-guided aspiration. *Gastroenterology* 1987; 93:1315–20.

157. Widdison AL, Alvarez C, Reber HA. Surgical intervention in acute pancreatitis: when and how. *Pancreas* 1991; 6(S1):S44–S51.

158. Bjornson HS. Pancreatic "abscess": diagnosis and management. *Pancreas* 1991; 6(S1):S31–6.

159. Buchler M. Malfertheiner P, Friess H *et al.* Human pancreatic tissue concentration of bactericidal antibiotics. *Gastroenterology* 1992; 103:1902–8.

160. Freeny PC. Radiology of acute pancreatitis: diagnosis, detection of complications and interventional therapy. In *Acute Pancreatitis: Experimental and Clinical Aspects of Pathogenesis and Management*. Edited by G Glazer, JHC Ranson. Baillière Tindall, London. 1988: 275–302.

161. Rotman N, Mathieu D, Anglade M-C, Fagniez P-L. Failure of percutaneous drainage of pancreatic abscesses complicating severe acute pancreatitis. *Surg Gynecol Obstet* 1992; 174:141–4.

162. Lee MJ, Rattner DW, Legermate DA *et al.* Acute complicated pancreatitis: redefining the role of interventional radiology. *Radiology* 1992; 1834:171–4.

163. Warshaw AL, Gongliang J. Improved survival in 45 patients with pancreatic abscess. *Ann Surg* 1985; 202:408–17.

164. Reber HA. Surgical intervention in necrotizing pancreatitis. *Gastroenterology* 1986; 91:479–81.

165. Beger HG, Bittner R, Block S, Bhchler M. Bacterial contamination of pancreatic necrosis. A prospective clinical study. *Gastroenterology* 1986; 91:433–8.

166. Bittner R, Block S, Bhchler M, Beger HG. Pancreatic abscess and infected pancreatic necrosis. *Dig Dis Sci* 1987; 32:1082–7.

167. Pederzoli P, Bassi C, Vesentini S, Campedell A. A randomized multicenter clinical trial of antibiotic prophylaxis of septic complications in acute necrotizing pancreatitis with imipenem. *Surg Gynecol Obstet* 1993; 176:480–3.

168. Kozaerk RA, Ball TJ, Patterson DJ, Freeny PC, Ryan JA, Traverso LW. Endoscopic transpapillary therapy for disrupted pancreatic duct and peripancreatic fluid collections. *Gastroenterology* 1991; 100:1362–70.

22

ERCP/EPT-induced pancreatitis: pharmacological prevention

*Ulricke von Arnim,
J. Enrique Dominguez-Muñoz & Peter Malfertheiner*

INTRODUCTION

Endoscopic retrograde cholangiopancreatography (ERCP) is a well established method in the diagnosis and treatment of biliary and pancreatic disorders. Although this procedure is considered to be safe, complications related to cannulation, contrast medium injection and sphincterotomy may appear. These complications include cholangitis, haemorrhage, perforation and acute pancreatitis. Pancreatitis is the most common of these complications. Clinically acute post-ERCP pancreatitis appears according to different series in 1–3% of patients[1-3]. These differences in incidence of post-ERCP pancreatitis are related to different definitions of the disease and to additional trauma such as endoscopic papillotomy (EPT). An asymptomatic increase of pancreatic enzymes in serum occurs in up to 70% of cases[4] and must be differentiated from post-ERCP pancreatitis characterized by abdominal pain and hyperamylasaemia. The mechanisms of pancreatic injury during ERCP are unknown but chemical, mechanical, enzymatic and possibly thermal injuries may be involved. These potential factors may act independently or in concert to induce post-ERCP pancreatitis. To prevent ERCP-induced pancreatitis a number of different agents have been used. This chapter reviews pharmacological agents that have been investigated in several studies to prevent post-ERCP/EPT pancreatitis.

DEFINITION OF POST-ERCP PANCREATITIS

An exact definition of post-ERCP pancreatitis seems to be difficult to draw, since in several studies restrictive to liberal definitions have been made. Most studies of ERCP-associated pancreatitis required a serum amylase that was elevated at least 2–3 times above the upper limit of normal, together with a variable duration of abdominal pain and tenderness. For the diagnosis of pancreatitis this very liberal definition does not allow classification into mild, moderate and severe pancreatitis. Cotton *et al.* suggested a grading system for the major complications of ERCP[2] that makes a differentiation according to severity (Figure 22.1).

In most cases, post-ERCP pancreatitis appears to be mild and self-limiting, but cases of death have been described as a consequence of this complication. Severe acute pancreatitis occurs after ERCP in an average of 0.5% of cases[5].

PHARMACOLOGICAL PREVENTION OF POST-ERCP/EPT PANCREATITIS

The pathophysiology of post-ERCP pancreatitis remains unknown. The following have been proposed as risk factors: increased intrapancreatic pressure caused by retrograde injection of contrast medium, with consequent damage of the acinar cells; a toxic component of contrast agents; and insufficient drainage of injected contrast media and pancreatic juice due to oedema of the papilla as a consequence of mechanical or thermal injury resulting from excessive coagulation during standard sphincterotomy, pre-cutting or poor orientation of the diathermy wire. Overinjection of contrast media, including a hydrostatic injury, has been proposed as the most common cause of pancreatitis following diagnostic ERCP [3,6]. Furthermore there is a correlation between the occurrence of post-ERCP pancreatitis and acinarization of the gland [7], and with the appearance of contrast medium in the renal outflow system, indicating absorption[8]. Since obstruction of both the bile duct and the pancreatic duct may be required for acute pancreatitis to occur, oedema of the papilla or even functional hypertension of the sphincter of Oddi due to manipulation probably plays a major pathophysiological role in post-ERCP pancreatitis. This could explain the cases of acute pancreatitis after manometry of the sphincter of Oddi, where a hydrostatic or chemical injury can be excluded.

	Mild	**Moderate**	**Severe**	**Figure 22.1** Grading system for post-ERCP pancreatitis (modified from Cotton *et al.*[2]).
Pancreatitis	Acute abdominal pain, amylase at least three times above normal more than 24h after ERCP, requiring admission or prolongation of planned admission to 2–3 days	Hospitalization of 4–10 days but without any major complication requring intensive care or surgery	Hospitalization for more than 10 days, or hospitalization in an intensive care unit, or necrotizing pancreatitis, pseudocyst, abscess or failure of one or more organs (respiratory or renal insufficiency, shock, coagulopathy, metabolic disturbance requiring therapy) related to pancreatitis	

Contrast medium

Contrast agents have been thought to be a source of irritation of the pancreatic duct and acinar cells. To evaluate the role of contrast agents, several studies have been performed comparing the incidence of post-ERCP pancreatitis using high- (ionic) or low- (non-ionic) osmolality contrast agents (Figure 22.2). The biggest prospective double-blind randomized controlled trial was performed by the Midwest Pancreaticobiliary Group[9] in 1995. A total of 1979 consecutive patients undergoing ERCP were enrolled and divided into subgroups according to the complexity of the procedure. They received injection of either non-ionic (low-osmolality) or standard ionic (high-osmolality) contrast media. Of the procedures, diagnostic ERCP had the lowest incidence of acute pancreatitis, while therapeutic ERCP and sphincter of Oddi manometry had higher rates. Using low-osmolality (non-ionic) contrast medium did not decrease the incidence of post-ERCP pancreatitis [9].

Pharmacological agents

Acute post-ERCP pancreatitis is an ideal clinical situation in which to study pharmacological agents that might be of some benefit in both prevention and therapy of acute pancreatitis. Numerous agents that are useful in experimental pancreatitis models, administered either prophylactically or after induction of the disease, have been clinically studied to determine whether their prophylactic administration might lower the incidence or severity of post-ERCP pancreatitis. In most of the studies the treatment was given prior to ERCP and then continued for a short time after the procedure. The role of various hormones such as glucagon[22], calcitonin[23] and somatostatin, as well as of other drugs such as corticosteroids, protease inhibitors and calcium antagonists, in preventing post-ERCP pancreatitis will be discussed in detail.

Somatostatin and octreotide

Somatostatin and its long-acting cyclic analogue octreotide exert a potent inhibition of both basal and stimulated exocrine pancreatic secretion[24–26]. In studies of experimentally induced pancreatitis in animals, somatostatin and octreotide have been shown to reduce the increase of serum pancreatic enzymes[27–30]. A concomitant histological improvement was seen in three of these studies [28–30]. Both somatostatin and octreotide have been evaluated in several clinical studies for the prevention of acute pancreatitis and elevation of serum pancreatic enzymes after ERCP (Figure 22.3).

Controlled studies evaluating the effect of somatostatin or octreotide on biochemical, clinical and morphological markers of pancreatitis associated with ERCP showed different results [31–43]. Most of these studies used small samples. Furthermore, comparisons between studies are difficult due to variability in drug administration (form of application, dosage and schedule), patient cohort composition (inclusion and exclusion criteria), and type of procedures performed during ERCP (diagnostic and therapeutic).

In Tulassay's study 29 patients received 0.1mg octreotide s.c. 45 min before ERCP[37]. All patients in the treatment group had a significantly smaller increase in serum amylase and lipase activities compared with 34 controls. Post-ERCP pancreatitis was not seen in either the octreotide group nor in the controls. An analysis of clinical parameters (abdominal pain and tenderness) was not performed.

A significant reduction in pain intensity and in maximum increase in pancreatic enzymes was seen in patients who received 0.1mg octreotide before and 4 hours after ERCP in a randomized double-blind study by Cicero et al.[32]. Bordas et al. performed a similarly designed clinical trial of 33 patients who received a bolus IV injection of natural somatostatin (4µg/kg body weight). This study showed a significant

Figure 22.2 Results of controlled studies comparing incidence of pancreatitis after ERCP according to the use of high-osmolality (ionic) or low-osmolality (non-ionic) contrast agents.

Author, year (ref)	High-osmolality contrast medium acute pancreatitis/ total patients	Low-osmolality contrast medium acute pancreatitis/ total patients
Osnes et al., 1975 (10)	0/12 (0%)	0/12 (0%)
Hamilton et al., 1982 (11)	0/33 (0%)	0/17 (0%)
Hannigan et al., 1985 (12)	0/32 (0%)	1/28 (3.6%)
Reimer-Jensen et al., 1985 (13)	0/28 (0%)	0/26 (0%)
Makela and Dean, 1986 (14)	0/44 (0%)	0/44 (0%)
Banerjee et al., 1986 (15)	5/25 (20%)	0/24 (0%)
Cunliffe et al., 1987 (16)	8/48 (16.6%)	2/46 (4.3%)
O'Connor et al., 1988 (17)	0/25 (0%)	0/25 (0%)
Barkin et al., 1991 (18)	3/15 (20%)	1/22 (4.5%)
Silverman et al., 1991 (19)	9/81 (11.1%)	11/75 (14.6%)
Rodriguez et al., 1991 (20)	2/25 (8%)	1/23 (4.3%)
Bedford et al., 1993 (21)	76/691 (11%)	76/700 (10.8%)
Johnson et al., 1995 (9)	86/830 (10.4%)	83/829 (10%)
Total	191/1889 (10.1%)	175/1871 (9.4%)

Figure 22.3 Somatostatin and octreotide in the prophylaxis of ERCP-induced pancreatitis.

Author, year (ref)	n	Drug	Effect
Borsch et al., 1984 (31)	20	Somatostatin	none
Cicero et al., 1985 (32)	38	Somatostatin	less enzyme rise, less pain
Bordas et al., 1988 (33)	33	Somatostatin	less enzyme rise, less pain
Saari et al., 1988 (34)	56	Somatostatin	none
Testoni et al., 1988 (35)	54	Somatostatin	none
Taylor et al., 1990 (36)	63	Octreotide	none
Tulassay and Papp, 1991 (37)	63	Octreotide	less enzyme rise, less pain
Guelrud et al., 1991 (38)	16	Somatostatin	less pancreatitis
Gambitta et al., 1991 (39)	34	Octreotide	less pancreatitis
Sternlieb et al., 1992 (40)	84	Octreotide	more pancreatitis
Binmoeller et al., 1992 (41)	245	Octreotide	none
Baldazzi et al., 1994 (42)	100	Octreotide	none
Testoni et al., 1996 (43)	60	Octreotide	less enzyme rise, less pain

reduction in abdominal pain and in pancreatic enzyme increase in this group compared with controls [33].

In a randomized trial of 16 patients with idiopathic recurrent pancreatitis who underwent an endoscopic sphincterotomy and afterwards hydrostatic balloon dilatation of the pancreatic part of the sphincter of Oddi, IV application of somatostatin at a dose of 250µg/h one hour before and 12 hours after dilatation reduced significantly the incidence of procedure-related acute pancreatitis[38]. In this study a particularly high-risk group of patients was evaluated. The overall incidence of acute pancreatitis was 43%. Prophylactic infusion of somatostatin resulted in an incidence of acute pancreatitis of 25% compared with 75% in the placebo group.

In a placebo-controlled study including 34 patients, 0.1mg octreotide was given s.c. 120 and 30 min before ERCP and 6 hours after ERCP[39]. Patients were followed up 3 days after ERCP. The treatment group showed no acute pancreatitis, whereas in the control group three cases of pancreatitis (diagnosed by persistent abdominal pain, tenderness and serum amylase elevation > 4000IU) were seen; they recovered under conservative treatment on the fourth day of hospitalization. Due to the low number of patients (17 in each group) and a liberal definition of post-procedure pancreatitis the results of this study are not conclusive.

Recently, a randomized controlled trial evaluated prophylactic long-term administration of octreotide in 60 consecutive patients undergoing EPT (56 patients) or ERCP (4 patients)[43]. Patients were randomly allocated to receive either 200µg octreotide t.i.d. for 3 days (30 cases) or placebo (30 controls). The study demonstrated a significantly lower increase in serum amylase activity in the treatment group compared to the placebo group at 4 and 8 hours after the procedure. Furthermore 'pancreatic-like' abdominal pain was significantly more often registered in controls. Acute oedematous pancreatitis was seen in three patients in the control group. The authors claimed, despite the relatively low number of patients investigated, that a 3-day prophylactic treatment with octreotide seems to be effective in reducing enzymatic changes after EPT/ERCP in especially 'risky' patients who have had previous episodes of acute pancreatitis, because amylase rise was more striking in those patients[43].

In contrast, several controlled studies have failed to show a protective effect of somatostatin or octreotide in ERCP/EPT-induced pancreatitis[34–36, 40–42]. A relatively small study including 20 patients showed no difference in the median rise of serum amylase between groups given somatostatin (250µg/h given before ERCP and continued for 24 hours) or placebo [31].

Another study of 56 patients randomized to somatostatin (250µg after contrast media emptying of the pancreatic duct) and placebo could not show a positive effect on hyperamylasaemia and adbominal pain [34]. The continuous infusion of somatostatin over 26 hours starting 2 hours before ERCP did not show significant reduction of serum amylase activity compared with a placebo group. All 54 patients in this study were undergoing endoscopic sphincterotomy [35].

Binmoeller et al.[41] evaluated the effect of octreotide on biochemical and clinical parameters of ERCP-induced pancreatitis in a randomized controlled study including 245 patients. Octreotide was given 0.1mg IV 5 min before ERCP and s.c. 45 min after ERCP. No significant differences in the median serum amylase and lipase levels were seen before ERCP and 8 and 24 hours after ERCP in the octreotide and placebo groups[41]. Acute pancreatitis was seen in five (2%) patients – three in the octreotide and two in the placebo group. A further 43 patients developed abdominal pain after ERCP – 21 in the octreotide and 22 in the placebo group. In the pancreatitis-like abdominal pain group, no significant differences were seen in serum amylase and lipase between treatment and placebo groups. Fifty-two procedures included therapeutic interventions; none of the patients involved developed pancreatitis. This study, with the largest number of patients recruited, suggests that octreotide may not protect against ERCP-induced pancreatitis.

A multicentre double-blind randomized clincal trial by Sternlieb et al.[40] was terminated because of an increase in pancreatitis in the octreotide group. Such a negative effect of the drug had never been observed before, either in humans or in animals. In the octreotide group, pancreatitis occurred significantly more often than in controls (35% versus 11%). This increased risk was observed only in the treatment group undergoing diagnostic ERCP (59% versus 6% in controls), and was not explained by known risk factors. The incidence of pancreatitis in the patients undergoing sphincterotomy was not significantly different in octreotide and control groups (15% versus 16%). Amylase levels in patients developing pancreatitis were significant lower after 24 hours in the group given octreotide. Furthermore, the time of hospitalization of pancreatitis patients in the octreotide group was significantly shorter (71% under 4 days versus 20% under 4 days in controls).

Considering the results of all studies dealing with the prophylactic administration of octreotide to prevent post-ERCP pancreatitis, it becomes clear that only a few studies, including few patients, could suggest a positive effect of the drug. Most of the studies showed neither an advantage nor a disadvantage of octreotide administration. The largest study, by Binmoeller and including 245 patients[41], showed no exception from that overall result. It can be concluded that neither somatostatin nor octreotide can prevent ERCP-induced pancreatitis.

Corticosteroids

Corticosteroids affect a number of factors involved in the process of tissue inflammation. Corticosteroids elevate functional C1 esterase inhibitor levels, which have been shown to suppress trypsin activation within the pancreas. Once trypsin is activated it is able to activate many other enzymes such as kallikrein, thrombin, elastase and phospholipase A2 [44]. Phospholipase A2 itself is inhibited by a protein called lipomodulin; synthesis of this protein is induced by corticosteroids. Since corticosteroids have been shown to increase the activity of selected protease inhibitors, especially C1 esterase inhibitor[45], they are able indirectly to inhibit phospholipase A2 activity[44]. This mechanism could alter the cascade of autodigestion leading to pancreatitis.

Based on this hypothesis a retrospective study was performed by Weiner et al. of the use of corticosteroids in preventing post-ERCP pancreatitis[46]. A total of 824 patients with a history of iodine hypersensitivity were treated with corticosteroids (651 with oral steroids and 173 with IV steroids) just before ERCP to prevent allergic reactions. These patients were studied retrospectively and compared with two control groups. Control group I consisted of 1000 patietns undergoing ERCP during the same time period (1984 to 1993). Control group II consisted of 1950 patients previously reported by the Midwest Pancreaticobiliary Group who were involved in a contrast media study[21]. Further, each group was subdivided into patients who received either diagnostic or therapeutic ERCP. There was no significant difference among the groups undergoing diagnostic ERCP in the incidence of pancreatitis. Comparing the patient groups who underwent therapeutic ERCP with or without sphincterotomy, the incidence of pancreatitis was significantly lower in the corticosteroid group. An explanation for this may be that corticosteroids reduce the oedema of the papilla. This retrospective study was not controlled for the number of cannulations, the amount of injected contrast media, and the radiological incidence of acinarization, which are known to be predisposing factors for post-ERCP pancreatitis.

The role of corticosteroids as pancreatitis-preventing drugs was also evaluated in another retrospective study including 36 patients [47]. In this study a standard dose of 50mg hydrocortisone as an IV bolus and 100mg as an IV infusion was administered and compared to controls matched for age and sex distribution. Numbers of diagnostic and therapeutic ERCP were similar in both groups. This study could show no positive effect of a preprocedure application of corticosteroids in decreasing the incidence of pancreatitis.

A further study evaluated the intrapancreatic instillation of dexamethasone in preventing sphincterotomy-induced pancreatitis in a canine model [48]. This invasive method also did not show a positive effect on the incidence of pancreatitis.

A definite conclusion on the role of corticosteroids in preventing acute post-ERCP pancreatitis based on the reported studies is not possible. A prospective randomized controlled trial including a sufficient number of patients is therefore warranted to evaluate the use of corticosteroids prior to ERCP procedures.

C1 inhibitor (C1-INH) and protease inhibitor (FOY)
C1 inhibitor is a serine protease inhibitor with great specificity to the first component of the human complement cascade, which itself has a key role in the control of the contact system. This system has important inflammatory activity through release of the vasoactive peptide bradykinin. The inhibition of ongoing complement and contact system activation by C1-INH has been reported to improve the outcome of a septic shock[49]. Activation of the contact system, along with release of other proteases, is involved in the course of acute pancreatitis[50]. Studies of experimental pancreatitis in animals have shown that the infusion of C1-INH prevents kallikrein activation, improves the outcome of the disease[51] and also reduces the extent of massive necrosis and the mortality rate regardless of the dosage[52]. This is the background to a study performed by Testoni et al.[53]. They tested the C1 inhibitor in the prevention of hyperamylasaemia in 40 patients undergoing endoscopic sphincterotomy for common bile duct stones or benign papillary stenosis. Twenty patients were given either C1-INH or placebo before the intervention. Serum amylase

levels 2, 4 and 8 hours after sphincterotomy showed significant differences between the two groups. The levels were significantly higher in the placebo group than in the pretreated patients. In this study no acute pancreatitis occurred in any of the two groups and therefore one cannot draw any conclusion concerning prevention of this complication by C1 inhibitor. These data demand further studies evaluating the prophylactic use of C1-INH. Moreover, in contrast to other antiproteases, which have to be administered by continuous infusion to reach effective serum levels, the C1-INH levels remained elevated throughout the observation period (24 hours) after a single IV infusion before the endoscopic procedure.

Gabexate-mesilate (FOY) is a synthetic protease inhibitor endowed with a potent inhibitory action against a broad spectrum of proteases. In experimental studies in animals a positive effect of protease inhibitors was shown by an improvement in the histological picture, especially when given prophylactically. This led to a randomized double-blind multicentre trial[54]. Frulloni et al. evaluated the efficacy of FOY in the prevention of serum amylase elevation and acute pancreatitis in the course of ERCP and/or EPT. A total of 424 patients (237 ERCP and 137 EPT with or without ERCP) were recruited. Of these, 213 received treatment with FOY by continuous infusion of 1g starting 30–90 min before performing the endoscopic intervention, while 211 were treated with placebo. Rising mean serum amylase activity 4, 8 12 and 24 hours after ERCP was significantly lower in the FOY group. Pain was reported by 12 patients in the treatment and 29 in the placebo group; this was a significant difference. Concerning the incidence of acute pancreatitis (definition: at least 5-fold increase in enzyme above normal limits associated with abdominal pain), three patients (1.4%) in the FOY group developed the disease compared to 19 (9%) in the placebo group. The results of this multicentre study proved evidence of an efficacy of FOY in reducing pancreatic damage after ERCP.

Nifedipine (calcium antagonist)
Nifedipine is known to relax the sphincter of Oddi; in response to the idea of a possible sphincter of Oddi spasm induced by cannulation during ERCP, the use of nifedipine for preventing acute post-ERCP pancreatitis was examined [55]. A total of 166 patients undergoing ERCP were randomized to receive three doses of either placebo or nifedipine 20mg at 8-hour intervals during the day of ERCP, in a double-blind manner. Six patients (4%) developed clinical pancreatitis, three from each group. Severe acute pancreatitis with necrosis was seen in three patients, two (2%) in the nifedipine and one (1%) in the placebo group. No difference was noted in serum amylase activity at 12 and 24 hours in the two groups. Nifedipine may significantly decrease the need for pain medication after ERCP (30% nifedipine and 50% placebo group). No preventive effect of nifedipine on post-ERCP acute pancreatitis was demonstrated, but nifedipine does appear to reduce epigastric pain induced by ERCP. One possibility for the effect on pain may be a decrease in contractility and basal pressure of the sphincter of Oddi[56] and a reduction in spontaneous gall bladder contractions[57].

References

1. Bilbao MK, Dotter CT, Lee TG, Kanton RM. Complications of endoscopic retrograde cholangiopancreatography (ERCP) - a study of 10,000 cases. *Gastroenterology* 1976; 70:314–20.

2. Cotton PB, Lehman G, Vennes J, Geenen JE, Russell RCG, Meyers WC, Liquory C, Nickl N. Endoscopic sphincterotomy complications and their management: an attempt at consensus. *Gastrointest Endosc* 1991; 37:383–93.

3. Sherman S, Lehman GA. ERCP and endoscopic sphincterotomy-induced pancreatitis. *Pancreas* 1991; 6:350–67.

4. Skude G, Wehlin L, Maruyama T, Ariyama J. Hyperamylasemia after duodenoscopy and retrograde cholangio-pancreatography. *Gut* 1976; 17:127–32.

5. Nordback I, Airo I. Post-ERCP acute necrotizing pancreatitis. *Ann Chir Gynecol* 1988; 77:15–20.

6. King CF, Kalvaris I, Sninsky CA. Pancreatitis due to endoscopic biliary manometry: proceed with caution. *Gastroentrology* 1988; 94:A227.

7. Hamilton I, Lintott DHJ, Rothwell J, Axon ATR. Acute pancreatitis following endoscopic retrograde cholangio-pancreatography. *Clin Radiol* 1983; 34:543–6.

8. Roszler MH, Campbell WL. Post-ERCP pancreatitis: association with urographic visualization during ERCP. *Radiology* 1985; 157:595–8.

9. Johnson GK, Geenen JE, Bedford RA, Johanson J, Cass O, Sherman S, Hogan WJ, Ryan M, Silverman W, Edmundowicz S, Payne M *et al*. A comparison of nonionic versus ionic contrast media: results of a prospective multicenter study. *Gastrointest Endosc* 1995; 42:312–16.

10. Osnes M, Skjennald A, Larsen S. A comparison of a new nonionic (metrizanide) and a dissociable (metrizoate) contrast medium in endoscopic retrograde pancreatography (ERP). *Scand J Gastroenterol* 1975; 12:821–5.

11. Hamilton T, Lintott D, Rothwell J, Axon A. Metrizamide as contrast medium in endoscopic retrograde cholangio-pancreatography. *Clin Radiol* 1982; 33:293–5.

12. Hannigan B, Keeling P, Slavin B, Thompson R. Hyperamylasemia after ERCP with ionic and non-ionic contrast media. *Gastrointest Endosc* 1985; 31:109–10.

13. Reimer-Jensen A, Malchow-Moller A, Matzen P *et al*. A randomized trial of iohexol versus amidotrizoate in endoscopic retrograde pancreatography. *Scand J Gastroenterol* 1985; 1:83–6.

14. Makela P, Dean P. The frequency of hyperamylasemia after ERCP with diatrizoate and iohexol. *Eur J Radiol* 1986; 6:303–4.

15. Banerjee A, Grainger S, Manners R, Thompson R. Safer endoscopic retrograde pancreatography? *Gut* 1986; 27:A601.

16. Cunliffe W, Cobden I, Lavelle M, Lendrum R, Tait N, Venahles C. A randomized prospective study comparing two contrast media for ERCP. *Endoscopy* 1987; 20 (suppl):126–7.

17. O'Connor H, Ellis W, Manning A, Lintott D, McMahon M, Axon A. Iopamidol as contrast medium in endoscopic retrograde pancreatography: a randomized comparison with diatrizoate. *Endoscopy* 1988; 20:244–7.

18. Barkin J, Casal G, Reiner D, Goldberg R, Phillips R, Kaplan S. A comparative study of contrast agents for endoscopic pancreatography. *Am J Gastroenterol* 1991; 86:1437–41.

19. Silverman W, Ruffolo T, Rogers D, Hawes R, Earlo D, Lehman G. Post ERCP pancreatitis (PEP); frequency with ionic and non-ionic contrast media in high risk patients. *Am J Gastroenterol* 1991; 86:A192.

20. Rodriguez J, Stoltenberg P, Avots A *et al*. A prospective randomized comparison of the safety and efficiacy of iohexol 180 and ditrizoate 60% as contrast agents for ERCP. *Gastroenterology* 1991; 100:A297.

21. Bedford RA, Johnson GK, Geenen JE *et al*. Ionic versus non-ionic contrast media: does stepwise therapy influence the incidence of post-ERCP pancreatitis. *Gastroenterology* 1993; 104(suppl):A294.

22. Silvis SE, Vennes JA. The role of glucagon in endoscopic cholangiopancreatography. *Gut* 1975; 17:127–32.

23. Odes HS, Bovis BN, Barbezat GO, Bank S. Effect of calcitonin on the serum amylase levels after endoscopic retrograde cholangiopancreatography. *Digestion* 1977; 16:180–4.

24. Creutzfeldt W, Lembcke B, Fölsch UR, Schleser S, Koop I. Effect of somatostatin analogue (SMS 201-995, Sandostatin) on pancreatic secretion in humans. *Am J Med* 1987; (Suppl 5B):49–54.

25. Kohler E, Beglinger C, Dettwiler S, Whitehouse I, Gyr K. Effect of a new Somatostatin analogue on pancreatic function in healthy volunteers. *Pancreas* 1986; 1:154–9.

26. Lembcke B, Creutzfeldt W, Schleser S, Ebert R, Shaw C, Koop I. Effect of somatostatin analogue sandostatin (SMS 201-995) on gastrointestinal, pancreatic and biliary function and hormone release in normal men. *Digestion* 1987; 36:108–24.

27. Lankisch PG, Koop, H, Winckler K, Fölsch UR, Creutzfeldt W. Somatostatin therapy of acute experimental pancreatitis. *Gut* 1977; 18:713–16.

28. Schwedes U, Althoff PH, Klempa I, Leuschner U, Mothes L, Raptis S *et al*. Effect of somatostatin on bile-induced acute haemorrhagic pancreatitis in the dog. *Horm Metab Res* 1979; 11:655–61.

29. Mann NS, Mauch MJ. Inhibitory effect of cycloheximide, somatostatin and 5-AZA cytidine on acute experimental pancreatitis. *Am J Proctol* 1981; 32:24–32.

30. Baxter JN, Jenkins SA, Day DW, Roberts NB, Cowell DC, Mackie CR *et al*. Effects of somatostatin and a long-acting somatostatin analogue on the prevention and treatment of experimentally induced acute pancreatitis in the rat. *Br J Surg* 1985; 72:382–5.

31. Borsch G, Bergbauer M, Nebel W, Sabin G. Effect of somatostatin therapy on amylase level and pancreatitis rate following ERCP. *Med Welt* 1984; 35:109–12.

32. Cicero GF, Laugier R, Sahel J, Mancanero M, Sarles H. Effects of somatostatin on clinical, biochemical and morphological changes after ERCP. *Ital J Gastroenterol* 1985; 17:265–8.

33. Bordas JM, Toledo V, Mondelo F, Rodes J. Prevention of pancreatic reactions by bolus somatostatin injection in patients undergoing endoscopic retrograde cholangiopancreatography and endoscopic sphincterotomy. *Horm Res* 1988; 29:106–8.

34. Saari A, Kivilaasko E, Schroder T. The influence of somatostatin on pancreatic irritation after pancreatography. An experimental and clinical study. *Surg Res Comm* 1988; 24:271–8.

35. Testoni PA, Masci E, Bagnalo F, Tittobello A. Endoscopic papillosphincterotomy: prevention of pancreatic reaction by somatostatin. *Ital J Gastroenterol* 1988; 20:70–3.

36. Taylor DH, Brodmerkel GJ, Alleheny FACG. Role of octreotide in ERCP associated pancreatitis. *Am J Gatroenterol* 1990; 85:1261(abstract).

37. Tulassay Z, Papp J. The effect of long acting somatostatin analogue on enzyme changes after endoscopic pancreatography. *Gastrointest Endosc* 1991; 37:48–50.

38. Guelrud M, Mendoza S, Viera L, Gelrud D. Somatostatin prevents acute pancreatitis after pancreatic duct sphincter hydrostatic dilatation in patients with idiopathic recurrent pancreatitis. *Gastrointest Endosc* 1991; 37:44–7.

39. Gambitta P, Grosso C, Marotta F, Rossi A, Arcidiacono R. Efficacy of Octreotide in the prevention of post-ERCP pancreatitis: a preliminary report. *Gastroenterology* 1991; 100:A272.

40. Sternlieb J, Aronchick C, Retig J, Dabeyeis M, Saunder F, Goosenberg R *et al*. A multicenter, randomized, controlled trial to evaluate the effect of prophylactic octreotide on ERCP-induced pancreatitis. *Am J Gastroenterol* 1992; 87:1561–6.

41. Binmoeller KF, Harris AG, Dumas R, Grimaldi C, Delmont JP. Does the somatostatin analogue octreotide protect against ERCP induced pancreatitis? *Gut* 1992; 33:1129–33.

42. Baldazzi G, Conti C, Spotti EG, Arisi GP, Scevola M, Gobetti F, Agliardi CM, Galasso P, Bonomi E, Bianchi F. Profilassi della pancreatite acuta post ERCP con octreotide. *Giornale Chir* 1994; 15:359–62.

43. Testoni PA, Lella F, Bagnolo F, Caporuscio S, Cattani L, Colombo E, Buizza M. Long-term prophylactic administration of octreotide reduces rise in serum amylase after endoscopic procedures on Vater's papilla. *Pancreas* 1996; 13:61–5.

44. Bettinger JR, Grendel JH. Intracellular events in the pathogenesis of acute pancreatitis. *Pancreas* 1991; 6(suppl):S2–6.

45. Lasser EC, Lang JH, Lyon SG, Hambln AE, Howard M. Glucocorticoid-induced elevation of C1-esterase inhibitor: a mechanism for protection against lethal dose range contrast challenge in rabbits. *Invest Radiol* 1981; 16:20–3.

46. Weiner GR, Geenen JE, Hogan WJ, Catalano MF. Use of corticosteroids in the prevention of post-ERCP pancreatitis. *Gastrointest Endosc* 1995; 42:579–83.

47. Kulkarni A, Thomas A, Bekal P, Brodmerkel GJ Jr, Agrawal RM. The role of corticosteroids in the prevention of post-ERCP pancreatitis. *Gastrointest Endosc* 1996; 43:409 (abstract).

48. Pasricha PJ, Hill SJ, Huang RL, Aggarwal R, Maggee CA, Kalloo AN. Intrapancreatic dexamethasone does not prevent sphincterotomy-induced pancreatitis in a canine model. *Gastrointest Endosc* 1996; 43:391 (abstract).

49. Hack CE, Ogilvie AC, Eisele B, Eerenberg AJM, Wagstaff J, Thijs ZG. C1-Inhibitor substitution therapy in septic shock and in the vascular leak syndrome induced by high doses of interleukin-2. *Intensive Care Med* 1993; 19(suppl):S19–28.

50. Uehara S, Honjyo K, Furukawa S, Hiramaya A, Sakamoto W. Role of kallikrein–kinin system in human pancreatitis. *Adv Exp Med Biol* 1989; 247B:643–8.

51. Ruud TE, Aasen AO, Pillgram-Larsen J, Stadaas JO. Effects on peritoneal proteolysis and haemodynamics of prophylactic infusion of C1-inhibitor in experimental pancreatitis. *Scand J Gastroenterol* 1986; 21:1018–24.

52. Vesentini S, Renetti I, Bassi C *et al*. Effects of C1-esterase inhibitor in experimental acute pancreatitis in rats: preliminary results. *Int J Pancreatol* 1993; 13:217–20.

53. Testoni PA, Cicardi M, Bergmanschini L, Guzzoni S, Cugno M, Buizza M, Bagnolo F, Agostoni A. Infusion of C1-Inhibitor plasma concentrate prevents hyperamylasemia induced by endoscopic sphincterotomy. *Gastrointest Endosc* 1995; 42:301–4.

54. Frulloni L, Cavallari A, Tittobello A and the Gruppo italiano gabesato endoscopia digestiva (GRIGED). Gabexate mesilate (FOY) in the prevention of pancreatic damage to endoscopic manoeuvres on the Vater's papilla. Results of an Italian randomised double-blind multicentre trial. *Endoscopy* 1995; 27:S25 (abstract).

55. Sand J, Nordback I. Prospective randomized trial of the effect of nifedipine on pancreatic irritation after endoscopic retrograde cholangiopancreatography. *Digestion* 193; 54:105–11.

56. Guelrud M, Mendoza S, Rossiter G, Ramirez L, Barkin J. Effect of nifedipine on sphincter of Oddi motor activity: Studies in healthy volunteers and patients with biliary dyskinesia. *Gastroenterology* 1988; 95:1050–5.

57. Clas D, Hould FS, Rosenthall L, Arzoumanian A, Fried GM. Nifedipine inhibits cholecystokinin-induced gallbladder contraction. *J Surg Res* 1989; 46:479–83.

Index

Abbreviations: CT, computed tomography; ER(C)P, endoscopic retrograde (cholangio)pancreatography; EBS, endoscopic biliary sphincterotomy; EPS, endoscopic pancreatic sphincterotomy; EUS, endoscopic ultrasonography; PD, pancreatic duct.

Note: 'Cancer' means pancreatic or pancreatobiliary cancer unless specifically noted otherwise.

Abbreviations: CT, computed tomography; ERCP, endoscopic retrograde (cholangio)pancreatography; EBS, endoscopic biliary sphincterotomy; EPS, endoscopic pancreatic sphincterotomy; EUS, endoscopic ultrasonography; PD, pancreatic duct.

Note: 'Cancer' means pancreatic or pancreatobiliary cancer unless specifically noted otherwise.

Abbreviations: CT, computed tomography; ER(C)P, endoscopic retrograde (cholangio)pancreatography; EBS, endoscopic
biliary sphincterotomy; EPS, endoscopic pancreatic sphincterotomy; EUS, endoscopic ultrasonography; PD, pancreatic duct.

Note: 'Cancer' means pancreatic or pancreatobiliary cancer unless specifically noted otherwise.

Abbreviations: CT, computed tomography; ERCP, endoscopic retrograde (cholangio)pancreatography; EBS, endoscopic biliary sphincterotomy; EPS, endoscopic pancreatic sphincterotomy; EUS, endoscopic ultrasonography; PD, pancreatic duct.

Note: 'Cancer' means pancreatic or pancreatobiliary cancer unless specifically noted otherwise.

Abbreviations: CT, computed tomography; ER(C)P, endoscopic retrograde (cholangio)pancreatography; EBS, endoscopic
  biliary sphincterotomy; EPS, endoscopic pancreatic sphincterotomy; EUS, endoscopic ultrasonography; PD, pancreatic duct.

Note: 'Cancer' means pancreatic or pancreatobiliary cancer unless specifically noted otherwise.